CW00549470

Lysosomal Storage Disorders

A Practical Guide

EDITED BY

Atul Mehta

Clinical Director, Lysosomal Storage Disorders Unit
Professor of Haematology, University College London
Royal Free Hospital
London, UK

Bryan Winchester

Emeritus Professor of Biochemistry
UCL Institute of Child Health at Great Ormond Street Hospital
University College London
London, UK

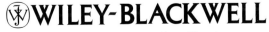
WILEY-BLACKWELL
A John Wiley & Sons, Ltd., Publication

This edition first published 2012, © 2012 by John Wiley & Sons, Ltd.

Wiley-Blackwell is an imprint of John Wiley & Sons, formed by the merger of Wiley's global Scientific, Technical and Medical business with Blackwell Publishing.

Registered Office
John Wiley & Sons, Ltd, The Atrium, Southern Gate, Chichester, West Sussex, PO19 8SQ, UK

Editorial Offices
9600 Garsington Road, Oxford, OX4 2DQ, UK
The Atrium, Southern Gate, Chichester, West Sussex, PO19 8SQ, UK
111 River Street, Hoboken, NJ 07030-5774, USA

For details of our global editorial offices, for customer services and for information about how to apply for permission to reuse the copyright material in this book please see our website at www.wiley.com/wiley-blackwell

The right of the author to be identified as the author of this work has been asserted in accordance with the UK Copyright, Designs and Patents Act 1988.

All rights reserved. No part of this publication may be reproduced, stored in a retrieval system, or transmitted, in any form or by any means, electronic, mechanical, photocopying, recording or otherwise, except as permitted by the UK Copyright, Designs and Patents Act 1988, without the prior permission of the publisher.

Designations used by companies to distinguish their products are often claimed as trademarks. All brand names and product names used in this book are trade names, service marks, trademarks or registered trademarks of their respective owners. The publisher is not associated with any product or vendor mentioned in this book. This publication is designed to provide accurate and authoritative information in regard to the subject matter covered. It is sold on the understanding that the publisher is not engaged in rendering professional services. If professional advice or other expert assistance is required, the services of a competent professional should be sought.

The contents of this work are intended to further general scientific research, understanding, and discussion only and are not intended and should not be relied upon as recommending or promoting a specific method, diagnosis, or treatment by physicians for any particular patient. The publisher and the author make no representations or warranties with respect to the accuracy or completeness of the contents of this work and specifically disclaim all warranties, including without limitation any implied warranties of fitness for a particular purpose. In view of ongoing research, equipment modifications, changes in governmental regulations, and the constant flow of information relating to the use of medicines, equipment, and devices, the reader is urged to review and evaluate the information provided in the package insert or instructions for each medicine, equipment, or device for, among other things, any changes in the instructions or indication of usage and for added warnings and precautions. Readers should consult with a specialist where appropriate. The fact that an organization or Website is referred to in this work as a citation and/or a potential source of further information does not mean that the author or the publisher endorses the information the organization or Website may provide or recommendations it may make. Further, readers should be aware that Internet Websites listed in this work may have changed or disappeared between when this work was written and when it is read. No warranty may be created or extended by any promotional statements for this work. Neither the publisher nor the author shall be liable for any damages arising herefrom.

Library of Congress Cataloging-in-Publication Data

Lysosomal storage disorders : a practical guide / edited by Atul Mehta, Bryan Winchester.
     p. ; cm.
  Includes bibliographical references and index.
  ISBN 978-0-470-67087-3 (pbk. : alk. paper)
  I. Mehta, Atul B.   II. Winchester, Bryan.
  [DNLM: 1. Lysosomal Storage Diseases. 2. Lysosomes–pathology. WD 205]
  571.6'55–dc23

2012017385

A catalogue record for this book is available from the British Library.

Wiley also publishes its books in a variety of electronic formats. Some content that appears in print may not be available in electronic books.

Set in 9.25/11.5 pt Minion by SPi Publisher Services, Pondicherry, India

1 2012

Contents

Contributors

Andrea Ballabio, MD

Director, TIGEM (Telethon Institute of Genetics and Medicine)
Naples, Italy;
Professor, Department of Molecular and Human Genetics
Baylor College of Medicine
Houston, TX, USA;
Jan and Dan Duncan Neurological Research Institute
Texas Children's Hospital
Houston, TX, USA;
Medical Genetics
Department of Pediatrics
Federico II University
Naples, Italy

Michael Beck

Children's Hospital
University of Mainz
Mainz, Germany

David J. Begley, BSc, PhD

Senior Lecturer in Physiology
Kings College London
London, UK

Erik J. Bonten, PhD

Department of Genetics
St. Jude Children's Research Hospital
Memphis, TN, USA

Thomas Braulke, PhD

Department of Biochemistry
Children's Hospital
University Medical Center Hamburg-Eppendorf
Hamburg, Germany

T. Andrew Burrow, MD

Assistant Professor
The Division of Human Genetics
University of Cincinnati Department of Pediatrics and
Cincinnati Children's Hospital Medical Center
Cincinnati, OH, USA

Joe T.R. Clarke, MD, PhD

Professor Emeritus (Pediatrics)
University of Toronto
Toronto, ON, Canada
Professor d'ensiegnement clinique
Centre Hospitalier Universitaire
Sherbrooke, QC, Canada

Jonathan D. Cooper, BSc(Hons), PhD

Professor of Experimental Neuropathology
Pediatric Storage Disorders Laboratory, Neuroscience
Centre for the Cellular Basis of Behaviour
King's Health Partners Centre for Neurodegeneration Research
James Black Centre
Institute of Psychiatry
King's College London
London, UK

Timothy M. Cox, MD, FMedSci

Professor of Medicine
University of Cambridge
Addenbrooke's Hospital
Cambridge, UK

Alessandra d'Azzo, PhD

Member and Endowed Chair
Department of Genetics
St. Jude Children's Research Hospital
Memphis, TN, USA

Robert J. Desnick, PhD, MD

Dean for Genetic and Genomic Medicine
Professor and Chairman Emeritus
Department of Genetics and Genomic Sciences
Mount Sinai School of Medicine
New York, NY, USA

Graciana Diez-Roux

Telethon Institute of Genetics and Medicine
Naples, Italy

Deborah Elstein, PhD

Clinical Research Coordinator
Gaucher Clinic
Shaare Zedek Medical Center
Jerusalem, Israel

Volkmar Gieselmann, MD

Professor of Biochemistry
Institut fuer Biochemie und Molekularbiologie
Rheinische-Friedrich-Wilhelms Universitaet
Bonn, Germany

Roberto Giugliani, MD, PhD

Professor, Department of Genetics,
Federal University of Rio Grande do Sul
Director, WHO Collaborating Centre
Medical Genetics Service, HCPA
Porto Alegre, RS, Brazil

Gregory A. Grabowski, MD

The A. Graeme Mitchell Chair in Human Genetics
Professor and Director, Human Genetics
Cincinnati Children's Hospital Medical Center
University of Cincinnati
Cincinnati, OH, USA

Carla E.M. Hollak, MD, PhD

Internist, Professor of Inherited Metabolic Diseases in Adults
Department of Endocrinology and Metabolism
Academic Medical Center
Amsterdam, The Netherlands

John J. Hopwood, AM, FAA, PhD

Lysosomal Diseases Research Unit
SA Pathology at Women's and Children's Hospital
North Adelaide, SA, Australia

Alastair Kent

Director
Genetic Alliance UK
London, UK

Ingeborg Krägeloh-Mann, MD

Professor of Pediatrics
Director, Pediatric Neurology and
   Developmental Medicine
University Children's Hospital
Tübingen, Germany

Christine Lavery, MBE

Chief Executive
Society for Mucopolysaccharide Diseases
Amersham, Buckinghamshire, UK

Gabor E. Linthorst, MD, PhD

Internist-Endocrinologist
Department of Internal Medicine, Endocrinology and
   Metabolism
Academic Medical Center
Amsterdam, The Netherlands

Dag Malm, MD, PhD

The Tromsø Centre of Internal Medicine (TIS)
Tromsø, Norway

Jeremy Manuel, OBE

Chairman
European Gaucher Alliance
Dursley, Gloucestershire, UK

Atul Mehta

Clinical Director
Lysosomal Storage Disorders Unit
Department of Haematology, University College London
Royal Free Hospital
London, UK

Matthew C. Micsenyi

The Dominick P. Purpura Department of Neuroscience
Albert Einstein College of Medicine
Bronx, NY, USA

Øivind Nilssen

Professor
Department of Clinical Medicine-Medical Genetics
University of Tromsø; Department of Medical Genetics
University Hospital of North-Norway
Tromsø, Norway

Marc C. Patterson, MD, FRACP

Chair, Division of Child and Adolescent Neurology
Professor of Neurology, Pediatrics and
   Medical Genetics
Mayo Clinic
Rochester, MN, USA

Sandra Pohl, PhD
Department of Biochemistry
Children's Hospital
University Medical Center Hamburg-Eppendorf
Hamburg, Germany

Annick Raas-Rothschild, MD
Associate Professor of Genetics
Department of Human Genetics and Metabolic Diseases
Hadassah Hebrew University Medical Center
Ein Kerem
Jerusalem, Israel

Uma Ramaswami, MBBS, MSc, MD, FRCPCH
Consultant Metabolic Paediatrician
The Willink Biochemical Genetics Unit
Genetic Medicine
St Mary's Hospital
Manchester, UK

Arnold J.J. Reuser
Department of Clinical Genetics
Center for Lysosomal and Metabolic Diseases
Erasmus MC University Medical Center
Rotterdam, The Netherlands

Paul Saftig, PhD
Biochemical Institute
Christian-Albrechts-University Kiel
Kiel, Germany

Maurizo Scarpa
Department of Paediatrics
University of Padova
Padova, Italy

Edward H. Schuchman, PhD
Genetic Disease Foundation – Francis Crick Professor
Vice Chairman for Research
Department of Genetics and Genomic Sciences
Mount Sinai School of Medicine
New York, NY, USA

Michael Schwake, PhD
Biochemical Institute
Christian-Albrechts-University Kiel
Kiel, Germany

Hilde Monica F. Riise Stensland, DrSc
Senior Scientist
Department of Medical Genetics
University Hospital of North-Norway
Tromsø, Norway

Ans T. van der Ploeg
Department of Pediatrics
Center for Lysosomal and Metabolic Diseases
Erasmus MC University Medical Center
Rotterdam, The Netherlands

Marie T. Vanier, MD, PhD
Director of Research (Emeritus)
Institut National de la Santé et de la Recherche Médicale
and Hospices Civils de Lyon
Lyon, France

Steven U. Walkley, DVM, PhD
Director, Rose F. Kennedy Intellectual and Developmental
  Disabilities Research Center
Professor of Neuroscience, Pathology and Neurology
Albert Einstein College of Medicine
Bronx, NY, USA

Melissa P. Wasserstein
Department of Genetics and Genomic Sciences
Mount Sinai School of Medicine
New York, NY, USA

David A. Wenger, PhD
Professor of Neurology
Thomas Jefferson University, Jefferson Medical College
Philadelphia, PA, USA

Ruth E. Williams
Department of Paediatric Neurology
Evelina Childrens Hospital
Guy's and St Thomas' NHS Foundation Trust
London, UK

Bryan Winchester
Biochemistry Research Group
UCL Institute of Child Health at Great Ormond Street Hospital
University College London
London, UK

J. Edmond Wraith, MBChB, FRCPCH
Professor of Paediatric Metabolic Medicine
Manchester Academic Health Sciences Centre;
Willink Biochemical Genetics Unit
Royal Manchester Children's Hospital
Manchester, UK

Ari Zimran, MD
Gaucher Clinic
Shaare Zedek Medical Center
The Hebrew University – Hadassah Medical School
Jerusalem, Israel

Preface

The concept of a lysosomal storage disorder is now almost 50 years old – an appropriate time, we feel, for a new review of the subject.

The term lysosome was coined by Christian de Duve [1], the discoverer of this organelle, to reflect its role as the major intracellular site for the enzymatic 'lysis' of macromolecules so that they may be recycled. The concept of a lysosomal storage disorder was first proposed by H G Hers [2], following the discovery that one of the glycogen storage diseases (Pompe disease, acid maltase deficiency) was due to deficiency of a lysosomal enzyme. The concept of 'cross-correction', formulated by Elizabeth Neufeld [3] and her group after the discovery that co-cultured fibroblasts derived from two patients with different lysosomal storage disorders mutually corrected each other, led to the notion of 'enzyme replacement therapy' (ERT). Roscoe Brady not only discovered the enzymatic basis for Gaucher disease and Fabry disease but also pioneered ERT for humans [4,5].

The last two decades, however, have seen a huge expansion in research in this area which has substantially extended our understanding of both the scientific and the clinical basis of lysosomal storage disorders [6]. Thus, at a scientific level it is now very well recognised that lysosomes are part of an endosomal/lysosomal network which plays a critical role in a whole range of cellular processes including the recycling of membrane and other organelles, the turnover of molecules and ingested matter through endocytosis and phagocytosis, and an emerging role in apoptosis and autophagy. At a clinical level successful treatments have been employed which reduce substrate accumulation or promote substrate degradation but it is increasingly recognised that the protean multi-system manifestations of these conditions result from pathologic processes over and above simple lysosomal storage and damage.

This book is the fruit of an ambitious project which aims to review both the scientific and the clinical aspects of lysosomal storage disorders. We perceive a need for an accessible volume giving an up to date overview of the subject. Even when effective treatments are available, there remains an urgent need to highlight awareness of the diseases so that early and appropriate treatment may be sought [7]. Furthermore, in a rapidly changing world, there is a real need to improve access to expensive treatments. The first section of the book reviews current understanding of the physiology and pathophysiology of lysosomal storage disorders and we again to attempt to classify the conditions. The second part of the book reviews individual diseases, and gives perspectives from patients and experts looking towards future therapeutic directions. The book is aimed at a wide audience including scientists, clinicians, health care workers and administrators, those working in the pharmaceutical industry, patients and their organisations.

We are highly indebted to Christine Lavery, the Founder and Chief Executive of the Society for Mucopolysaccharidosis Diseases (MPS Society, UK). Christine has been an integral part of the project from the very beginning, a partner during its production and a driver towards its completion. The extremely high regard in which she is held internationally has allowed us to assemble a glittering array of distinguished contemporary scientists and clinicians working in this area.

Furthermore, all contributors and the editors have donated their royalties to the MPS society, which is dedicated to promote research into these diseases and to the support of patients and families who suffer from them. We are also grateful to Shire HGT which has made the project possible through an unrestricted educational grant given to the MPS Society. The Editors and contributors take full responsibility for the contents of the book and confirm that Shire HGT, the MPS Society and Wiley-Blackwell have not had any role in influencing the content of the work.

We would also like to thank Elisabeth Dodds, Production Manager, Nick Godwin and Rob Blundell at Wiley-Blackwell who have helped us at every stage of the project. Our distinguished contributors have made time in their busy schedules to prepare and revise their contributions and we thank them for their patience, timeliness, clarity and charity in delivering their chapters to us.

We would each like to acknowledge some, of our many, academic mentors. For Atul this has to be Lucio Luzzatto, a clinician and scientist who guided his early academic career, emphasising the need for meticulous and reflective observation and record. Atul would also like to thank Victor Hoffbrand, who has provided invaluable encouragement during his career as a clinician, academic – and as a writer. Bryan would like to thank Don Robinson for introducing him to lysosomal storage diseases and giving him his first job, and Bob Jolly, who taught him the importance of linking pathology and biochemistry through the study of animal models. Finally, we would both like to thank our respective wives and families for their continuing forbearance and support.

Atul Mehta
Bryan Winchester

References

1 de Duve C, Pressman B, Gianetto R, Wattiaux R, Appelmans F. Tissue fractionation studies: Intracellular distribution patterns of enzymes in rat-liver tissue. *Biochem J* 1955;**64**:604–617.

2 Hers HG. Alpha glucosidase deficiency in generalised glycogen storage disease (Pompe Disease). *Biochem J* 1963; **86**:11–16.

3 Fratantoni JC, Hall CW, Neufeld EF. The defect in Hurler and Hunter Syndromes II deficiency of specific factor involved in mucopolysaccharide degradation. *Proc Nat Acad.Sci USA* 1969; **64**:360–366.

4 Barton NW, Furbish FS, Murray GJ, Garfield M, Brady RO. Therapeutic response to intravenous infusions of glucocerebrosidase in a patient with Gaucher disease. *Proc Natl Acad Sci USA.* 1990;**87**:1913–6.

5 Brady RO. Enzyme replacement therapy for lysosomal diseases *Annu Rev Med* 2006; **57**: 283–296.

6 Cox TM, Cachon-Gonzales MB. The cellular pathology of lysosomal diseases. *J Pathol* 2012; **226**:241–254.

7 D'Aco K, Underhill L, Rangachani L *et al.* Diagnosis and treatment trends in mucopolysaccharidosis I; findings from the MPS I registry. *Eur J Pediatr* 2012: Advance online publication.

Foreword

Soon after the discovery of metabolic abnormality in Gaucher disease, a recommendation was made to examine the potential benefit of enzyme replacement therapy for patients with hereditary enzyme deficiency disorders [1]. A search for a suitable source of the requisite enzymes was initiated. Because of the possibility of sensitizing recipients to a foreign protein, one wished to avoid the administration of an enzyme obtained from a non-human source. Eventually it occurred to me that human placental tissue might be an appropriate starting material and an effort to isolate glucocerebrosidase, the enzyme that is deficient in Gaucher patients, was begun.

Because of its high hydrophobicity, and lack of experience in the handling of such a protein, much difficulty was encountered in obtaining useful quantities of the requisite enzyme. Eventually a small amount of sufficiently purified glucocerebrosidase was obtained and administered to a patient with Type 3 Gaucher disease and a second with Type 1 Gaucher disease [2]. There was a 26% reduction of glucocerebroside in the liver of both patients, as well as a striking reduction in the quantity of glucocerebroside associated with circulating erythrocytes in the recipients. Another long delay was encountered before consistent clinical benefit of enzyme replacement therapy was demonstrated in a cohort of patients with Gaucher disease [3].

This book is a timely review of this rapidly developing field. The Editors are to be congratulated on securing contributions from so many distinguished scientists and clinicians. The benefits, as well as the disappointments, of enzyme replacement therapy (ERT) in various sphingolipid and mucopolysaccharide storage disorders are discussed in individual chapters devoted to these topics. Despite the remarkable successes of ERT with regard to the systemic manifestations of metabolic storage disorders, one is still confronted with the disappointing inability to achieve comparable benefit with regard to the central nervous system manifestations of these conditions. This area is under active investigation and ultimately success in this endeavor is anticipated. Several additional approaches are under consideration. One is the use of small molecules, such as molecular chaperones, to enhance the stability and delivery of mutated enzymes to lysosomes where they can function. Another is to determine the effect of histone deacetylase inhibitors on the quantity and function of mutated enzymes. Eventually an ultimate goal is the development of effective gene therapy to provide permanent cures for patients with lysosomal storage disorders.

Finally, I would like to endorse the work of the MPS Society, which is devoted to research to improve the lives of sufferers and their families. The editors and authors have donated their royalties to this valuable charitable cause and I very much hope this book will succeed in raising awareness of these diseases.

Roscoe O. Brady, MD

References

1 Brady RO. The sphingolipidoses. *N Engl J Med* 1966; **275**: 312–318.
2 Brady RO, Pentchev PG, Gal AE, Hibbert SR, Dekaban AS. Replacement therapy for inherited enzyme deficiency: use of purified glucocerebrosidase in Gaucher's disease. *N Engl J Med* 1974; **291**: 989–993.
3 Barton NW, Brady RO, Dambrosia JM, et al. Replacement therapy for inherited enzyme deficiency — macrophage-targeted glucocerebrosidase for Gaucher's disease. *N Engl J Med* 1991; **324**: 1464–1470.

PART 1

General Aspects of Lysosomal Storage Diseases

CHAPTER 1

The Lysosomal System: Physiology and Pathology

Matthew C. Micsenyi and Steven U. Walkley

The Dominick P. Purpura Department of Neuroscience, Albert Einstein College of Medicine, Bronx, NY, USA

Introduction

The lysosome and its constituent parts – what has been referred to as the *greater lysosomal system* [1] – constitute a major metabolic regulatory network in eukaryotic cells. This system includes secretory streams transporting newly synthesized enzymes and other proteins to lysosomes, endosomal and retrosomal streams contributing to signal transduction and related processing, autophagic streams delivering intracellular material for lysosomal degradation, and salvage streams facilitating egress of lysosomal degradation products to other sites in the cell for reutilization. Operating in close parallel are additional proteolytic mechanisms such as the ubiquitin–proteasome system (UPS), which assists in efficient protein turnover. The central coordinator of this remarkable intracellular network is ultimately the lysosome itself, an acidic membrane-bound organelle that functions to degrade and reprocess a vast array of cellular material. Hydrolytic enzymes localized to the lysosomal lumen are optimally active at an acidic pH and have the capacity to degrade most macromolecules including proteins, carbohydrates, lipids, RNA and DNA. Following the breakdown of this material, the resultant amino acids, sugars, simple glycolipids, cholesterol and nucleotides are salvaged by transport through the lysosomal membrane with the aid of specific transporter proteins for delivery to other cell organelles and membranes for subsequent use in biosynthetic processes. Although traditionally depicted as a terminal compartment, this role in recycling molecular precursors brings the importance of the lysosome full circle. Taken as a whole, the greater lysosomal system therefore functions at the very hub of cellular metabolic homeostasis. With the recent discovery of an overarching gene regulatory network referred to as CLEAR (Coordinated Lysosomal Expression and Regulation) and its master gene transcription factor EB (TFEB), many components of the greater lysosomal system have been shown to be linked at the transcriptional level [2]. Indeed, these studies further establish the lysosomal system as a highly efficient and coordinated network. As such, proper lysosomal function is essential since failure of this system leads, inexorably, to catastrophic consequences for cells, organs, and individuals, with nearly 60 different types of lysosomal diseases documented to date (see Classification in Chapter 5).

The greater lysosomal system

Our understanding of the lysosome and its role in cells has evolved significantly since its discovery by Christian de Duve more than 50 years ago. This organelle and the constituent streams or pathways to which it is linked comprise a processing and recycling centre essential to all cells. While each component is typically defined separately, it is important to conceptualize the various parts functioning as a highly orchestrated cellular mechanism (Figure 1.1).

Endocytosis

The endolysosomal pathway consists of the major delivery streams and molecular machinery necessary for the internalization of cell surface and extracellular material linking

Lysosomal Storage Disorders: A Practical Guide, First Edition. Edited by Atul Mehta and Bryan Winchester.
© 2012 John Wiley & Sons, Ltd. Published 2012 by John Wiley & Sons, Ltd.

The Greater Lysosomal System

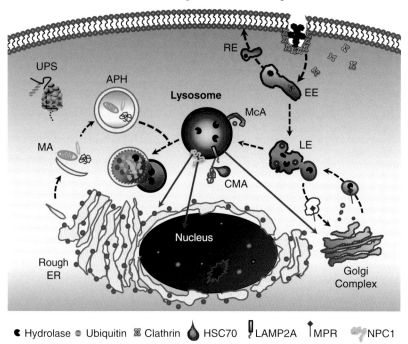

❤ Hydrolase ● Ubiquitin ▩ Clathrin 🌢 HSC70 ▯LAMP2A ↑MPR ⟿NPC1

Figure 1.1 Schematic highlighting the major pathways and mechanisms contributing to the greater lysosomal system including: the secretory pathway involved in targeting of acid hydrolases from the Golgi complex to late endosomes/lysosomes; the endocytic pathway where extracellular components are internalized; the autophagic pathway – macroautophagy (MA), chaperone-mediated autophagy (CMA), and microautophagy (McA) – where intracellular proteins and organelles are targeted for degradation; and the ubiquitin-proteasome system (UPS) which is allied with the autophagic/lysosomal system in maintaining proteolytic quality control. Salvage streams are depicted as solid red lines where simple molecular products are transported out of lysosomes and trafficked to organelles throughout the cell to be reutilized. (APH, autophagosome; EE, early endosome; LE, late endosome; RE, recycling endosome; MPR, mannose 6-phosphate receptor; NPC1, Niemann–Pick type C1 protein).

cells with their external environment. The full scope of the complexity of the endocytic system continues to evolve with the characterization of diverse forms of endocytosis and the elucidation of key molecular components associated with these pathways. Endocytic processes are often grouped by the morphological characteristics of the invagination of the membrane. Clathrin-mediated endocytosis (CME) is defined by clathrin-coated pits localized to the plasmalemma that internalize receptor/cargo complexes into vesicles that are sorted and targeted to various intracellular locations. In the CNS, neurons rely on CME for the cycling of neurotransmitter receptors regulating signaling and activity-dependent neuroplasticity. Clathrin-independent endocytosis has also been described and most often occurs at flask-like invaginations along the plasmalemma called caveolae. Caveolae are long-lived plasma membrane microdomains composed of caveolins,

cholesterol, sphingolipids including glycosphingolipids (GSLs) and sphingomyelin, GPI-anchored proteins and various receptor proteins. Such specialized membrane structures which are ultimately processed by the endolysosomal system are known to play a critical role as platforms for cell signalling and as regulators of lipid components within the plasmalemma.

The canonical endocytic pathway progresses along an increasing lumen-acidic gradient from early endosomes retrogradely trafficked from the plasma membrane, to multivesicular bodies or late endosomes, and finally to perinuclear-localized lysosomes. Deviating from this pathway, early endosomes can be recruited back to the plasmalemma or to other organelles as sorting/recycling endosomes. These divergent streams allow for the recycling and reinsertion of cell surface receptors, delivery of signaling ligands throughout the cell, and internalization of membrane components to be reorganized. Such carefully orchestrated processing and its related signal transduction events may be interrupted in diseases of the lysosomal system in which endocytosed components including cholesterol and GSLs accumulate. While this accumulation is typically associated with late endosomes and lysosomes, recent evidence has emerged suggesting additional involvement of early endosomal compartments [3], raising the likelihood that the consequences of lysosomal disease extend well beyond the lysosome itself.

Autophagy

In addition to endocytic pathways, autophagic streams feed into the lysosome and are involved in targeting intracellular material including effete organelles, long-lived proteins and pathogens for degradation [4]. Autophagy, which is often activated following starvation stress, is divided into three distinct subtypes – microautophagy, chaperone-mediated autophagy (CMA) and macroautophagy – defined by the delivery method of substrate to lysosomes. Microautophagy involves the direct engulfment of cytosolic material by the lysosome either by direct invagination of the lysosomal membrane, or projected arm-like extensions that sequester material into intralysosomal vesicles. CMA is selective for soluble monomeric proteins containing the peptide signalling motif Lys-Phe-Glu-Arg-Gln (KFERQ). This motif allows for binding by the heat shock cognate 70 protein (HSC70). HSC70 and co-chaperones then promote protein unfolding and translocation across the lysosomal membrane via the lysosome-associated membrane protein type 2A (LAMP2A). Macroautophagy has been traditionally characterized as a vesicle-mediated bulk degradation mechanism activated in response to nutrient deprivation. Recently, however, it has been shown that macroautophagy is also constitutively active and selective. When macroautophagy is stimulated, double membrane vesicles known as autophagosomes form to engulf cytosolic material. This material, including dysfunctional organelles and oligomerized proteins, is selectively recognized by chaperone complexes and adapter molecules including heat-shock proteins (HSPs), ubiquitin, and p62/SQSTM1 (p62) which allow for the specific uptake of these substrates within autophagosomes. To date several lysosomal diseases have been found to exhibit alterations in autophagy, however the downstream consequences for disease progression remain unclear. Of particular interest is evaluating how impaired autophagy contributes to neurodegenerative processes.

Salvage

Degradation products resulting from lysosomal processing must be efficiently removed from the organelle for utilization elsewhere in the cell. This salvage process involves numerous lysosomal membrane proteins that act as transporters, including cystinosin, sialin, cobalamin transporter and NPC1 protein (see Chapter 17). For example, a defect in the salvage of cobalamin (also known as vitamin B12) leads to cobalamin F-type disease, a disorder characterized in children by megaloblastic anaemia, failure to thrive and neurological deficits [5]. The inability of cobalamin to leave the lysosome and enter the cytosol means that it is unavailable for conversion into enzyme cofactors methylcobalamin and adenosylcobalamin, which are critical for multiple metabolic processes. Another example of salvage compromise involves the reutilization of lysosomal degradation products directly in synthetic pathways in the Golgi and elsewhere in the cell. In Niemann–Pick type C disease (NPC), lack of the NPC1 protein and the resulting compromise in egress of unesterified cholesterol to other sites in the cell is known to cause compensatory increases in cholesterol synthesis [6] and a similar phenomenon involving glycosphingolipids (GSLs) may occur following sequestration of GM2 and GM3 gangliosides [3]. Following synthesis in the Golgi and transport to the plasmalemma, GM1 and other complex gangliosides are eventually endocytosed and degraded in lysosomes. Salvage of simple gangliosides (e.g., GM2 and GM3) from lysosomes and their transport back to the Golgi allows for efficient production of complex gangliosides without the need for complete de novo synthesis from ceramide. Even in other lysosomal disease caused by defects in degradation rather than egress – such as Sandhoff disease in which GM2 accumulates following absence of β-hexosaminidase – neurons may similarly be deprived of this precursor for complex ganglioside synthesis. Reutilization of simple molecular components derived from lysosomal degradation would be energetically favourable over full de novo synthesis. What storage may lead to in terms of cell energy consumption and altered regulatory processing is only now beginning to be explored in depth. Thus, while lysosomal diseases have been historically viewed as states of overabundance of non–degraded material, it is only logical to assume that they are also likely deficiency diseases in which critical components for multiple metabolic pathways are in reduced supply.

Ubiquitin–Proteasome System (UPS)

In addition to pathways directly feeding into and out of the lysosome, the lysosomal system includes mechanisms functionally allied in maintaining proteolytic quality control, namely the UPS. As the primary degradative pathway for most soluble short-lived proteins, the UPS plays a pivotal role in cellular regulatory processes, including the endoplasmic reticulum associated degradation system (ERAD). The ERAD system is responsible for turning over aberrantly misfolded proteins immediately following their translation thereby serving as a quality control check-point. Additionally, the UPS has been found to coordinate proteolysis with the autophagic/lysosomal system in certain instances. For example, UPS inhibition promotes the upregulation of macroautophagy in an apparent effort to redirect and sustain efficient protein degradation through the lysosome. Furthermore, the UPS and autophagic/lysosomal systems rely on several of the same key molecules – most notably ubiquitin and p62 – selectively targeting substrates for degradation. This complementation is limited, however, as the UPS only has the ability to degrade monomeric proteins that have been properly unfolded and fed into the proteasome catalytic core, while macroautophagy is capable of bulk degradation of organelles and oligomerized proteins. In lysosomal disease states in which the degradative capacity of the lysosome is compromised it is conceivable that the UPS may be employed to compensate for some of the proteolytic load, although the molecular machinery and sequence of events involved in this cross-talk is largely unknown. Finally, it is unclear whether there is a threshold at which the UPS may too become overwhelmed, perhaps contributing to ER stress and thereby causing complete proteolytic failure in lysosomal disease states.

Lysosomal diseases

After more than a half century of clinical recognition and classification, lysosomal storage diseases were conceptualized as disorders resulting from deficiencies in single lysosomal hydrolases followed by the subsequent accumulation of a specific substrate for that enzyme [7]. Today, lysosomal diseases are known to include nearly 60 monogenic disorders with a combined frequency of approximately 1: 7000 live births. They are known to be caused by deficiencies not only in lysosomal hydrolases, but also in other lysosomal and non-lysosomal proteins including enzymes, soluble non-enzymatic proteins, and membrane-associated proteins critical for proper function of the greater lysosomal system [8]. Categorizing lysosomal disorders is not completely straightforward as several diseases exhibit significant overlap of pathological features, storage material, and so forth. However, grouping lysosomal diseases based on the traditional biochemical

nature of the primary storage material is often preferred; these include the lipidoses, mucopolysaccharidoses (MPSs), glycogenoses, neuronal ceroid lipofuscinoses (NCLs), mucolipidoses (MLs), glycoproteinoses and others (see Classification in Chapter 5).

In general, most lysosomal diseases afflict children. Age of onset and clinical course can vary significantly, but nearly all lysosomal diseases have a delayed non-congenital onset, and progressive course ultimately leading to premature death. Even as our grasp of the genetic, molecular and biochemical bases of these disorders has advanced in recent years there are still many gaps in our understanding as to pathogenic mechanisms and the reversibility of disease-induced cell damage. Some of the most important questions in this regard involve the brain.

CNS Involvement (See also Chapter 21) Adding to lysosomal disease complexity is the broad systemic involvement of multiple tissues and organs. Clinical presentation often involves bone, muscle, liver, kidney and spleen, while nearly two-thirds of these disorders also exhibit extensive neurological impairment (see Chapter 2). Intellectual disability, dementia, seizures, motor system deficits, visual impairment and hearing loss are common manifestations associated with several lysosomal diseases. The progressive clinical and pathological course presented in these disorders highlights the indispensible role of the lysosome, especially in postmitotic neurons which are predominately affected. Interestingly, this vulnerability becomes manifest in a highly specified manner with different neuronal subtypes and brain regions exhibiting distinct pathophysiological changes.

One of the more perplexing phenomena associated with lysosomal disease is neurodegeneration. While many of these disorders exhibit some degree of patterned neuronal loss, the question remains why some neurons appear more vulnerable to this fate than others and what effect neurodegeneration has on disease course. A common theme implicated in motor system impairment is Purkinje cell (PC) death. PC death in mice with NPC begins early and progresses in an anterior to posterior lobe pattern within the cerebellum. This cell loss is severe and nearly total, with the conspicuous exception of lobule X (flocculonodular lobe in humans) where PCs are well preserved. Remarkably, almost identical patterns of PC loss occur across a wide spectrum of lysosomal diseases, including mucolipidosis type IV and the gangliosidoses. It should also be noted that in the case of NPC disease that both PCs and cerebrocortical neurons exhibit extensive pathological storage of cholesterol and ganglioside, however unlike PC degeneration, cortical neuron death is often not as conspicuous in the early stages of the disease.

CNS inflammation is an additional feature of lysosomal diseases that in many cases has been shown to be spatially and temporally correlated with neuronal dysfunction and neurodegeneration. Of particular interest is how this initial protective response to disease may become deleterious with chronic induction, ultimately leading to secondary damage and exacerbation of pathogenic processes. In the normal brain, microglia play an essential house-keeping role intimately coupled to neuronal function. As the resident macrophage of the CNS, microglia are also critical for synapse maintenance, axon and spine pruning, clearing extracellular debris and apoptotic cells, glutamate and trophic factor regulation, and probing their surroundings for homeostatic deviations in the extracellular environment. Conversely, during disease/injury activated microglia proliferate, and, along with infiltrating macrophages, can generate cytotoxic components including reactive oxygen species, nitric oxide and pro-inflammatory cytokines. Microglia and macrophages exhibit altered morphological states in many lysosomal diseases, while activated astrocytes are also a prominent feature contributing to the pathological landscape in the CNS. Some NCLs, gangliosidoses, MPSs, MLs and neuronopathic Gaucher disease exhibit neuroinflammatory features. A study in Sandhoff disease mice showed that microglial activation precedes neuronal cell death, and that bone marrow transplantation ameliorates the expansion of microglia and neurodegeneration [9]. Interestingly, however, this improvement did not coincide with any significant decrease in GM2 ganglioside storage, suggesting that microglial activation is a significant component of neuronal death independent of storage. As such, the use of anti-inflammatory drugs to treat lysosomal diseases may be a relevant therapeutic strategy for providing benefit in certain instances. Future efforts to decipher the protective roles of microglial activation and inflammation from pathogenic stimulating events, and to determine the temporal window for using anti-inflammatory drugs in the treatment of lysosomal disease states, will be critical.

Intracellular storage

Ever since the concept of lysosomal disease was developed by H.G. Hers, intracellular storage material has been a defining characteristic of these disorders. As the complexity of this pathological feature has evolved well beyond the original single enzyme/single substrate

theory, research has focused on understanding how storage contributes to pathogenic cascades. The relationship between primary and secondary storage warrants clarification. Primary storage may be defined as the lysosomal buildup of biochemical components that accumulate as a direct result of a failure of degradation within, or egress of, degradation products from the lysosomal system. Secondary storage is material accumulating from subsequent downstream compromise in lysosomal function. Given a number of lysosomal diseases caused by proteins of unknown or poorly understood function, however, the classification of specific storage material as primary or secondary continues to evolve. Neuronal storage is often found in perinuclear regions of the perikarya, although it may extend into dendrites and the axon hillock. Large swellings in the latter are known as meganeurites (described below).

At its simplest, the buildup of primary storage material probably further compromises the degradative capacity of lysosomes and thereby exacerbates the accumulation of secondary storage components in a deleterious cycle. More complex is the question of how storage may affect the lysosomal system as a whole through such expanding downstream events. These include the regulation of appropriate lysosomal pH, proper coordination of fusion events between autophagosomes, endosomes and lysosomes, unabated signal transduction along the endocytic pathway, and efficient and appropriate lysosomal salvage for regulating biosynthetic processes. Like selective neurodegeneration, differences in storage can also occur in distinct neuronal populations with regional specificity. For example, in mucolipidosis (ML) IV mice, different gangliosides accumulate throughout the CNS; in the hippocampus, however, gangliosides appear to be confined to specific regions – storage of GM3 occurs in the CA3 region, while GD3 is found in the CA1–CA2 regions only [10]. What this region-dependent storage represents remains unknown.

Determining whether lysosomal storage *per se* is a fundamental cause of neuronal dysfunction remains an important question. Studies in NCL disease have shown no direct correlation between the accumulation of saposins A and D and subunit c of mitochondrial ATP synthase (SCMAS) and neuron loss (Figure 1.2). In fact, storage pathology in NCL and other lysosomal diseases is typically prevalent long before the onset of any behavioural phenotype in animal models [8]. Similarly, neurons in many lysosomal diseases present significant storage pathology early, and yet survive for extended periods of time (decades) suggesting that accumulation is

SCMAS storage in the *CLN2⁻ᐟ⁻* mouse model

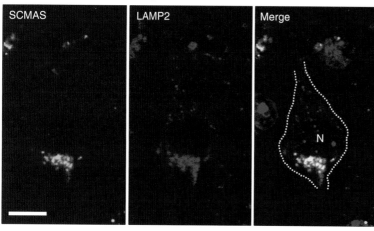

Figure 1.2 Storage accumulation of subunit c of mitochondrial ATP synthase (SCMAS) in a cortical pyramidal neuron of the *Cln2⁻ᐟ⁻* mouse model of classic late-infantile NCL disease. Image by confocal immunofluorescence microscopy of a single plane from a z-series showing SCMAS colocalization with the late endosomal/lysosomal marker LAMP2. Merged image stained with the nuclear marker DAPI (N; nucleus). Scale bar represents 10 μm.

not immediately cytotoxic. Yet this does not mean that neurons remain functionally normal. Indeed, as described below, given the presence of metabolic compromise and of axonal, dendritic and synaptic abnormalities, it is highly likely that affected neurons are not optimally functioning even from early time points in the storage process. Eventually the presence of such variously malfunctioning neurons in given neural networks would be anticipated to reach a *tipping-point* at a systems level, with clinical disease emanating as a result, even in the absence of frank neurodegeneration. Such clinical deficits would be solidified, and possibly worsened, with the eventual death of neurons that participate in these neural circuits. It is essential to understand these issues in the face of emerging therapies that may rescue the storage phenotype long after it has been established, but before neuron death. Interestingly, substrate reduction therapy either aimed at inhibiting the biosynthesis of GSLs in gangliosidoses [11], or at enhancing the egress of cholesterol and GSLs in NPC disease, has proven effective in delaying clinical onset and increasing life-span [12]. These studies clearly indicate that reducing storage is beneficial in lysosomal disorders but reveal little about the precise link between storage and brain dysfunction.

In contrast to a primary role in disease pathogenesis, storage may have a more indirect and broader influence on hindering metabolic homeostasis in cells. Impairment in lysosomal salvage probably represents a progressive and deleterious metabolic burden forcing cells to expend energy synthesizing simple molecules to replace those trapped within residual lysosomes. Owing to its tight

regulation of peripheral energy stores via the hypothalamus, as well as to additional local support from astrocytes, the brain in general, and neurons in particular, are considered resistant to starvation events. Lysosomal diseases, however, may represent a unique pathophysiological state within the CNS characterized by chronic energy depletion. This could perhaps explain why neurons which need to sustain high levels of activity are particularly susceptible in these disorders. It is also interesting to consider how this scenario might be further compounded in lysosomal disorders that have been speculated to involve suboptimal mitochondrial function (e.g. NCL disorders and MLIV), and whether this could be a cause, or a result, of chronic energy strain. Once again, clues as to how storage correlates with CNS dysfunction and why specific neuronal subtypes are more susceptible to pathological changes in lysosomal diseases may lie in the different metabolic requirements of individual neuronal populations. These so-called *metabolic signatures* may determine a cell's vulnerability to downstream deleterious events like starvation stress, oxidative stress, ER stress and even the capacity to tolerate protein aggregates and storage accumulation.

In addition to interfering with metabolic homeostasis, lysosomal storage may inhibit the destined function of the stored material within the cell. For instance, glycosaminoglycans (GAGs) are the predominant storage material in MPS diseases. Normally, mature proteoglycans are decorated with GAG side chains and localized to the outer leaflet of the plasma membrane to function in intercellular signalling cascades. Specifically, proteoglycans play a significant role in CNS development during axon guidance

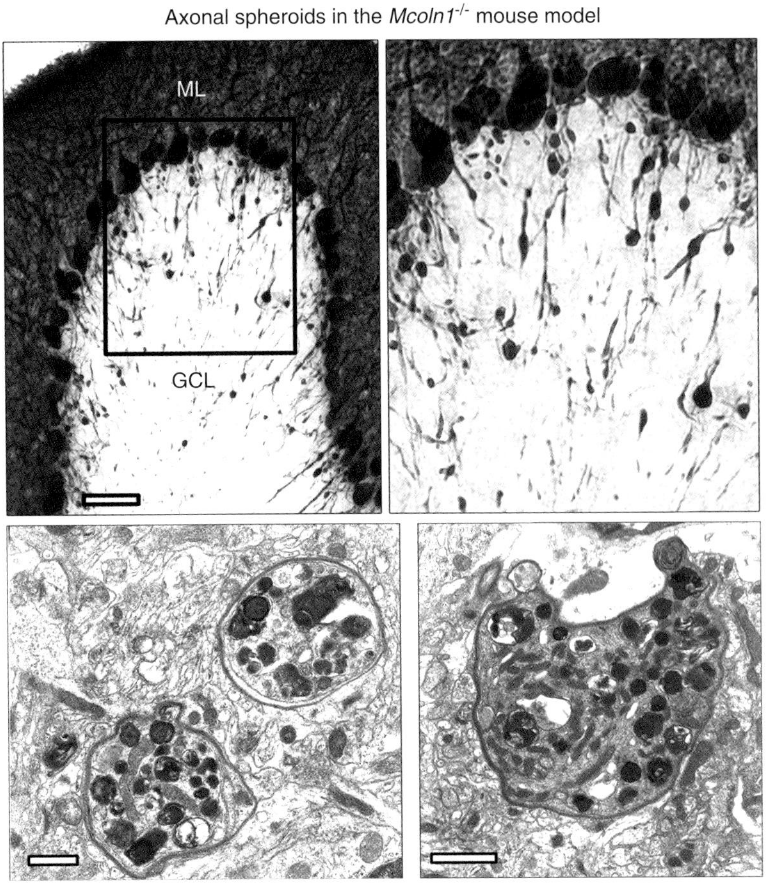

Axonal spheroids in the *Mcoln1*$^{-/-}$ mouse model

Figure 1.3 Axonal spheroid pathology in the cerebellum of the *Mcoln1*$^{-/-}$ mouse model of MLIV disease by immunohistochemistry (IHC) and electron microscopy (EM). For IHC, tissue sections were labelled with a primary antibody to calbindin D-28 K and stained with 3, 3′-diaminobenzidine (DAB) substrate kit for peroxidase (Vector Laboratories). Staining shows calbindin labelling of Purkinje cells, their dendritic arbors in the molecular layer (ML), and axonal spheroids in the granule cell layer (GCL). Boxed region is magnified at right. Electron micrographs show examples of spheroids in the *Mcoln1*$^{-/-}$ mouse with elongated mitochondria, dense bodies, and tubulovesicular profiles. Scale bar(s) for IHC represents 50 μm; for EM 1 μm.

and synapse formation through their interaction with growth factors and other extracellular components. Although MPS disorders, like other lysosomal diseases, are not believed to be associated with abnormal brain development *per se*, it is conceivable that the buildup of GAGs in MPS disease may over time hinder appropriate signalling events – eventually reaching a tipping-point for neuron and neural circuit dysfunction as described above.

Axonal spheroids

Neuroaxonal dystrophy, also known as axonal spheroid formation, occurs in a wide spectrum of lysosomal diseases, from the gangliosidoses to the glycoproteinoses [8]. Notably, this feature appears to occur predominantly in γ-aminobutyric acid (GABA)ergic neurons, particularly PCs in the cerebellum (Figure 1.3). Morphologically, spheroids are characterized as focal swellings along axons where mitochondria, multivesicular and dense bodies, tubulovesicular profiles and possibly autophagic vacuoles

accumulate. Interestingly, this material is ultrastructurally similar across different lysosomal diseases, yet distinct from the storage found in neuronal cell bodies. Given the large surface area of neurons and their highly polarized nature, functional anterograde and retrograde trafficking is essential. Spheroids appear to reflect a compromise in such transport and may as a result hinder critical growth factor support for the development, maintenance, and survival of target neurons. They are also large enough to impact normal action potential propagation and thereby contribute to neuronal dysfunction. Indeed, the incidence of spheroids appears to correlate with the onset and progression of CNS impairment in animal models, suggesting a similar, significant role in human clinical neurological disease [8].

Calcium signalling

Calcium plays a critical role as a second messenger involved in a wide range of cellular functions, and altered calcium homeostasis and signalling have provided clues to lysosomal disease mechanisms. Indeed, calcium is critical for intraorganellar fusion events along the endocytic and autophagic pathways. Not surprisingly, several lysosomal diseases show defects in endosome/autophagosome/lysosome fusion that may be attributed in part to abnormal calcium homeostasis. A number of diseases have been characterized by elevated neuronal intracellular calcium levels as a result of aberrant ER calcium channel function affected by storage accumulation. In NPC1, sphingosine storage has been reported to lead to reduction in lysosomal calcium stores, altered pH, trafficking defects and the storage of cholesterol, sphingomyelin and GSLs [13]. Altered calcium homeostasis may also be linked to the excitotoxic stress seen in NCL disease, with cortical excitatory neurons unable to recover from depolarization due to high intracellular levels of calcium.

Meganeurites and ectopic dendritogenesis

The buildup of storage within the basilar region of neurons can extend into the axon hillock resulting in the aberrant formation of a meganeurite. This striking feature can be visualized by silver or Golgi stains, for example, in cerebral cortex in ganglioside storage diseases. A clear functional consequence of meganeurites is the distal displacement of the axonal initial segment rich in sodium channels (the action potential trigger zone) away from the cell body. This displacement may result in inappropriate action potential initiation, with serious repercussions for neuronal function. Notably, meganeurites are morphologically distinct from axonal spheroids. Whereas meganeurites occur at the axon hillock proximal to the initial segment and contain storage bodies characteristic of a particular lysosomal disease, spheroids occur distal to the initial segment in the axon proper and contain a generic accumulation of organelles and other structures as described earlier [8].

Ectopic dendritogenesis, which often is seen in conjunction with meganeurite formation, is a phenomenon in which a subset of excitatory cortical pyramidal neurons exhibit new dendrite and synapse formation [8]. This unprecedented event is both mislocalized to the axon hillock and occurs distinctively after the normal temporal window of dendritogenesis during early development. Ectopic dendritogenesis has been documented in several lysosomal diseases, all of which are characterized by primary or secondary storage of gangliosides. The precise relationship, however, between ectopic dendritogenesis, endosomal/lysosomal dysfunction and GSL metabolism remains to be determined.

Autophagy dysfunction

Autophagy dysfunction marked by a buildup of autophagosomes in brain tissue has been closely linked to neurodegeneration, and not surprisingly several lysosomal diseases have been found to exhibit alterations in this critical homeostatic mechanism [14]. This buildup can represent a pathogenic failure in autophagosome degradation, a physiological induction in macroautophagy flux, or, in some cases, both a blockage and induction. Given the primary disease defect and general compromise of the lysosome, impaired autophagosome maturation is a predicted downstream consequence of lysosomal storage accumulation. Trafficking and fusion deficits between autophagosomes and lysosomes, as well as failures in degrading autophagic material, have been attributed to the observed increases in autophagosomes in specific disorders. The presence of autophagosomes implies that the molecular machinery for macroautophagy initiation is intact and functional, while later steps in the pathway are compromised. Danon disease, which is caused by a deficiency in LAMP2, represents a classic example of failure in autophagosome maturation [14]. Studies in mice have found LAMP2 to be critical for the fusion of autophagosomes and lysosomes, resulting in significant accumulation of autophagic vacuoles in disease tissue. Also worth noting is the importance of the LAMP2A isoform in mediating CMA, although potential dysfunction along this pathway in Danon disease has not been thoroughly explored.

Evidence of an induction or overactive macroautophagy is also commonly seen in many lysosomal diseases, although the reason for this response is not entirely clear. Perhaps most relevant to consider is an upregulation of macroautophagy in an effort to counter energy deprivation stress incurred within cells due to salvage failure. In Pompe disease, a deficiency of α-glucosidase and the consequent failure to breakdown glycogen in lysosomes stimulates macroautophagy, while the buildup of storage concomitantly impedes autophagosome maturation. This resulting accumulation of autophagosomes in Pompe disease severely hinders muscle contraction and contributes to muscle deterioration [14]. Interestingly, overactive autophagy in type-II muscle fibres is believed to interfere with enzyme replacement therapy in Pompe, where recombinant enzyme is taken up in accumulating autophagosomes, preventing efficient trafficking to the lysosome. Significantly, studies have shown that suppression of macroautophagy in skeletal muscle corrects enzyme delivery deficits and attenuates glycogen storage in mouse models of Pompe disease. Several other lysosomal diseases have shown evidence of upregulated

(a)

p62 accumulation in *Npc1^{-/-}* Purkinje cell

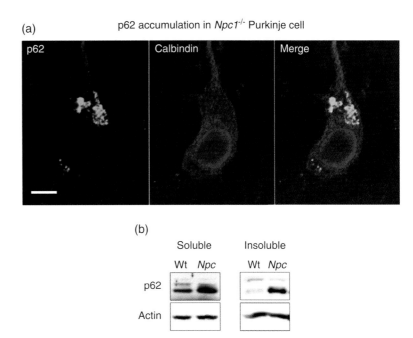

Figure 1.4 p62 accumulation in end-stage cerebellum of the *Npc1^{-/-}* mouse model. (a) Confocal immunofluorescence image of lobule X Purkinje cell from *Npc1^{-/-}* cerebellum showing p62 aggregates. Scale bar represents 10 μm. (b) Western blot probed for p62 in soluble and SDS-insoluble fractions from cerebellar homogenate of wildtype and *Npc1^{-/-}* showing increases in both protein fractions. β-actin was used as a loading control.

macroautophagy, but whether this initial response is detrimental or protective remains unknown.

An additional scenario to consider in regard to autophagy impairment is a failure to initiate the macroautophagy pathway or target appropriate cargo to autophagosomes. As opposed to inefficiencies late in autophagosome maturation and flux, the accumulation of oligomerized proteins and effete organelles is suggestive of general proteolytic compromise and failures in constitutive macroautophagy initiation. Several lysosomal diseases (MPS IIIA, MSD, NPC, MLIV, several NCLs and several gangliosidoses) have been found to exhibit increased levels of proteins preferentially degraded by macroautophagy, most notably the autophagosome adaptor protein p62 (Figure 1.4). Often interpreted simply as an indirect marker of autophagy function, the accumulation of cytosolic p62-positive aggregates may more appropriately signify a deficiency in autophagosome formation and/or engulfment of material by autophagosomes. These p62 aggregates are widely distributed throughout the CNS in both neuronal and glial cell populations depending on the disease. It remains unclear however, what role aggregates play and how they contribute to the pathological milieu of lysosomal disorders. In addition to aggregate formation, macroautophagy initiation impairment and cargo recognition failure directly result in the inefficient turnover of damaged

mitochondria, also known as mitophagy. Accumulation of dysfunctional mitochondria can have a significant deleterious effect on cells including altered calcium homeostasis and the generation of reactive oxygen species (ROS). Most importantly, dysfunctional mitochondria can stimulate the release of cytochrome c initiating intrinsic apoptotic cell death pathways. Several lysosomal diseases are associated with mitochondrial abnormalities, although how mitophagy deficits contribute to this phenotype remains unclear. Future studies will need to focus on whether alterations in autophagy are consistent with an induction or blockage in a given disease state, what the repercussions are for protein aggregate accumulation, and importantly how compromise of mitophagy may contribute to neurodegeneration. In addition to evaluating how lysosomal compromise affects pathways that feed into the lysosome, it will also be prudent to consider how systems allied in maintaining proteolytic quality control, like the UPS, may be affected downstream in lysosomal disease pathogenesis. To date, little is known about this relationship.

Concluding remarks

Delineation of the pathogenic cascades underlying lysosomal diseases continues to reveal the intricate nature of the *greater lysosomal system* and its role in cell homeostasis. Novel genes and proteins contributing to lysosome function continue to be identified and the list of lysosomal and lysosomal-associated diseases continues to grow. Studies of the molecular and cellular pathogenesis of lysosomal diseases have also never been more compelling, and are progressively opening up new avenues for therapy. Furthermore, parallels across groups of traditionally unrelated neurological disorders have emerged, providing insight into CNS dysfunction and reshaping the way we think about the role of the lysosomal system in neuron function. Indeed, in recent years pathophysiological boundaries have blurred between lysosomal diseases and other neurological disorders including both early-onset neurogenetic diseases like Angelman syndrome [15], to late-onset neurodegenerative diseases like Alzheimer's [16] and Parkinson's [17]. Emerging commonalities in lysosomal dysfunction and their links across this spectrum of conditions may indeed provide valuable insights toward the goal of developing therapeutic strategies for a host of presently untreatable neurological conditions.

References

1 Walkley SU. Pathogenic cascades in lysosomal disease – Why so complex? *J Inherit Metab Dis* 2009; **32**(2): 181–189.

2 Sardiello M, Palmieri M, di Ronza A, *et al.* A gene network regulating lysosomal biogenesis and function. *Science* 2009; **325**(5939): 473–477.

3 Zhou S, Davidson C, McGlynn R, *et al.* Endosomal/lysosomal processing of gangliosides affects neuronal cholesterol sequestration in Niemann-Pick disease type C. *Am J Pathol* 2011; **179**(2): 890–902.

4 Klionsky DJ. Autophagy: from phenomenology to molecular understanding in less than a decade. *Nat Rev Mol Cell Biol* 2007; **8**(11): 931–937.

5 Ruivo R, Anne C, Sagne C, Gasnier B. Molecular and cellular basis of lysosomal transmembrane protein dysfunction. *Biochim Biophys Acta* 2009; **1793**(4): 636–649.

6 Xie C, Turley SD, Pentchev PG, Dietschy JM. Cholesterol balance and metabolism in mice with loss of function of Niemann-Pick C protein. *Am J Physiol* 1999; **276**(2 Pt 1): E336–344.

7 Hers HG. Inborn lysosomal diseases. *Gastroenterology* 1965; **48**: 625–633.

8 Platt FM, Walkley SU. *Lysosomal Disorders of the Brain: Recent Advances in Molecular and Cellular Pathogenesis and Treatment.* Oxford: Oxford University Press, 2004; xxvii, 447 pp.

9 Wada R, Tifft CJ, Proia RL. Microglial activation precedes acute neurodegeneration in Sandhoff disease and is suppressed by bone marrow transplantation. *Proc Natl Acad Sci USA* 2000; **97**(20): 10954–10959.

10 Micsenyi MC, Dobrenis K, Stephney G, *et al.* Neuropathology of the Mcoln1(-/-) knockout mouse model of mucolipidosis type IV. *J Neuropathol Exp Neurol* 2009; **68**(2): 125–135.

11 Zervas M, Somers KL, Thrall MA, Walkley SU. Critical role for glycosphingolipids in Niemann-Pick disease type C. *Curr Biol* 2001; **11**(16): 1283–1287.

12 Davidson CD, Ali NF, Micsenyi MC, *et al.* Chronic cyclodextrin treatment of murine Niemann-Pick C disease ameliorates neuronal cholesterol and glycosphingolipid storage and disease progression. *PLoS One* 2009; **4**(9): e6951.

13 Lloyd-Evans E, Morgan AJ, He X, *et al.* Niemann-Pick disease type C1 is a sphingosine storage disease that causes deregulation of lysosomal calcium. *Nat Med* 2008; **14**(11): 1247–1255.

14 Lieberman AP, Puertollano R, Raben N, *et al.* Autophagy in lysosomal storage disorders. *Autophagy* (in press)

15 Stromme P, Dobrenis K, Sillitoe RV, *et al.* X-linked Angelman-like syndrome caused by Slc9a6 knockout in mice exhibits evidence of endosomal-lysosomal dysfunction. *Brain* 2011; **134**(11): 3369–3383.

16 Lee JH, Yu WH, Kumar A, *et al.* Lysosomal proteolysis and autophagy require presenilin 1 and are disrupted by Alzheimer-related PS1 mutations. *Cell* 2010; **141**(7): 1146–1158.

17 DePaolo J, Goker-Alpan O, Samaddar T, *et al.* The association between mutations in the lysosomal protein glucocerebrosidase and parkinsonism. *Mov Disord* 2009; **24**(11): 1571–1578.

CHAPTER 2

Clinical Aspects and Clinical Diagnosis

J. Edmond Wraith[1] and Michael Beck[2]

[1] Willink Biochemical Genetics Unit, Royal Manchester Children's Hospital, Manchester, UK
[2] Children's Hospital, University of Mainz, Mainz, Germany

Introduction

For clinicians managing patients with lysosomal storage disease (LSD), the early years of the 21st century have been characterized by the introduction of a number of new, disease specific, therapies. Initial results from the use of these treatments all suggest that the best results are obtained in patients that present early in the course of the disease before the development of irreversible organ damage. As a consequence, clinicians are under increasing pressure to make a timely diagnosis to allow their patients to benefit from these advances. In the absence of newborn screening for LSD early diagnosis has to depend on clinical acumen and as the disorders are remarkably variable this may involve a number of different specialists.

In some patients the presentation may be in the newborn period with hydrops foetalis, whereas in others, with the same enzyme deficiency (but a different genetic mutation), onset may be in late adulthood.

For many patients the onset of symptoms may be in the first months or years of life following an unremarkable early course. The first signs may be a slowing of development and other neurological abnormalities; in other patients, visceromegaly or coarse features may be present. Recognition of these clinical signs will assist in the choice of the most appropriate diagnostic tests (Figure 2.1). Increasingly LSDs are being diagnosed for the first time in adult life. In this group, presentation may be atypical and neuropsychiatric manifestations in the absence of dysmorphic features or visceromegaly are much more common in these patients.

Clinical presentation

Hydrops foetalis

Hydrops foetalis (HF) can be caused by a wide range of foetal, placental or maternal disorders. Foetal mortality is high and so every effort must be made to recognize those disorders that may be associated with an increased risk of recurrent hydrops. This area of prenatal presentation has been extensively reviewed [1]. Figure 2.2 illustrates a suggested diagnostic approach when presented with a hydropic pregnancy. Placental pathology is often very useful as the placenta may appear pale and bulky to gross examination, and lysosomal vacuolation is usually readily seen by light or electron microscopy in cases where the HF is secondary to LSD.

Dysmorphism

The facial appearance of patients with underlying LSDs associated with dysmorphism (Figure 2.1) is often labelled as "coarse" and is seen in its fully developed form in Mucolipidosis II (ML II, I-cell disease) when it may be noticed at birth (Figure 2.3). In most other disorders appearance is normal at birth and the facial phenotype that develops over the first year of life is characterized by a flattened, wide nasal bridge, frontal bossing, thickened gums and macroglossia. Infants affected by some LSDs (in particular, mucopolysaccharidoses) may be large at birth and growth may be normal for the first 2 or 3 years, but then slows. There is a characteristic skeletal dysplasia (dysostosis multiplex, described in more detail later), joint contractures and often both umbilical and inguinal hernias.

Lysosomal Storage Disorders: A Practical Guide, First Edition. Edited by Atul Mehta and Bryan Winchester.
© 2012 John Wiley & Sons, Ltd. Published 2012 by John Wiley & Sons, Ltd.

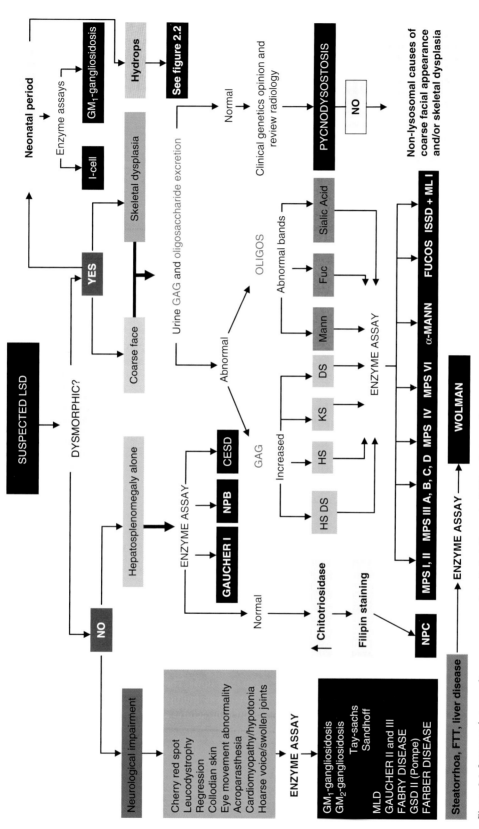

Figure 2.1 Lysosomal storage disease: an approach to clinical diagnosis. CESD – cholesterol ester storage disease, DS – dermatan sulfate, Fuc – fucosidosis, GAG – glycosaminoglycans, GSD – glycogen storage disease, HS – heparan sulfate, ISSSD – infantile sialic acid storage disease, KS – keratan sulfate, Mann – mannosidosis, ML – mucolipidosis, MLD – metachromatic leucodystrophy, MPS – mucopolysaccharidosis, OLIGOS – oligosaccharidosis, NPB – Niemann–Pick disease type B, NPC – Niemann–Pick disease type C.

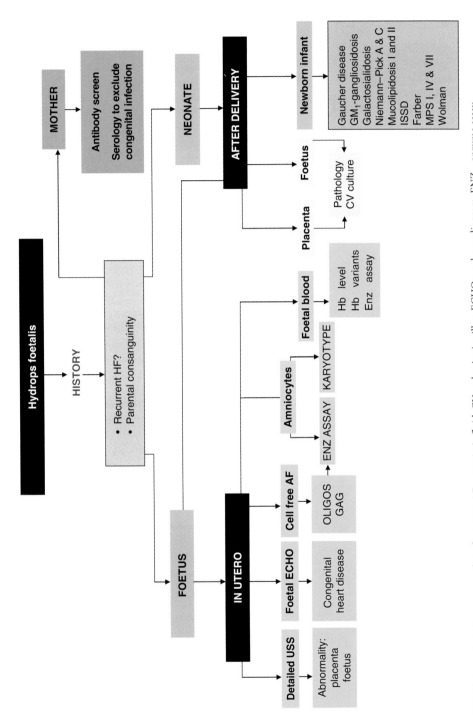

Figure 2.2 Hydrops foetalis: an approach to diagnosis. AF – amniotic fluid, CV – chorionic villus, ECHO – echocardiogram, ENZ – enzyme assay, GAG – glycosaminoglycan analysis, Hb – haemoglobin, HF – hydrops foetalis, ISSD – infantile sialic acid storage disease, OLIGOS – oligosaccharide analysis, USS – ultrasound scan.

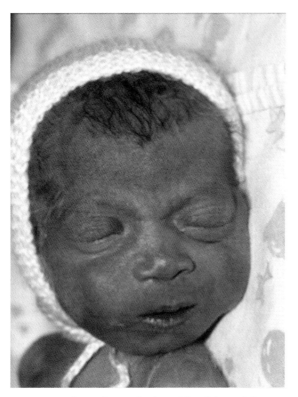

Figure 2.3 Infant with Mucolipidosis II (I-cell disease) day 1. Facial features of LSD already apparent.

Patients with acute neuronopathic Gaucher disease (GDII) can present with severe icthyosis ("collodian baby"), unusual facies, arthrogryposis, enlargement of the liver and spleen, and hernias. Another dermatological clue to the presence of underlying LSD is the abundant Mongolian blue spots seen in children with mucopolysaccharidoses.

Upper airway obstruction, deafness and frequent respiratory infections

Many infants with underlying LSD fail their neonatal hearing assessment. In those that go on to develop the characteristic facial dysmorphism, upper airway obstruction with obstructive sleep apnoea (OSA) and associated frequent upper respiratory infections are common. These patients may present to Ear, Nose and Throat (ENT) surgeons in the first year of life before underlying LSD has been considered, and infants that require ENT surgery in the first 12–18 months of life should be viewed as potential LSD patients and investigated appropriately [2]. In Mannosidosis deafness is a very early symptom and is observed in virtually all affected individuals.

Cardiac disease

In infantile Pompe disease (glycogen storage disease type II, acid maltase deficiency), cardiac failure, cardiac arrhythmia and cardiomegaly may all be present at birth. Indeed in a number of affected infants, cardiomegaly has been demonstrated on foetal ultrasounds performed in the last trimester of pregnancy. Affected infants also have macroglossia with a protruding tongue and are generally hypotonic. In addition to the cardiomyopathy demonstrated on echocardiography (usually hypertrophic, occasionally dilated) there is also elevation of liver enzymes and CPK on biochemical testing and the blood film will reveal vacuolated lymphocytes in the vast majority of affected patients.

Neonatal cardiomyopathy is a feature of other LSDs and is seen commonly in GM1-gangliosidosis, ML II (I-cell disease) and MPS IH (Hurler syndrome). In this group of patients coronary artery disease may also be present and episodes of ischaemia may go undetected unless specifically looked for by electro- and echocardiography [3].

In older patients with LSD, valve involvement (especially mitral and aortic) becomes common and in some older patients valve replacement surgery becomes necessary.

Specific cardiac involvement is a feature of other LSDs (for example, Fabry disease) and this is considered in more detail within the specific disease sections.

Hepatosplenomegaly and liver disease

Hepatosplenomegaly in the newborn period has very many different causes, and the common ones such as bacterial and viral infections or anatomical abnormalities need to be diagnosed quickly as specific treatment may be available.

A number of LSDs can also present with enlargement of the liver and spleen, and in a number of affected patients ascites will also be present. Careful clinical and radiological examination for other abnormalities may be helpful, and in some circumstances bone marrow or liver biopsy may suggest underlying LSD.

In contrast to this non-specific presentation, some infants with Niemann–Pick disease type C (NP-C) have a very typical clinical presentation with liver disease in the newborn period. In these affected infants (about a quarter of all patients with NP-C seen in our clinic) severe liver dysfunction often associated with conjugated hyperbilirubinaemia suggests a diagnosis of biliary atresia and a number of NP-C infants have had surgical procedures to exclude this diagnosis. A significant number of these patients will go on to develop liver failure and dic (about one-third) while others will slowly improve over months (and even years in some patients) and eventually make a full recovery from their liver disease only to present with the neurological manifestations of the disease often many years later.

Finally, in the newborn period, patients with early-onset lysosomal acid lipase deficiency (LAL deficiency, Wolman disease) present with severe failure to thrive due to fat malabsorption, liver disease (ultimately progressing to liver failure) and severe anaemia. Calcification of the adrenal glands visible on plain abdominal radiology is an important clue to the diagnosis.

Hepatosplenomegaly in older patients may be the presenting manifestation of Gaucher disease (types I and III), cholesterol ester storage disease and Niemann–Pick disease. There are often abnormal blood lipids as well as haematological abnormalities secondary to hypersplenism and bone marrow infiltration. Respiratory infiltration is often under-recognized in these patients who, on rare occasions, will present with respiratory failure.

Dysostosis multiplex

The radiological abnormalities associated with LSD are known as dysostosis multiplex and comprise a characteristic constellation of radiological abnormalities which are seen in the most fully developed form in patients with mucopolysaccharidoses (MPS). Typically the skull is scaphiocephalic and large. The odontoid process of C2 is often dysplastic and the lower vertebrae show anterior beaking, most commonly seen at the thoracolumbar junction and responsible for the gibbus abnormality that is often an early clinical clue to diagnosis [4]. The iliac bones are flared, with a flattened acetabulum and the long bones are short and broad. There is anterior expansion of the clavicles and ribs and the metacarpals are pointed proximally. Some of these general changes are illustrated in Figure 2.4(a) and (b) and have been recently reviewed in some detail [5].

In some disorders the radiological abnormalities are more specific. In MPS IV, for example, the odontoid is often very dysplastic and the vertebrae reveal generalized platyspondyly, with the anterior beaking characteristic of other MPS disorders not as noticeable. In ML II (I Cell disease) there are often intrauterine fractures and in some patients a very severe neonatal skeletal dysplasia is found in conjunction with biochemical evidence of hyperparathyroidism.

Bone disease is a late feature of other LSDs but can occasionally be the first sign of an underlying disorder such as Gaucher disease, where presentation with avascular necrosis or pathological fracture has been reported.

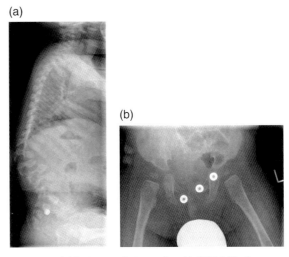

Figure 2.4 (a) Patient aged 18 months with MPS I (Hurler syndrome) gibbus deformity at thoracolumbar junction with anterior beaking of lumbar vertebrae. (b) Patient aged 12 months with MPS I (Hurler syndrome) acetabular dysplasia and coxa valga.

Neurological presentation

Unfortunately a great majority of LSDs have a significant neurological component, and in a number of disorders it is the dominating clinical effect of the disease (e.g. most sphingolipidoses), whereas in others it is merely one element of a more generalized disorder (e.g. mucopolysaccharidosis type I).

In infantile Tay–Sachs disease the onset of the neurological disorder can seem very acute, mimicking an encephalitic process, with an explosive onset of seizures starting towards the end of the first year of life in a patient initially thought to be following a normal pattern of development. Rapid neurodegeneration follows with visual loss, spasticity and eventually loss of all skills culminating in death before the age of 5 years in the most affected infants. In these patients clinical examination reveals the classical macular "cherry red spot" secondary to storage within the retinal cells (Figure 2.5). As the disease progresses, the cherry red spot disappears [6].

The typical developmental pattern seen in LSDs is one of regression. After a period of apparently uneventful progress, development slows and peers start to acquire skills at an increasingly faster rate. Eventually development reaches a plateau and acquired skills are then lost in a pattern. The most recently acquired skills are lost first, and eventually the child becomes dependent on its carers for all needs.

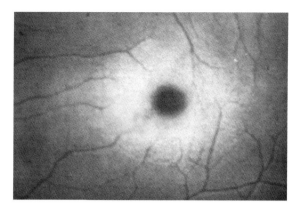

Figure 2.5 Cherry-red spot in 2-year-old infant with Tay–Sachs disease.

For some disorders characteristic patterns can be seen. In mucopolysaccharidosis type III (Sanfilippo syndrome) most of the affected children are normal until the age of 12 to 18 months, then fail to develop normal speech. Initially this is usually thought to be due to associated middle ear disease and deafness; however, when this is corrected speech fails to improve and developmental progress is further impaired. Children with this disorder have only mild somatic abnormalities and the facial features of an MPS disorder are often not appreciated. Diagnosis is usually established when the patients develop the characteristic challenging behaviour seen in MPS III. This is characterized by severe insomnia and often extreme hyperactivity, making management extremely difficult. As the disease progresses skills are lost and the children become unsteady and fall, and also develop neurological dysphagia. By their mid-teenage years most affected patients are dependent on their carers for all needs, before death occurs towards the end of the second or early in the third decade of life.

Neuronal Ceroid Lipofuscinosis (NCL) is a group of disorders said to be the commonest neurodegenerative disorder of childhood. The neurodegeneration occurs at a differing age of onset and speed of progression, depending on the type of NCL present. The group as a whole is characterized by seizures (often difficult to control) and progressive visual loss. Enzyme assay and DNA mutation analysis has made diagnosis of NCL more readily available.

Niemann–Pick disease type C (NP-C) can present with two unusual but specific neurological abnormalities. The first involves an abnormality of voluntary eye movement due to a failure to initiate ordinary saccades. This supra-nuclear gaze palsy initially affects vertical movements and affected patients often blink excessively in an attempt to initiate eye movement. This is often the first neurological abnormality detected in affected patients. Over time the horizontal movements are also affected and the eyes become virtually immobile. (In Gaucher disease type III, horizontal gaze palsy develops and in these patients rapid head movements (head thrusting) are used to stimulate eye movement.)

The second neurological abnormality seen commonly in NP-C is cataplexy, a sudden transient loss of muscular tone precipitated by emotion, usually humour. Patients have bouts of laughter culminating in sudden hypotonia and will fall to the ground if not supported. The attacks last seconds but can recur in bouts and be very disabling. Cataplexy is closely related to narcolepsy, which is another neurological complication seen in NP-C patients. It is important to recognize cataplexy for what it is and not diagnose the episodes as epilepsy. Cataplexy does not usually respond to standard anticonvulsants and is most responsive to tricyclic antidepressants such as imipramine.

Adult-onset disease

A number of LSDs are well recognized as adult disorders. Examples would include Gaucher disease type 1, Fabry disease, and late-onset acid maltase deficiency. For some conditions features may be present in childhood but misinterpreted. In the classical male Fabry patient, for instance, presentation in childhood with acroparasthesia or abdominal pain is usual, but the diagnosis is rarely made at this time. These patients may attend rheumatology, gastroenterology or pain clinics for many years before the correct diagnosis is made, often decades later, when a more serious complication of the disease is recognized.

All of the disorders presenting typically in childhood have attenuated variants that only become apparent in late childhood or adulthood. These disorders may present to many different specialists. For example, in MPS I, patients with the attenuated Scheie variant may present to a rheumatology clinic with an apparent non-inflammatory arthropathy [7] and other LSDs may have prominent musculoskeletal symptoms presenting to either orthopaedic or rheumatology specialists [8]. Occasionally corneal clouding or heart valve abnormalities will be additional clues to the correct underlying diagnosis.

The childhood neurological LSDs also have attenuated variants that can be difficult to identify and diagnose correctly. Often cognitive impairment is not an early feature and a range of other neurological abnormalities may be present such as slowly progressive spasticity, ataxia, dystonia or neuropathy. Other conditions, for example, Niemann–Pick disease type C (NP-C), may present to mental health services with prominent psychiatric disturbance (for example, acute psychosis) with neurological abnormalities only revealed by careful examination [9].

Making a diagnosis

The introduction of a number of disease-specific therapies has highlighted the need for a timely diagnosis of LSD in an affected individual. The clinical approach and tests performed depend on the age of the patient, the chronology of symptoms and the clinical signs present on examination. An approach to diagnosis is illustrated in Figure 1.1 and investigations will usually include urine and blood testing as well as the use of plain radiology and specialized imaging. For some disorders skin fibroblast cultures will be necessary (e.g., NP-C and Mucolipidosis I, Neuraminidase deficiency).

The laboratory diagnosis is considered further in Chapter 3.

References

1 Staretz-Chacham O, Lang TC, LaMarca ME, et al. Lysosomal storage disorders in the newborn. *Pediatrics* 2009; **123**(4): 1191–1207.
2 Simmons MA, Bruce IA, Penney S, et al. Otorhinolaryngological manifestations of the mucopolysaccharidosis. *Int J Pediatr Otorhinolaryngol* 2005; **69**: 589–595.
3 van den Broek L, Backx AP, Coolen H, et al. Fatal coronary artery disease in an infant with severe mucopolysaccharidosis type I. *Pediatrics* 2011; **27**: e1343–1346.
4 Mundada V, D'Souza N. Lumbar gibbus: early presentation of dysostosis multiplex. *Arch Dis Child* 2009; **94**: 930–931.
5 Rasalkar DD, Chu WCW, Hui J, et al. Pictorial review of mucopolysaccharidosis with emphasis on MRI features of brain and spine. *Br J Radiol* 2011; **84**: 469–477.
6 Kivlin JD, Sanborn GE, Myers GG. The cherry-red spot in Tay–Sachs and other storage diseases. *Ann Neurol* 1985; **17**: 356–360.
7 Cimaz R, Coppa GV, Kone-Paut I, et al. Joint contractures in the absence of inflammation may indicate mucopolysaccharidosis. *Pediatr Rheumatol Online J* 2009 Oct 23; **7**: 18.
8 Manger B, Mengel E, Schaefer RM. Rheumatologic aspects of lysosomal storage diseases. *Clin Rheumatol* 2007; **26**: 335–341.
9 Sevin M, Lesca G, Baumann N, et al. The adult form of Niemann–Pick disease type C. *Brain* 2007; **130**: 120–133.

CHAPTER 3

Laboratory Diagnosis of Lysosomal Storage Diseases

Bryan Winchester

Emeritus Professor of Biochemistry, UCL Institute of Child Health at Great Ormond Street Hospital, University College London, London, UK

There is no currently available universal diagnostic test for lysosomal storage diseases. The route to a definitive diagnosis is based upon the clinical presentation (see Chapter 2) and a panel of laboratory tests on blood and urine. Most laboratories specializing in the diagnosis of the LSDs follow a similar flexible algorithm (Figure 3.1) [1, 2]. It is important to be aware of the considerable clinical and genetic heterogeneity seen within this group of disorders and within individual disorders. Sometimes the results of initial biochemical studies appear normal but this may not mean the absence of disease, especially if the clinical indication is strong. Further investigations using cultured fibroblasts or lymphoblastoid cells and occasionally a tissue biopsy are essential for diagnosis of some diseases and are often necessary to resolve cases with an atypical presentation.

Referral to specialist laboratory

Upon suspicion of a lysosomal storage disease, the clinician should arrange for a blood sample containing an anticoagulant and, in some cases, a urine sample to be sent to a laboratory specializing in the diagnosis of LSDs. The use of dried blood spots is increasing because of the convenience of collection and transport, the interest in newborn screening and the development of suitable methods [3]. The clinician should provide as much clinical information as is possible on the request form and highlight the main symptoms and signs, e.g. hepatosplenomegaly, dysmorphic features, neurological symptoms and, if possible, indicate whether a particular type of LSD is suspected, e.g. MPS (see Chapter 2). Close collaboration between clinicians and laboratory scientists is essential if the diagnosis is to be made in a rapid, efficient and affordable manner.

Preliminary screening tests on urine or blood

The definitive diagnosis of most LSDs will be based upon demonstrating a deficiency of a specific lysosomal enzyme activity or loss of function of a lysosomal protein in cells. However, an indication of the type of storage disease or even a specific disorder can be obtained from preliminary screening tests on blood and urine samples. These tests consist either of the measurement or detection of storage products or detection of abnormal levels of serum/plasma proteins e.g. chitotriosidase (Table 3.1). For some disorders the preliminary test in blood or urine is an essential first step in the diagnosis e.g. the quantitative and qualitative analysis of urinary glycosaminoglycans for the diagnosis of a mucopolysaccharidosis (MPS). Traditionally TLC, electrophoresis or HPLC has been used to measure metabolites, but increasing use is being made of tandem mass spectrometry [4].

Lysosomal Storage Disorders: A Practical Guide, First Edition. Edited by Atul Mehta and Bryan Winchester.
© 2012 John Wiley & Sons, Ltd. Published 2012 by John Wiley & Sons, Ltd.

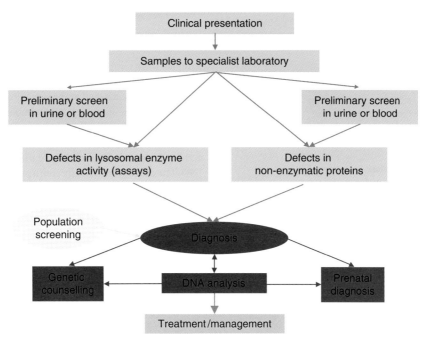

Figure 3.1 Algorithm for diagnosis of new cases of lysosomal storage diseases. Screening may be in newborns or in targeted populations (see Chapter 23). If the patient is from a family with a known LSD, the diagnosis may be made directly by enzyme assay, genetic analysis or quantitative metabolite analysis.

Table 3.1 Preliminary screening tests in blood or urine.

Disease or group of diseases	Test	Technique
(a) Biochemical tests		
MPS	Urinary glycosaminoglycans and derived oligosaccharides	Quantitative precipitation and qualitative electrophoresis or TLC; tandem mass spectrometry
Glycoproteinoses	Urinary oligosaccharides	TLC, GC-MS, tandem mass spectrometry
Sialic acid storage disease and sialidosis	Urinary free and total sialic acid	Colorimetric assay, tandem mass spectrometry
Glycosphingolipidoses	Urinary glycolipids	Tandem mass spectrometry
Pompe disease	Urinary oligosaccharides	Tandem mass spectrometry
Cobalmin-F transporter	Homocysteine and methylmalonic acid in blood and urine	Tandem mass spectrometry
(b) Histochemical tests		
Gaucher	Gaucher cells, foamy macrophages and sea-blue histiocytes in bone marrow smears	Staining of bone marrow aspirate
Metachromatic leukodystrophy	Metachromatic granules (sulfatide) in urine	Stained urinary sediment
GM1-gangliosidosis (type 1), Galactosialidosis, sialic acid storage, sialidosis, fucosidosis, α-mannosidosis, I-cell disease, CLN3	Numerous large and bold vacuoles in lymphocytes	Stained blood film
Niemann–Pick type A, Pompe, Wolman	Small discrete vacuoles in lymphocytes	Stained blood film
MPS VI & VII, multiple sulphatidosis	Alder granulation of neutrophils	Stained blood film
(c) Serum/plasma proteins		
Gaucher disease, other lipidoses and neurodegenerative disorders	Chitotriosidase	Enzyme assay
Pompe disease	Creatine kinase	Enzyme assay
Mucolipidosis IV	Gastrin	Immunoassay

Table 3.2 Enzymes that can be assayed initially in plasma*.

Enzyme	Disease
Arylsulfatase A[†]	I-cell
Aspartylglucosaminidase	Aspartylglucosaminuria
α-Fucosidase[†]	Fucosidosis
α-N-acetylgalactosaminidase	Schindler
α-Galactosidase[†]	Fabry
β-Glucuronidase[†]	MPS VII
Total β-hexosaminidase[†]	Sandhoff
β-Hexosaminidase A[†]	Tay–Sachs / B1 variant
α- and β-Mannosidases	α- and β-Mannosidosis
Chitotriosidase[§]	All children under 1 year and all with hepatosplenomegaly

*Usually plasma but activities can be measured in serum
[†]Pseudodeficiency of enzyme reported
[§]Common null allele

Diagnosis of lysosomal enzyme defects

There is a deficiency of a specific lysosomal hydrolase in about 60% of the LSDs (see Classification in Chapter 5), which account for about 85–90% of the cases diagnosed. The diagnosis of a lysosomal enzyme defect is made by demonstrating a deficiency of a specific enzyme activity in white blood cells, lymphocytes or dried blood spots. Cultured fibroblasts are not used routinely as the primary source of enzyme activity unless the activity cannot be measured reliably in white blood cells, e.g. neuraminidase. Some enzyme deficiencies can be demonstrated reliably in plasma (Table 3.2). The enzymes are usually assayed in groups or panels (Table 3.3), according to the clinical indications (see Chapter 2) and the results of the preliminary tests. Some laboratories assay a large number of enzymes routinely, whereas others are very selective. Most lysosomal enzymes can be assayed using synthetic substrates, such as derivatives of the flurophore, 4-methylumbelliferone or the chromophore, paranitrophenol to increase the sensitivity and simplify the procedure. Novel substrates have been developed for use in mass spectrometric assays. They increase the sensitivity, permit simultaneous assay of several enzymes (multiplexing) and are particularly useful for measuring activity in dried blood spots [3, 5]. To validate a diagnosis another lysosomal enzyme must be assayed in the same sample at the same time to check the viability of the sample.

Samples from a known case of the specific LSD (positive control) and from a normal control (negative control) should always be assayed at the same time under the same conditions. The activities are compared to reference ranges obtained under the same conditions. A complete deficiency or a very low amount of a specific enzyme activity is considered a definitive diagnosis of a specific LSD. The diagnosis is usually confirmed by DNA analysis. Some variant forms of LSD with a later onset and/or slower course have measurable residual enzyme activity with synthetic substrates. Their diagnosis can be confirmed by genetic testing because most variants are associated with specific mutations. Diagnostic laboratories should regularly participate in external quality assurance schemes [6, 7].

There are several complications with the diagnosis of enzyme defects that require special attention and experience.

Pseudodeficiencies

A polymorphism that lowers the enzymatic activity without causing disease can lead to a pseudodeficiency of a lysosomal enzyme activity and a false-positive diagnosis or ambiguous result. A pseudodeficiency has been found for at least nine lysosomal enzymes (listed in Classification in Chapter 5) but is particularly frequent for the arylsulfatase A enzyme, a deficiency of which causes metachromatic leukodystrophy (MLD) (see Chapter 9). Analysis of the patient's DNA can distinguish between mutations causing MLD and the pseudodeficiency, which can also occur on the same chromosome as a disease-causing mutation. Discrepancies between the clinical indication and an apparent enzyme deficiency should alert the laboratory to the possibility of a pseudodeficiency.

Sphingolipid activator proteins defects

In contrast normal activity is sometimes found when attempting to diagnose a sphingolipidosis with synthetic substrates, despite strong clinical indications or manifestation of storage in preliminary tests. This could be due to a defect in a sphingolipid activator protein or SAP (see Chapters 6, 8 and 9). Five SAPs have been described: GM2 activator protein and saposins A–D derived from a common precursor, prosaposin. Whereas lysosomal hydrolases require a SAP to act on many glycolipids *in vivo*, they can act on soluble synthetic substrates in the absence of the saposin *in vitro* to give a false negative result if a SAP is defective. Variant forms of GM2-gangliosidosis, Gaucher disease, Krabbe disease and metachromatic leukodystrophy resulting from SAP

Table 3.3 Panels of enzymes assayed in blood according to clinical indication (see Chapter 2). The groups of enzymes in each panel may vary and are not prescriptive.

A. *Hydrops foetalis* (see Figure 2.2)

Disease	Enzyme Tests
MPS VII (very common)	β-Glucuronidase
Sialidosis (ML I)	α-Neuraminidase
Galactosialidosis	α-Neuraminidase/β-galactosidase
GM1-gangliosidosis	β-galactosidase
Gaucher	β-glucosidase
MPS I (Hurler)	α-Iduronidase
Wolman	Acid lipase
Niemann–Pick A	Sphingomyelinase
MPS IVA (Morquio A)	Galactosamine-6-sulfatase
Farber	Ceramidase
ML II (I-cell disease)	Multiple deficiencies in fibroblasts or increases in plasma
	Other tests
Infantile sialic acid storage	Sialic acid in amniotic fluid or urine
Niemann–Pick C	Cholesterol esterification

Plasma chitotriosidase is assayed in all cases

B. *Dysmorphic*

Disease	Enzyme
G_{M1}-gangliosidosis	β-galactosidase
Multiple sulphatidosis	Arylsulfatase A
Fucosidosis	α-Fucosidase
α-Mannosidosis	α-Mannosidase
Sialidosis	α-Neuraminidase
I-cell disease	I-cell screen
β-Mannosidosis	β-Mannosidase
MPS VII	β-Glucuronidase
Schindler	α-*N*-acetylgalactosaminidase
Aspartylglucosaminuria	Aspartyl *N*-acetylglucosaminidase

The preliminary test for a dysmorphic child is urinary GAG analysis.
Plasma chitotriosidase is assayed in all infants under 1 year of age.

C. *Dysostosis multiplex*

If urinary GAGs are elevated enzymes defective in MPS are assayed.
If urinary oligosaccharides are elevated enzymes defective in glycoproteinoses are assayed.

D. *Cardiomyopathy*

Disease	Enzyme
ML II (I-cell)	I-cell screen, multiple deficiencies
MPS I (Hurler)	α-Iduronidase
MPS II (Hunter)	α-Iduronidate-2-sulfatase
MPS VI (Maroteaux-Lamy)	Arylsulfatase B
Fabry	α-Galactosidase
Glycogen storage disease type 2 (Pompe)	α-Glucosidase
GM1-gangliosidosis	β-galactosidase

(*Continued*)

Table 3.3 (*Cont'd*)

E. *Hepatosplenomegaly*

Disease	Enzyme
GM1-gangliosidosis	β-galactosidase
Sialidosis	α-Neuraminidase
Galactosialidosis	α-Neuraminidase/β-galactosidase
Gaucher	β-Glucocerebrosidase
Niemann–Pick A and B	Sphingomyelinase
Wolman	Acid lipase
Fucosidosis	α-Fucosidase
α-Mannosidosis	α-Mannosidase
β-Mannosidosis	β-Mannosidase
MPS VII-Sly	β-Glucuronidase
I-cell disease	I-cell screen
	Other tests
Niemann–Pick C	Cholesterol esterification

Plasma chitotriosidase is assayed in all cases

F. *Neurodegenerative disease including leukodystrophy*

Disease	Enzyme
GM1-gangliosidosis	β-Galactosidase
GM2-gangliosidoses:	
Tay Sachs/B1 variant	Hexosamindase A
Sandhoff	Total hexosaminidase
Krabbe leukodystrophy	Galactocerebrosidase
Metachromatic leukodystrophy	Arylsulphatase A
Fucosidosis	α-Fucosidase
α-Mannosidosis	α-Mannosidase
β-Mannosidosis	β-Mannosidase
Schindler	α-*N*-Acetylgalactosaminidase
MPS VII-Sly	β-Glucuronidase
I-Cell disease	I-Cell screen, multiple deficiencies

G. *More specific indications*

Angiokeratoma

Disease	Enzyme
Fabry	α-Galactosidase
Fucosidosis	α-Fucosidase
Sialidosis	α-Neuraminidase
Galactosialidosis	α-Neuraminidase/β-galactosidase
Adult GM1-gangliosidosis	β-galactosidase
α-Mannosidosis	α-Mannosidase
β-Mannosidosis	β-Mannosidase
Schindler	α-*N*-acetylgalactosaminidase
Aspartylglucosaminuria	Aspartylglucosaminidase

Table 3.3 (*Cont'd*)

Cherry-red spot (see figure 2.5)

Disease	Enzyme
GM1-gangliosidosis	β-Galactosidase
GM2-gangliosidoses:	
Tay–Sachs / B1 variant	Hexosamindase A
Sandhoff	Total hexosaminidase
Krabbe leukodystrophy	Galactocerebrosidase
Niemann–Pick A	Sphingomyelinase
Sialidosis	α-Neuraminidase
Galactosialidosis	α-Neuraminidase/β-galactosidase

deficiencies and a neurovisceral storage disease resulting from a deficiency of prosaposin have been described (see Classification in Chapter 5). A functional test, immuno-detection of the SAP and/or a molecular genetic test are carried out to confirm the diagnosis.

Genetic defects in the processing or transport of lysosomal enzymes.

A defect in the post-translational processing of sulfatases by the Cα-formylglycine-generating enzyme (SUMF1) leads to the deficiency of several lysosomal and non-lysosomal sulfatases in the disorder, multiple sulfatase deficiency (MSD). Therefore if a deficiency of a specific sulfatase is detected when testing for MPS, it is very important to assay another lysosomal sulfatase to distinguish between a genuine single sulfatase deficiency, as in MPS II, IIIA, IIID, IV or VI, and multiple sulfatase deficiency.

A multiple deficiency of lysosomal hydrolases is found in fibroblasts (and other cells) but not white blood cells from patients with mucolipidosis II and III owing to a defect in the intracellular transport of the enzymes to the lysosomes. Mutations in the genes encoding the α/β and γ subunits of the enzyme, N-acetylglucosamine phospho-transferase, prevent the formation of the lysosomal targeting motif, mannose-6-phosphate, and the transport of enzymes to lysosomes in certain cells. This leads to an increase in the levels of the enzymes in plasma and the preliminary diagnosis of ML II and III is often made by detecting grossly elevated levels of several lysosomal enzymes in plasma. The diagnosis is confirmed by the demonstration of a deficiency of several enzymes (but not β-glucocerebrosidase) in cultured fibroblasts and by DNA analysis.

A combined deficiency of β-galactosidase and α-neuraminidase occurs in galactosialidosis due to a defect in the protective protein, cathepsin A. Again, if a deficiency of either of these enzymes is found in an enzyme screen, the activity of the other should be checked to eliminate the possibility of galactosialidosis. α-Neuraminidase is measured in cultured cells because of the presence of other sialidases in white blood cells.

A severe deficiency of β-glucocerebrosidase activity in cultured skin fibroblasts but normal activity in leukocytes is found in a deficiency of the lysosomal membrane protein, LIMP-2, which is believed to be involved in the intracellular sorting pathway of β-glucocerebrosidase. Although there is storage in the brain of poorly character-ized material, this disorder is called "action myoclonus-renal failure syndrome" (AMRF) because of the dominant clinical features.

LSDs due to defects in non-enzymatic proteins

Lysosomal membrane transporter defects

Three LSDs result from defects in the transporters of metabolites across the lysosomal membrane, cystinosis, sialic acid storage disease (SSSD) and the very rare cobal-amin F disease. A preliminary indication of SSSD and cobalamin F disease can be obtained by the detection of urinary oligosaccharides/sialic acid and methylmalonic acid, respectively. In all three disorders diagnosis is made by measuring the levels of the accumulating metabolites in cells and/or mutation analysis of the relevant gene. Tandem mass spectrometry is being used increasingly to measure the accumulating metabolites. As a large dele-tion in the cystinosin gene accounts for ~60% of the cases of classic cystinosis, genetic testing is productive at an early stage if the clinical suspicion of cystinosis is strong.

Other lysosomal/endosomal protein defects

The trafficking of cellular cholesterol and glycolipids is disrupted in Niemann–Pick disease type C (NPC). Both NPC1 and 2 can be diagnosed by demonstrating the characteristic accumulation of unesterified cholesterol and glycolipids in the lysosomal/late endosomal system by staining living cells with filipin. This test requires considerable experience, especially for the detection of variant phenotypes.

Mucolipidosis IV (MLIV) is due to mutations in *MCOLN1*, which encodes for mucolipin-1, a member of the transient receptor potential (TRP) cation channel family. Diagnosis is based upon observation of membrane- and non-membrane-bound cytoplasmic inclusions by electron microscopy. Most patients have an elevated level of gastrin in their blood. About 70–80% of the cases of MLIV occur in the Ashkenazi Jewish population [8] and two mutations account for about 95% of the disease-causing alleles in this population.

Danon disease is a rare X-linked disorder due to a deficiency of the lysosomal membrane protein, LAMP-2, which appears to be involved in the trafficking of lysosomal hydrolases. After the discovery of autophagic material and glycogen in skeletal and cardiac muscle, diagnosis can be made in males by demonstrating a deficiency of the LAMP-2 protein immunochemically in various tissues including leukocytes [9]. Females have to be diagnosed by DNA analysis, which is also used to confirm the diagnosis in males.

Neuronal ceroid lipofuscinoses (NCLs)

The NCLs (see Chapter 18) are characterized by the progressive accumulation of autofluorescent lipopigment, which is responsible for the characteristic histopathology of neuronal cells in the 10 different types of NCL. The morphology of the inclusions in biopsies or lymphocytes provides a preliminary diagnosis for the different types of NCL [10]. The gene products in CLN1, 2 and 10 are soluble lysosomal proteases, which can be assayed in white blood cells or dried blood spots using synthetic substrates to make a biochemical diagnosis, which can be confirmed by genetic testing. Confirmation of the diagnosis of the other forms is by molecular genetic testing. The occurrence of a large deletion in the *CLN3* gene

in ~80% of NCL3 patients facilitates genetic diagnosis of this form. A combination of the clinical features and pathological, biochemical and genetic tests provides an effective diagnostic protocol for children presenting with symptoms suggestive of NCL.

Molecular genetic testing

Genetic testing is used to confirm a biochemical diagnosis, to clarify the effect of a pseudodeficiency of an enzyme and to make the diagnosis for those disorders for which there is no straightforward biochemical test, e.g. several forms of NCL. LSDs are inherited in an autosomally recessive manner except Danon, Fabry and Hunter diseases, which are X-linked (see Chapter 4). The genes relevant to the diagnosis of the vast majority of LSDs have been cloned, permitting the identification of the underlying mutations in most patients. DNA is isolated from a blood sample or fibroblasts from the patient and the target gene analysed for mutations. Many methods are available for mutation detection [2] and a diagnostic laboratory will use a range of methods to detect nonsense and missense mutations, small deletions and insertions, large gene alterations and mutations that affect the amount and nature of the messenger RNA. Rapid sequencing of a gene may supersede all other methods in the future. Sequence changes found in the gene may correspond to known disease-causing mutations or be novel putative mutations, which have to be evaluated for their pathological potential. LSDs are very heterogeneous genetically with many "private" family mutations. Recurrent mutations for some genes occur in ethnic groups and in regional populations. The initial testing for recurrent mutations in an appropriate patient can sometimes expedite the diagnosis, e.g. NCL3, classic cystinosis and Hurler syndrome.

Once the mutation(s) have been established in the proband, a specific test, either an existing one for a known mutation or one devised for the novel mutation, can be used to offer genetic counselling to the proband's family. Carriers can only be diagnosed reliably by genetic testing and this is particularly so for the X-linked disorders because of random inactivation of the X-chromosome. Genetic testing can be used for prenatal diagnosis when the pregnancy is at risk for known mutation(s). The patient's genotype is sometimes useful for predicting the course and outcome of the disease and for selecting patients for treatment. Molecular genetic testing has become an integral part of the diagnostic algorithm.

Prenatal diagnosis

Once the diagnosis is confirmed in the index case and the carrier status of the parents established, prenatal diagnosis in a foetus at risk for a LSD can be achieved using similar tests to those used to make the diagnosis in the index case [11, 12]. Chorionic villus sampling (CVS) has largely superseded amniocentesis because a diagnosis can be made in the first trimester. The CVS must be examined rigorously to exclude maternal contamination before use in direct enzyme assays, extraction of DNA for mutation analysis and for ultrastructural examination [13]. If a pregnancy is at risk for known mutations, i.e. the mutations have been identified in the index case and parents and the likely phenotype for the foetal genotype is understood, mutation analysis has become the preferred method for prenatal diagnosis. However, a functional enzyme or protein assay is often still performed to support the genetic diagnosis. When attempting an enzymatic diagnosis, it is essential to assay the activity in material, preferably CVS, from an affected case and ideally from at least two unaffected cases at the same time as the foetal cells. Striking changes in the trophoblast occur in some LSDs and ultrastructural examination of the villi can be an important aspect of prenatal diagnosis of the NCLs. For certain diseases, e.g. Niemann–Pick type C or saposin defects, a culture of cells is established from the villus sample for specific tests. Diagnostic tests can also be performed on cultured amniotic fluid cells and amniotic fluid can be analysed for storage products, e.g. glycosaminoglycans in MPS, or for secreted lysosomal enzymes in I-cell disease. It is possible to carry out tests on foetal blood, even stored as a dried blood spot [14]. Pre-implantation genetic diagnosis, which permits identification of unaffected embryos prior to *in vitro* fertilization, has been applied to couples at risk for several lysosomal storage diseases (see Chapter 22) [12]. The detection of specific mutations in foetal cells and cell-free foetal DNA in the maternal circulation may provide a less invasive and risky prenatal diagnosis in the future (see Chapter 22 in reference [12]). There has been a decline in requests for prenatal diagnosis of those diseases for which treatment is available.

Prospects

The laboratory diagnosis of LSDs is at a watershed. The search for biomarkers to monitor treatment is yielding sensitive screening tests for storage products and disease-specific proteins, which will speed up and broaden the preliminary stage in the diagnostic pathway. The use of dried blood spots as the source of enzymatic activity is increasing because of improved conventional assays [15], multiplexed assays using substrates suitable for mass spectrometry [4] and the interest in newborn screening (see Chapter 22). Protein profiling based on immuno-quantification or proteomic analysis of lysosomal proteins may lead to generic testing for LSDs as well as newborn screening [16]. Molecular genetic testing will increase both to confirm an enzyme-based diagnosis and as the primary diagnostic test as disease-specific DNA chips and rapid, affordable, high throughput sequencing of DNA become more widely available. Dried blood spots are also a good source of DNA for analysis. Digital microfluidics will permit more enzyme assays to be carried out on a single dried blood spot [17] and the same technology can be used for immunodetection of proteins and DNA analysis. However, these technological advances will still require skilled and experienced laboratory staff to interpret the data to make the diagnosis.

Acknowledgements

The author is very grateful to Elisabeth Young, Jan-Eric Månnson and Ed Wraith for their helpful comments after reading the manuscript. He acknowledges the dedication, experience and friendship of his colleagues in the Enzyme Diagnostic Laboratory at Great Ormond Street Hospital, London, with whom he worked for many years and without whom this chapter could not have been written.

References

1 Meikle PJ, Fietz MJ, Hopwood JJ. Diagnosis of lysosomal storage disorders: current techniques and future directions. *Expert Rev Mol Diagn* 2004; **4**: 677–691.

2 Filocamo M and Morrone A Lysosomal storage disorders: molecular basis and laboratory testing. *Hum Genom* 2011; **5**: 156–169.

3 Gelb MH, Turecek F, Scott CR, Chamoles NA. Direct multiplex assay of enzymes in dried blood spots by tandem mass spectrometry for the newborn screening of lysosomal storage disorders. *J Inherit Metab Dis* 2006; **29**: 397–404.

4 Mills K, Morris P, Lee P, *et al.* Measurement of urinary CDH and CTH by tandem mass spectrometry in patients hemizygous and heterozygous for Fabry disease. *J Inherit Metab Dis* 2005; **28**: 35–48.

5 Zhang XK, Elbin CS, Turecek F, *et al.* Multiplex lysosomal enzyme activity assay on dried blood spots using tandem mass spectrometry. *Methods Mol Biol* 2010; **603**: 339–350.

6 Ruijter GJ, Boer M, Weykamp CW, *et al*. External quality assurance programme for enzymatic analysis of lysosomal storage diseases: a pilot study. *J Inherit Metab Dis* 2005; **289**: 79–90.

7 De Jesus VR, Zhang XK, Keutzer J, *et al*. Development and evaluation of quality control dried blood spot materials in newborn screening for lysosomal storage disorders. *Clin Chem* 2009; **55**: 158–164.

8 Bach G, Zeevi DA, Frumkin A, Kogot-Levin A. Mucolipidosis type IV and the mucolipins. *Biochem Soc Trans* 2010; **38**: 1432–1435.

9 Fanin M, Nascimbeni AC, Fulizio L. *et al*. Generalized lysosome-associated membrane-2-defect explains multisystem clinical involvement and allows diagnostic screening in Danon disease *Am J Pathol* 2006; **168**: 1309–1320.

10 Williams RE, Aberg L, Autti T, *et al*. Diagnosis of the neuronal ceroid lipofuscinoses: an update. *Biochim Biophys Acta* 2006; **1762**: 865–872.

11 Lake BD, Young EP, Winchester BG. Prenatal diagnosis of lysosomal storage diseases. *Brain Path* 1998; **8**: 133–149.

12 Milunsky A, Milunsky JM (eds.). Chapters 12, 14, 16, 19, 29 and 30 in *Genetic Disorders and the Fetus: Diagnosis, Prevention and Treatment*. Wiley–Blackwell, Chichester, UK, 2010.

13 Fowler DJ, Anderson G, Vellodi A, *et al*. Electron microscopy of chorionic villus samples for prenatal diagnosis of lysosomal storage disorders. *Ultrastruct Pathol* 2007; **31**: 15–21.

14 Burin MG, Ribeiro E, Mari J, *et al*. Prenatal diagnosis of mucopolysaccharidosis VI by enzyme assay in a dried spot of fetal blood: a pioneering case report. *Prenat Diagn* 2010; **30**: 89–90.

15 Oemardien LF, Boer AM, Ruijter GJ, *et al*. Hemoglobin precipitation greatly improves 4-methylumbelliferone-based diagnostic assays for lysosomal storage diseases in dried blood spots. *Mol Genet Metab* 2011; **102**: 44–48.

16 Fuller M, Tucker JN, Lang DL, *et al*. Screening patients referred to a metabolic clinic for lysosomal storage disorders. *J Med Genet* 2011; **48**: 422–5.

17 Millington DS, Sista R, Eckhardt A, *et al*., Digital microfluidics: a future technology in the newborn screening laboratory? *Semin Perinatol* 2010; **34**: 163–169.

CHAPTER 4

Genetics of Lysosomal Storage Disorders and Counselling

John J. Hopwood

Lysosomal Diseases Research Unit, SA Pathology at Women's and Children's Hospital, Adelaide, Australia

Introduction

Lysosomal storage disorders (LSDs) comprise a group of more than 50 inherited, clinically progressive disorders that lead to a spectrum of physical and/or mental disabilities, and often premature death. Over the past 20 years, and particularly in the past 10 years, translation of laboratory research has delivered advances in diagnostic capabilities and introduced therapies into clinical practice for the treatment of many of the major LSDs. Currently, most LSDs are detected following clinical presentation from which detailed genetic or biochemical diagnosis can be made. The clinical heterogeneity of all LSDs is the major issue when it comes to interpreting genetic data and the ability to provide accurate counselling to patients and families.

Progressive lysosomal accumulation of undegraded metabolites results in generalized cell and tissue dysfunction from multisystemic pathology. Storage may begin early in embryonic development, and clinical presentation can vary from an early and rapidly developing clinical phenotype to late-onset with slowly developing disease. Until recently, biochemical diagnosis of LSD involved the analysis of urinary metabolites as a first-line screen to suggest relevant enzymatic and molecular genetical tests to identify the specific LSDs and causative mutations. With this information counselling may include prediction of the possible clinical phenotype, identification of carriers in the family, options for treatment and the possibility of prenatal testing in subsequent pregnancies. When genotype–phenotype correlations are available

[this is not always possible], they can be helpful in prognosis and in making decisions about therapy.

Recent observations supporting early commencement of therapies have accelerated improvements in diagnostic technology and driven the development and recent introduction of population screening programs to identify LSD individuals at birth, often before symptoms are apparent. Early diagnosis will enable treatment options to be considered much earlier than has previously been possible. However, because LSD patients present and develop within a wide clinical spectrum of characteristics such as age of onset and rate of disease progression, the option to treat before symptoms are apparent introduces a major challenge – the dilemma of whether or when to treat and with what particular therapy. Clearly, these issues need to be addressed and are under intense research.

Genes, proteins, stored substrates, clinical phenotypes and diagnosis

Most LSD patients have functional deficiencies of single lysosomal proteins or, in a few cases, from the involvement of non-lysosomal factors that contribute to lysosomal biogenesis or lysosomal protein maturation/activation. New LSDs continue to be recognized and defined clinically, genetically and biochemically. Also, as clinical presentations of known LSDs continue to be redefined – particularly as late-onset forms are identified – the mechanism(s) by which lysosomal dysfunction leads to clinical problems is becoming better appreciated.

Lysosomal Storage Disorders: A Practical Guide, First Edition. Edited by Atul Mehta and Bryan Winchester.
© 2012 John Wiley & Sons, Ltd. Published 2012 by John Wiley & Sons, Ltd.

Besides its 'classical' involvement in the cyclic digestion of most macromolecules in the cell and its matrix, the lysosome is also connected, through the endosome-network, to other cellular processes such as recycling, autophagy, exocytosis, matrix remodeling, cholesterol homeostasis and pathogen defence. Dysfunction or variable functioning of this endosome-lysosome-network may also directly cause, contribute to, or modify the nature and the rate of phenotype development of all LSDs. Not all LSDs result from a deficiency of a protein activity in the lysosome: for example, ceroid lipofuscinosis, neuronal disease 8 (CLN8) results from a reduction in a gene-directed protein in the endoplasmic-reticulum-Golgi, whereas CLN4 (adult dominant Parry disease) results from reduced synaptic activity consequent to a deficient cysteine-string protein (see Classification). Other examples include: lysosome-related organelle biogenesis disorders like the Hermansky–Pudlak and Chediak–Higashi syndromes [not in Table 4.1 but see Classification in Chapter 5 and Chapter 19]; a Golgi enzyme that mediates the second step in the synthesis of the mannose phosphate lysosomal targeting signal on lysosomal enzymes leads to persistent stuttering (Mucolipidosis Stuttering variant, see Table 4.1 and Chapter 19). These, and other examples, highlight a current dilemma of what defines an LSD.

LSDs share common biochemical characteristics that lead to storage of substrates within the endosome-lysosome-network. This storage results from a mutation(s) in a different gene and a consequent deficiency of an enzyme/protein, mostly in the endosome-lysosome-network. The nature of the substrate, its contribution to the pathological cascade, or its organ/cell type location/site(s) varies with each LSD. Often, the type of storage has grouped LSDs into broad categories: for example, the ceroid lipofuscinoses neuronal (CLN); the mucopoly-saccharidoses (MPS); and the sphingolipidoses (see Classification). Despite this attempt to group and simplify LSDs on biochemical grounds, clinical features such as organomegaly, skeletal-dysplasia and CNS-dysfunction are common across all LSDs.

The CLN, which involve at least 10 different genes – 8 with known function and 2 under investigation (see Table 4.1 and Chapter 18) – are challenging in terms of establishing accurate diagnoses. Although practical to view the CLN as one group, sharing common storage profile characteristics, considerable care is required to reach a specific diagnosis and to accurately counsel patients/families. Interpretation of genetic information to predict a CLN phenotype is complicated by the possible location and function of CLN proteins in the endoplasmic reticulum, Golgi or the endosome-lysosome-network. Previously, diagnosis of adult recessive CLN (Kufs disease) would often require an invasive biopsy; now a screen for CLN6 mutations would be considered first if Kufs disease is suspected [1]. Similarly, if a dominant Kufs disease (Table 4.1) is suspected, mutations in the *DNAJC5* gene could be used to identify CLN4 (adult dominant Parry disease) [10]. On the other hand, the diagnosis, genetics and counselling of patients with one of seven MPS syndromes (11 genes are involved in lysosomal degradation of mucopolysaccharide-substrates) are relatively well defined and counselling options are less complicated despite the phenotypic complexity of this group of disorders.

Most LSDs are inherited as autosomal recessive disorders. The exceptions are Hunter syndrome (MPS II; X-linked recessive), Danon disease (X-linked dominant), Fabry disease (which, with a high proportion of clinically affected females, is best described as X-linked recessive) and the Parry type of Kufs disease (CLN4), which is auto-somal dominant [11]) (see Classification). Genomic imprinting has been observed in Niemann–Pick A/B where one mutant allele in the sphingomyelinase gene is preferentially expressed over the other normal allele in a carrier individual to give 15% sphingomyelinase activity and a disease phenotype [16] (see Chapter 10).

Virtually all LSDs have been classified into clinical subtypes (for example, infantile–juvenile to adult forms of Pompe disease; neuronopathic and non-neuronopathic Gaucher disease; neuronopathic MPS I (Hurler syndrome) or non-neuronopathic MPS I (Scheie syndrome)). Importantly, it is now recognized that all LSDs display a broad continuum of clinical severity. This continuum is reflected in the rate of clinical progression – from rapid, with symptoms at birth leading to death within a few years, to a much slower progression with clinical onset in adult or elderly years. For many LSD cases, this broad clinical phenotypic spectrum has seriously complicated and slowed the process of obtaining a diagnosis, and hindered or even prevented accurate prognosis. This has also made it likely that many late-onset LSD patients remain undiagnosed.

Residual enzyme activity is one of many factors that affect the clinical outcome of individual LSD patients. Rapid progression of pathology is likely in patients with null enzyme activity. Different epigenetic factors, genetic variability in the synthesis of the stored substrate, and the overall functional efficiency and control of an individual

Table 4.1 Prevalence of lysosomal storage disorders.

Disease	OMIM No.	Incidence[a]/Prevalence[b] 1:000's			
		Australia [8]	Czech Republic [14]	The Netherlands [13]	Northern Portugal [12]
α-N-Acetylgalactosaminidase deficiency				500	
Type I Schindler	#609241				
Type II Kanzaki	#609242				
Acid lipase deficiency	#278000	528	330		
Cholesterol ester storage disease (Wolman)					
Action myoclonus-renal failure	#254900				
Aspartylglucosaminuria	#208400	2111		769	58
Ceroid Lipofuscinosis, neuronal	#256730	60[c]	526		588
CLN1 disease Santavuori–Haltia					
Ceroid Lipofuscinosis, neuronal	#204500	60[c]	278		1,429
CLN2 disease Jansky–Bielschowsky					
Ceroid Lipofuscinosis, neuronal	#204200	60[c]	370		208
CLN3 disease Vogt–Spielmeyer, Spielmeyer–Sjogren					
Ceroid Lipofuscinosis, neuronal	#204300				
Adult recessive Kufs disease					
Ceroid Lipofuscinosis, neuronal	#162350				
CLN4 disease Parry disease					
CeroidLipofuscinosis, neuronal	#256731		470		
CLN5 disease Finnish variant					
Ceroid Lipofuscinosis, neuronal	#601780		5,000		70
CLN6 disease					
Ceroid Lipofuscinosis, neuronal	#610951		118		
CLN7 disease					
Ceroid Lipofuscinosis, neuronal	#600143				
CLN8 disease					
Finland, Northern epilepsy	#610003				
Ceroid Lipofuscinosis, neuronal	%609055				
CLN9 disease					
Ceroid Lipofuscinosis, neuronal	#610127				
CLN10 disease					
Cystinosis, nephropathic	#219800	Combined			
Cystinosis, nephropathic	#219900	192			
Cystinosis, non-nephropathic	#219750				
Danon	#300257				
Fabry	#301500	117[d]	100[d]	476[d]	833[d]
Farber	#228000				
Fucosidosis	#230000	>2,000		2,000	
Galactosialidosis	#256540			2,500	130
Goldberg syndrome					
Gaucher Type I	#230800	Combined 57	Combined 89	Combined 86	Combined 74
Type II	#230900				
Type III	#231000				
Gaucher Saposin C deficiency	#610539				
Gaucher Prosaposin deficiency	#611721				

(Continued)

Table 4.1 (*Cont'd*)

Disease	OMIM No.	Incidence[a]/Prevalence[b] 1:000's			
		Australia [8]	Czech Republic [14]	The Netherlands [13]	Northern Portugal [12]
Globoid cell leukodystrophy Krabbe disease	#245200	Combined 201	Combined 250	Combined 74	Combined 82
Globoid cell leukodystrophy Saposin A deficiency	#611722				
Glycogen storage disease II Pompe	#232300	Combined 146		Combined 50	Combined 588
GM1-gangliosidosis Type I	#230500	Combined 384	Combined 385	Combined 243	Combined 161
Type II	#230600				
Type III	#230650				
GM2-gangliosidosis Tay–Sachs disease, AB variant	#272750				
GM2-gangliosidosis Tay–Sachs disease, B variant	#272800	Combined 201		Combined 243	Combined 32
GM2-gangliosidosis, Sandhoff disease, O variant	#268800	Combined 384	Combined 526	Combined 294	Combined 67
α-Mannosidosis	#248500	1,056	263	1,111	833
β-Mannosidosis	#248510		625	769	833
Metachromatic leukodystrophy	#250100	Combined 92	Combined 148	Combined 70	Combined 54
Metachromatic leukodystrophy Saposin B deficiency	#249900				
Mucolipidosis I Sialidosis	#256550		1,400	2,000	
Mucolipidosis II α/β I-cell disease	#252500	325	Combined 455	416	37
Mucolipidosis III α/β Pseudo-Hurler polydystrophy	#252600				
Mucolipidosis III γ Iranian variant	#252605				
Mucolipidosis Stuttering variant	%609261				
Mucolipidosis IV	#252650		5,000		
Mucopolysaccharidosis I Hurler	#607014	Combined 88	Combined 139	Combined 84	Combined 75
Hurler–Scheie	#607015				
Scheie	#607016				
Mucopolysaccharidosis II Hunter	#309900	136[d]	121[d]	149[d]	92[d]
Mucopolysaccharidosis IIIA Sanfilippo A	#252900	114	213	86	
Mucopolysaccharidosis IIIB Sanfilippo B	#252920	211	5,000	238	139
Mucopolysaccharidosis IIIC Sanfilippo C	#252930	1,407	238	476	833
Mucopolysaccharidosis IIID Sanfilippo D	#252940	1,056		1,000	
Mucopolysaccharidosis IVA Morquio A	#253000	169	141	455	167
Mucopolysaccharidosis IVB Morquio B	#253010		5,000	714	
Mucopolysaccharidosis VI Maroteaux-Lamy	#253200	235	2,000	666	238
Mucopolysaccharidosis VII Sly	#253220	2,111	5,000	416	
Mucopolysaccharidosis IX	#601492				
Multiple sulfatase deficiency	#272200	1,407	385	2,000	208
Niemann–Pick A	#257200	Combined	Combined	Combined	Combined 167
Niemann–Pick B	#607616	248	303	189	
Niemann–Pick C1	#257220	211		286	45

Table 4.1 (*Cont'd*)

Disease	OMIM No.	Incidence[a]/Prevalence[b] 1:000's			
		Australia [8]	Czech Republic [14]	The Netherlands [13]	Northern Portugal [12]
Niemann–Pick C2	#607625				
Prosaposin deficiency (see Gaucher)	#611721				
Pycnodysostosis Cathepsin K deficiency	#265800				
Sialic acid storage disease	#269920	528		1,428	
Salla disease	#604369				

[a] Incidence in Australia defined as the total number of cases diagnosed within a certain period of time divided by the total number of births in the same period, expressed as 000's of births per diagnoses.

[b] Birth prevalence in The Netherlands, the Czech Republic and Portugal defined as the total number of diagnosed cases born within a certain period of time divided by the total number of births in the same period, expressed as 000's of births per diagnoses.

[c] Combined incidence of CLN1, CLN2 and CLN3 [8].

[d] Values for hemizygotes only.

OMIM indicated Online Mendelian Inheritance in Man (www.ncbi.nlm.nih.gov/omim).

patient's endosome-lysosome-network are other factors that may influence clinical outcome.

Arylsulfatase A (ARSA) mutations that result in low activity (between 5 and 20% of normal) are common in European, American and other populations but are believed not to cause "classical" clinical presentation of metachromatic leukodystrophy. They have been referred to as pseudo-deficiencies (see Chapter 9). However, genotype–phenotype analysis of these individuals suggests that ARSA pseudodeficiencies may contribute to the clinical severity of metachromatic leukodystrophy [19], multiple sclerosis [3] and possible onset of neuropsychological and non-verbal learning disabilities [20, 21].

Although mucolipidosis IV is a pan-ethnic neurodegenerative disorder, with most patients of Ashkenazi Jewish origin (see Chapter 17), its frequency may be much greater than currently appreciated because its common presentation as a cerebral palsy-like encephalopathy may lead to misdiagnosis, particularly with "'milder" patients. The problem of accurately defining some LSD phenotypes is further illustrated by mutations (and so-called polymorphisms) in the ß-glucocerebrosidase gene, which result in Gaucher disease but are also associated with Parkinson disease. Over the coming years it is likely that many other genes/proteins will be identified as causing dysfunction of the endosome-lysosome-network with yet to be defined clinical outcomes.

Incidence and prevalence

LSD incidence, defined as the total patient number divided by total births in the same period of time, has been reported in a number of countries (Table 4.1). Major difficulties associated with obtaining accurate epidemiological data involve the individual rarity of these disorders and the numerous diagnostic centres that often use different diagnostic methods. Most LSD patients are diagnosed after clinical presentation, and this is often the basis upon which to evaluate the likely genetic and biochemical tests required to fully define the LSD and its likely prognosis.

Importantly, if the studies have missed a diagnosis considerable differences may result to a calculated prevalence for an extremely rare disease; care should therefore be exercised to estimate inheritance risk from this data. Further, when comparing in Table 4.1 data that have been collected from different studies, the nature of the methods used to calculate birth prevalence and incidence values must be considered. For instance, the Australian study [8], based on clinical diagnoses between 1980 and 1996, assumed that late-onset patients who were diagnosed during this period were representative of late-onset patients born within the study dates but yet to present clinically; whereas in The Netherlands [13] the period used to calculate birth prevalence was based on the patient's age, with the assumption that patients born prior to the last patient in the subgroup were identified. Both methods have limitations and it is likely that the identification of late-onset patients has been underestimated. In Australia, Pompe disease has a clinical incidence of 1 in 146,000 births, whereas, based on carrier detection studies in the USA and The Netherlands, an incidence as high as 1 in 40,000 is likely [2, 7], suggesting that adult Pompe patients may be under-detected in the Australian population.

In recent times the observed discrepancy between the measured LSD incidence and the predicted carrier rates suggests that LSD cases are substantially under-diagnosed in the general population. For instance, an under-diagnosis rate may be particularly high among individuals with LSD gene mutations that lead to disease characterized by psychotic symptoms or stroke and cardiac problems. Newborn screening for LSD has identified much higher incidences of some LSDs – for example, Fabry disease – than previously estimated based on classical Fabry syndrome presentation alone (see "Populations at a high-risk" and "Population screening and diagnostic methods" below and Chapter 23). Thus, the LSD overall (and specific disease) incidence may be much higher than currently appreciated.

Retrospective data collected in Australia (from 1980 to 1996) reported 470 diagnoses representing 27 different LSDs (Table 4.1). The incidence ranged from 1 in 57,000 for Gaucher to 1 in 4,222,000 for Mucolipidosis type I. The combined incidence of all LSDs, with prenatal diagnoses included, was 1 in 7,700 births [8].

In The Netherlands, 963 LSD patients were diagnosed between 1970 and 1996, giving an incidence of 1 in 7,100 births, with glycogen storage disease II the most prevalent at 1 in 50,000 [13]. Between 1975 and 2008, 478 LSD patients were reported in the Czech Republic with 34 different LSDs and an overall LSD prevalence of 1 in 8,000 births, with Gaucher being most prevalent at 1 in 89,000 [14]. In Northern Portugal, 222 LSD patients were identified over approximately 20 years, giving an incidence of 1 in 2,500; 29 different LSD patients were reported with GM2-gangliosidosis, Niemann–Pick C and Gaucher being the most prevalent at 1 in 31,950, 45,450 and 74,070, respectively [12].

Populations at a high-risk

Most LSDs have a low incidence in most populations although there are a number of exceptions, particularly in communities that have been, or continue to be, genetically isolated either culturally or geographically: for example, Ashkenazi Jews are at high risk for Gaucher (1 in 855 births), Tay–Sachs and Niemann–Pick A diseases.

CLN incidence in Newfoundland is estimated to be 1 in 7,353 live births. The incidence of CLN2 was 9 per 100,000, or 1 in 11,161 live births, the highest reported in the world [10].

Recent population screening programs have suggested a high-prevalence of a late-onset form of Fabry disease where the "classical" Fabry presentation (1 in 117,000 in Australia [8]) is in the order of 40-fold less. For example, newborn screening in Italy and Taiwan has identified a high-incidence of α-galactosidase deficiency (~1 in 3,000 births) with a high proportion of mutations likely to cause cardiac or stroke in males in later life [6, 18]; screening of males in Belgian nephrology, cardiac and stroke clinics also detected previously undiagnosed Fabry patients [4].

Burden of illness

Although the overall impact of LSD on patients, families and the broader community is poorly documented, it is undoubtedly significant in financial, emotional and psychosocial terms. We are moving into a new era where effective therapies are becoming available and early detection through newborn/population screening is under consideration. Health care systems that are paying for these improved clinical outcomes are under increasing pressure to define and document individual and community burdens to effectively balance/prioritize the distribution of health resources. These economic pressures will continue to encourage cheaper treatments such as chaperone therapies to be developed, but are also likely to encourage the rationalization of the use of expensive treatments for patients who have an established disease, the downside of which may be that treatment may be less effective than if it had been started earlier. As a variety of therapies for individual LSD cases become clinically available, and as their long-term effectiveness and cost are documented, an overall appreciation of the burden to the community will be clearer. The introduction of population and newborn screening will also provide accurate prevalence data and assist the calculation of cost burden to public health systems.

Population screening and diagnostic methods

Technology using dried blood spot "Guthrie" cards has been developed to screen populations for single and multiple LSD (e.g. [5, 9, 15, 17, 22] – see also Chapter 23). Presymptomatic screening of newborns for a single LSD – for example Fabry, Krabbe and Pompe diseases – has identified higher incidences than previously estimated, based on clinical presentation alone. However, the impact of early diagnosis on patient outcome remains uncertain due to the variable phenotype of attenuated forms of LSD, since such patients may not present with symptoms until later in life and available therapies may not alter their clinical course. Therefore, it is critical that the clinical course and rate of disease progression are accurately determined for neonates and others identified in these screening programmes. Other important questions are when, should and how do we treat and monitor pre-symptomatic patients?

An objective of a truly effective population screen for LSD is to have closely linked confirmatory diagnostic and prognostic capacity that is amenable to samples that can be easily collected and transported – ideally, dried blood samples from the initial "Guthrie" screening card.

As each LSD has a broad clinical heterogeneity, the gathering of epidemiological data is a significant problem. This broad heterogeneity has led to missed diagnoses, diagnostic error and confusion, often leading to the collection of poor epidemiological data and an underestimation of the impact of LSD in the community. Accurate data is essential if both the specific and overall impact of LSD on families and the community are to be appreciated. Knowledge of prevalence and LSD carrier frequency is important for counselling. An appreciation of this data is also needed to justify the introduction of policies to effectively reduce the burden of these disorders.

Counselling issues

For counselling, it is important to understand the nature of LSD pathology. Once an individual's LSD protein deficiency and/or genotype are known, genetic counselling should ideally include the prediction of likely clinical phenotype, identification of carriers in the family and those at risk, knowledge of the availability and efficacy of therapies and prediction of clinical progression in patients diagnosed before obvious symptoms are apparent. One final but critical question is whether the CNS is likely to become involved.

Genetic counselling offers planning options to high-risk family members. Prenatal diagnosis may be performed on fresh or cultured chorionic villus cells or cultured amniotic fluid cells. The choice of test (enzymatic and/or molecular) is often based on the characteristics of the defect to be investigated. Prenatal testing is advantaged if the genotype of the family index case is known. Both

enzyme activity and molecular genetics, together with an assay to eliminate the potential for maternal contamination of the test sample, increase the reliability of the diagnostic procedure. The option of pre-implantation testing of IVF embryos should also be considered as an option for prenatal diagnosis for subsequent pregnancies.

References

1 Arsov T, Smith K, Damiano J, et al. Kufs disease, the major adult-form of neuronal ceroid lipofuscinosis, caused by mutations in CLN6. Am J Hum Genet 2011; 88: 566–573.

2 Ausems MG, Verbiest J, Hermans MP, et al. Frequency of glycogen storage disease type II in The Netherlands: implications for diagnosis and genetic counselling. Eur J Hum Genet 1999; 7: 713–716.

3 Baronica KB, Minac K, Ozretic, et al. Arylsulfatase a gene polymorphisms in relapsing remitting multiple sclerosis: genotype-phenotype correction and estimation of disease progression. Coll Antropol 2011; 35 (Suppl 1): 11–16.

4 Brouns R, Thijs V, Eyskens F, et al. Belgian Fabry study: prevalence of Fabry disease in a cohort of 1000 young patients with cerebrovascular disease. Stroke 2010; 41: 863–868.

5 Fuller M, Tucker JN, Lang DL, et al. Screening patients referred to a metabolic clinic for lysosomal storage disorders. J Med Genet 2011; 48: 422–425.

6 Lin HY, Chong KW, Hsu JH, et al. High incidence of the cardiac variant of Fabry disease revealed by newborn screening in the Taiwan Chinese population. Circ Cardiovasc Genet 2009; 2: 450–456.

7 Martinuk F, Chen A, Mack A, et al. Carrier frequency of glycogen storage disease type II in New York and estimates of affected individuals born with the disease. Am J Med Genet 1998; 79: 69–72.

8 Meikle PJ, Hopwood JJ, Clague, AE, et al. Prevalence of lysosomal storage disorders. JAMA 1999; 281: 249–254.

9 Meikle PJ, Grasby DJ, Dean CJ, et al. Newborn screening for lysosomal storage disorders. Mol Genet Metab 2006; 88: 307–301.

10 Moore SJ, Buckley DJ, MacMillan A, et al. The clinical and genetic epidemiology of neuronal ceroid lipofuscinosis in Newfoundland. Clin Genet 2008; 74: 213–222.

11 Nosková L, Stránecký V, Hartmannová H, et al. Mutations in DNAJC5, encoding cysteine-string protein alpha, cause autosomal-dominant adult-onset neuronal ceroid lipofuscinosis. Am J Hum Genet 2011; 89: 241–252.

12 Pinto R, Caseiro C, Lemos M, et al. Prevalence of lysosomal storage diseases in Portugal. Eur J Hum Genet 2004: 12: 87–92.

13 Poorthuis BJ, Wevers RA, Kleijer WJ, et al. The frequency of lysosomal storage disorders in The Netherlands. Hum Genet 1999; 105: 151–156.

14 Poupetová H, Ledvinová J, Berná L, *et al.* The birth prevalence of lysosomal storage disorders in the Czech Republic: comparison with data in different populations. *J Inherit Metab Dis* 2010; **33**: 387–386.

15 Reuser AJ, Verheijen FW, Bali D, *et al.* The use of dried blood spot samples in the diagnosis of lysosomal storage disorders – current status and perspectives. *Mol Genet Metab* 2011; **104**: 144–148.

16 Simonaro CM, Park J-H, Eliyahu E, *et al.* Imprinting at the *SMPD1* locus: implications for acid sphingomyelinase-deficient Niemann–Pick disease. *Am J Hum Genet* 2006: **78**: 865–870.

17 Spáčil Z, Elliott S, Reeber SL, *et al.* Comparative triplex tandem mass spectrometry assays of lysosomal enzyme activities in dried blood spots using fast liquid chromatography: application to newborn screening of Pompe, Fabry, and Hurler diseases. *Anal Chem* 2011; **83**: 4822–4828.

18 Spada M, Pagliardini S, Yasuda M, *et al.* High incidence of later-onset Fabry disease revealed by newborn screening. *Am J Hum Genet* 2006; **79**: 31–40.

19 Tinsa F, Caillaud C, Vanier MT, *et al.* An unusual homozygous arylsulfatase: a pseudodeficiency in a metachromatic leukodystrophy Tunisian patient. *J Child Neurol* 2010; **25**: 82–86.

20 Tylki-Szymańska A, Ługowska A, Chmielik J, *et al.* Investigations of micro-organic brain damage (MOBD) in heterozygotes of metachromatic leukodystrophy. *Am J Med Genet* 2002; **110**: 315–319.

21 Weber Byars AM, McKellop JM, Gyato K, *et al.* Metachromatic leukodystrophy and nonverbal learning disability: neuropsychological and neuroradiological findings in heterozygous carriers. *Child Neuropychol* 2001; **7**: 54–58.

22 Zhou H, Fernhoff P, Vogt RF. Newborn bloodspot screening for lysosomal storage disorders. *J Pediatr* 2011; **159**: 7–13.

CHAPTER 5

Classification of Lysosomal Storage Diseases

Bryan Winchester

Emeritus Professor of Biochemistry, UCL Institute of Child Health at Great Ormond Street Hospital, University College London, London, UK

Basis of classification of lysosomal storage diseases

Historically, the lysosomal storage diseases were classified on the basis of their storage products, e.g. lipidoses, mucopolysaccharidoses, glycoproteinoses, glycogen storage disease. This categorization brought together diseases with common symptoms reflecting disturbances in the lysosomal catabolic pathway for a particular group of metabolites. This is still the most informative classification for those diseases resulting from a block in a single enzymatic step in a catabolic pathway, as illustrated by defects in the catabolism of the glycosphingolipids, including those due to a defect in a sphingolipid activator protein (Figure 5.1) Other disorders did not appear to fit easily into this scheme, e.g. I-cell disease, cystinosis, mucolipidosis II/III and IV. The elucidation of the molecular basis of these and other non-enzymatic lysosomal disorders has permitted a new classification based on the nature of the molecular defect in the lysosomal system, e.g. the transport of molecules across the lysosomal membrane or within the endosomal-lysosomal system, post-translational modification and intracellular transport of lysosomal enzymes, formation of stabilizing complexes (Table 5.1). The mucolipidoses (MLs), which were originally defined as diseases that combined clinical features common to both mucopolysaccharidoses and glycosphingolipidoses can now be allocated to more appropriate subgroups: ML I to the glycoproteinoses, ML II and III to processing defects and ML IV to membrane defects. In contrast, the neuronal ceroid lipofuscinoses (CLNs), which arise by diverse defects in the lysosomal system, are classified together because they share characteristic clinical and pathological features, particularly the accumulation of autofluorescent material within the lysosome.

A classification based on molecular defects in the lysosomal system focuses attention on function, pathogenetic mechanisms and the development of logical forms of therapy. The pathophysiological boundaries between lysosomal disorders and other types of disease, e.g. some neurological disorders (see Chapter 1), have become blurred with dysfunction of the lysosomal system playing a wider role in disease processes. A scheme based on molecular cell defects can accommodate new classes of lysosomal disorders as they are recognized.

Acknowledgements

Members of the European Study Group on Lysosomal Diseases (ESGLD) are thanked for their comments on this Classification, which was presented for discussion at their meeting in Finland in September 2011.

Lysosomal Storage Disorders: A Practical Guide, First Edition. Edited by Atul Mehta and Bryan Winchester.
© 2012 John Wiley & Sons, Ltd. Published 2012 by John Wiley & Sons, Ltd.

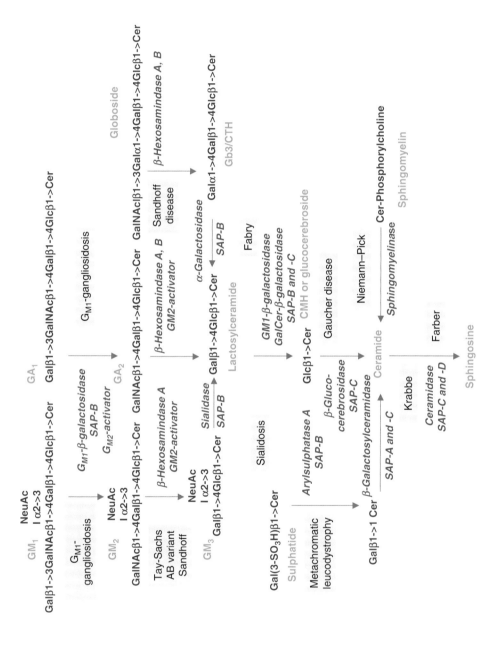

Figure 5.1 Lysosomal catabolism of some glycosphingolipids. (Reproduced from Winchester B. Primary defects in lysosomal enzymes. In: *Lysosomal Disorders of the Brain: Recent Advances in Molecular and Cellular Pathogenesis and Treatment*. Platt FM, Walkley SU (eds.). Oxford: Oxford University Press, 2004, with permission from Oxford University Press.)

Table 5.1 Classification of lysosomal storage diseases.

Sphingolipidoses including sphingolipid activator defects (Chapters 6–10)

Disease (OMIM phenotype number)	Enzyme/Protein deficiency	Storage material	Preliminary test	Diagnostic test ‡ §	Prenatal diagnosis*	Inheritance, gene symbol & location
GM1-gangliosidosis types I, II & III (230500, 230600, 230650)	β-Galactosidase	GM1, KS, oligos, glycolipids	Urinary oligos	Enzyme§ assay in WBC/DBS Genetic	Enzyme/genetic	AR GLB1 3p22.3
GM2-gangliosidosis Tay–Sachs B variant (272800) (Including B1 variant)	β-Hexosaminidase A (α polypeptide)	GM2, oligos globoside, glycolipids	?	Enzyme§ assay in WBC/DBS. Genetic	Enzyme/genetic	AR HEXA 15q23
Sandhoff O variant (268800)	β-Hexosaminidase A&B (β polypeptide)	GM2, oligos	Urinary oligos	WBC enzyme assay, Genetic	Enzyme/genetic	AR HEXB 5q13.3
GM2 activator defect AB variant (272750)	GM2 ganglioside activator	GM2, oligos	GM2 in CSF	Natural substrate assay in cells Genetic	Genetic	AR GM2A 5q33.1
Fabry disease (301500)	α-Galactosidase A	Galactosylated glycolipids	Urinary glycolipids	Enzyme§ assay in WBC/DBS‡, Genetic	Enzyme/genetic	X-LR GLA Xq22.1
Gaucher disease types I, II & III (230800, 230900, 231000)	β-Glucosidase	Glc-Cer	Plasma Chitotriosidase	Enzyme assay in WBC/DBS‡	Enzyme/genetic	AR GBA 1q21
Gaucher disease, atypical (610539)	Saposin C defect	Glc-Cer	Plasma Chitotriosidase	Genetic, western blotting	Genetic	AR PSAP 10q21–q22
Metachromatic leukodystrophy (MLD) (250100)	Arylsulfatase A	Sulfatide	Metachromatic granules/sulfatide in urine	Enzyme§ assay in WBC, Genetic	Enzyme/genetic	AR ARSA 22q13.33
Metachromatic leukodystrophy (MLD (249900)	Saposin B	Sulfatides	Metachromatic granules in urine	Genetic, western blotting	Genetic, western blotting	AR PSAP 10q21–q22

(Continued)

Table 5.1 (Cont'd)

Sphingolipidoses including sphingolipid activator defects (Chapters 6–10)

Disease (OMIM phenotype number)	Enzyme/Protein deficiency	Storage material	Preliminary test	Diagnostic test ‡§	Prenatal diagnosis*	Inheritance, gene symbol & location
Globoid cell leukodystrophy Krabbe disease (245200)	β-Galactocerebrosidase	Galactosylceramide	–	Enzyme assay in WBC/DBS‡. Genetic	Enzyme/genetic	AR GALC 14q31
Atypical Krabbe due to saposin A defect (611722)	Saposin A	Galactosyl-ceramide	–	Genetic, western blotting in WBC	Genetic, western blotting	AR PSAP 10q21–q22
Niemann–Pick A & B (257200 & 607616)	Sphingomyelinase	Sphingomyelin	Plasma chitotriosidase	Enzyme assay in WBC/DBS‡. Genetic	Enzyme/genetic	AR SPMD1 11p15.4
Farber (228000)	Acid ceramidase	Ceramide	–	Enzyme assay in WBC. Genetic	Enzyme/genetic	AR ASAH1 8p22
Prosaposin deficiency (611721)	Prosaposin	Non-neuronal glycolipids Ubiquitinated material in neuro-lysosomes	Urinary glycosphingo-lipids	Genetic, western blotting	Genetic, western blotting (not tested)	AR PSAP 10q21–q22

Mucopolysaccharidoses (MPS) (Chapter 12)

Disease (OMIM)	Enzyme/Protein deficiency	Storage material	Preliminary test	Diagnostic test ‡§	Prenatal diagnosis*	Inheritance, gene symbol & location
MPS I Hurler (MPS IH) (607014) Hurler/Scheie (MPS IH/S) (607015) Scheie (MPS IS) (607016)	α-L-iduronidase	DS, HS and oligos	Urinary GAGs	Enzyme§ assay in WBC/DBS‡ Genetic	Enzyme/genetic	AR IDUA 4p16.3

Disorder	Enzyme	Storage	Screening	Diagnosis	Test type	Inheritance/Gene/Locus
MPS II Hunter (309900)	Iduronate-2-sulfatase	DS, HS and oligos	Urinary GAGs	Enzyme assay in WBC/DBS‡ Genetic	Enzyme† and genetic	X-LR *IDS* Xq28
MPS IIIA Sanfilippo A (252900)	Heparan N-sulfatase	HS and oligos	Urinary GAGs	Enzyme assay in WBC. Genetic	Enzyme/genetic	AR *SGSH* 17q25.3
MPS IIIB Sanfilippo B (252920)	α-N-acetyl-glucosaminidase	HS and oligos	Urinary GAGs	Enzyme assay in WBC/DBS. Genetic	Enzyme/genetic	AR *NAGLU* 17q21.2
MPS IIIC Sanfilippo C (252930)	Acetyl CoA: α-glucosamine N-acetyl transferase	HS and oligos	Urinary GAGs	Enzyme assay in WBC. Genetic	Enzyme/genetic	AR *HGSNAT* 8p11.2
MPS IIID Sanfilippo D (252940)	N-acetylglucosamine-6-sulfatase	HS and oligos	Urinary GAGs	Enzyme assay in WBC. Genetic	Enzyme/genetic	AR *GNS* 12q14.3
MPS IVA Morquio A (253000)	N-acetylgalactosamine-6-sulfatase	KS and oligos	Urinary GAGs	Enzyme assay in WBC/DBS‡ Genetic	Enzyme/genetic	AR *GALNS* 16q24.3
MPS IVB Morquio B (253010) allelic to GM1-gangliosidosis	β-Galactosidase	KS and oligos	Urinary GAGs	Enzyme§ assay in WBC/DBS‡ Genetic	Enzyme/genetic	AR *GLB1* 3p22.3
MPS VI Maroteaux-Lamy (253200)	N-acetylgalactosamine-4-sulfatase (Arylsulfatase B)	DS, oligos	Urinary GAGs	Enzyme assay in WBC/DBS‡ Genetic	Enzyme/genetic	AR *ARSB* 5q14.1
MPS VII Sly (253220)	β-Glucuronidase	CS, DS, HS oligos	Urinary GAGs	Enzyme§ assay in WBC/DBS‡ Genetic	Enzyme/genetic	AR *GUSB* 7q11.21
MPS IX (601492)	Hyaluronidase	Hyaluronan	–	Zymography Enzyme assay in serum/plasma	Not tested	AR *HYAL1* 3p21.31

Table 5.1 (*Contd*)

Glycoproteinoses (Oligosaccharidoses) (Chapters 14 and 15)

Disease (OMIM)	Enzyme/Protein deficiency	Storage material	Preliminary test	Diagnostic test ‡§	Prenatal diagnosis*	Inheritance, gene symbol and location
Aspartylglucosaminuria (208400)	Aspartylglucosaminidase (glycosylasparaginase)	Glycosyl-asparagines	Urinary oligos	Enzyme assay in WBC. Genetic	Enzyme/genetic	AR *AGA* 4q34.3
Fucosidosis (230000)	α-L-Fucosidase	Oligos, glycopeptides, glycolipids	Urinary oligos	Enzyme§ assay in WBC. Genetic	Enzyme/genetic	AR *FUCA1* 1p36.11
α-Mannosidosis (248500)	α-D-Mannosidase	Oligos	Urinary oligos	Enzyme assay in WBC. Genetic	Enzyme/genetic	AR *MAN2B1* 19p13.2
β-Mannosidosis (248510)	β-D-Mannosidase	Oligos	Urinary oligos	Enzyme assay in WBC. Genetic	Enzyme/genetic	AR *MANBA* 4q24
Sialidosis I/II (Mucolipidosis I) (256550)	Neuraminidase (Sialidase1)	Oligos, glycopeptides	Urinary oligos Bound & free sialic acid	Enzyme assay in cultured cells Genetic	Enzyme/genetic test in cultured cells	AR *NEU1* 6p21.3
Schindler\Kanzaki (609241 & 609242)	α-N-acetyl-galactosaminidase (α-Galactosidase B)	Oligos	Urinary oligos	Enzyme assay in WBC. Genetic	Not tested?	AR *NAGA* 22q13.2
Galactosialidosis (PPCA deficiency) (256540)	Protective protein / cathepsin A (PPCA)	Sialylated oligos and glycopeptides	Urinary oligos	Enzyme assays in lymphocytes or cultured cells. Genetic	Enzyme assays in cultured cells Genetic	AR *CTSA* 20q13.12

Other enzyme defects (Chapters 13 and 19)

Disease (OMIM)	Enzyme/Protein deficiency	Storage material	Preliminary test	Diagnostic test ‡§	Prenatal diagnosis*	Inheritance, gene symbol & location
Glycogenoses (Chapter 13) **Glycogen storage disease type II (Pompe)** (232300)	α-Glucosidase (acid maltase)	Glycogen, oligos	Urinary oligos, creatine kinase	Enzyme§ assay in WBC/lympho/fibr DBS‡. Genetic	Enzyme/genetic	AR *GAA* 17q25.3

Lipidoses (Chapter 19)

Wolman, cholesterol ester storage disease (278000)	Acid lipase	Cholesterol esters	Vacuolated lymphocytes	Enzyme assay in WBC. Genetic	Enzyme/genetic	AR *LIPA* 10q23.31

Protease defects (Chapter 19) – see also galactosialidosis and CLN2 and 10

Papillon-Lefèvre	Cathepsin C Dipeptidyl peptidase I (DPP I)	–	Periodontitis	Enzyme assay in neutrophils Genetic	–	AR *CTSC* 11q14.2
Pycnodysostosis (265800)	Cathepsin K	Collagen, other bone proteins	Radiology	Radiology Genetic	Genetic	AR *CTSK* 1q21.3

Defects in post-translational processing of lysosomal enzymes (Chapters 16)

Disease (OMIM)	Enzyme/Protein deficiency	Storage material	Preliminary test	Diagnostic test ‡§	Prenatal diagnosis*	Inheritance, gene symbol & location
Multiple sulfatase deficiency, mucosulfatidosis (272200)	Formylglycine generating enzyme (SUMF1)	Sulfatides, GAGs, glycolipids	Urinary GAGs sulfatide	Sulfatase assays in WBC. Genetic	Enzyme assays / genetic	AR *SUMF1* 3p26.1
Mucolipidosis IIα/β (ML II or I-cell) (252500) Mucolipidosis IIIα/β (ML IIIA or pseudo-Hurler polydystrophy) (252600)	N-acetylglucosamine-1-phosphotransferase α/β subunit	Oligos, GAGs, lipids	Urinary oligos Sialyl oligos	Enzyme assays in plasma & cultured fibros	Enzyme assays in cultured cells & AF Genetic	AR *GNPTAB* 12q23.2
Mucolipidosis IIIγ (ML III variant) (252605)	N-acetylglucosamine-1-phosphotransferase γ subunit	Oligos, GAGs, lipids	Urinary oligos	Enzyme assays in plasma & cultured fibros	Enzyme assays in cultured cells & AF Genetic	AR *GNPTG* 16p13.3
Stuttering (STUT2) (609261)	N-acetylglucosamine-1-phosphotransferase α/β and γ subunits; N-acetylglucosamine-1-phosphodiester α-N-acetylglucosaminidase (uncovering enzyme)					*GNPTAB*§ 12q23.2 *GNPTG*§ 16p13.3 *NAGPA*§ 16p13.3

(Continued)

Table 5.1 (*Contd*)

Lysosomal membrane and transport defects (Chapters 11 and 17)

Disease (OMIM)	Enzyme/Protein deficiency	Storage material	Preliminary test	Diagnostic test [‡§]	Prenatal diagnosis*	Inheritance, gene symbol and location
Cystinosis (219800, 219000 & 219750)	Cystinosin (cystine transporter)	Cystine	Urinary sediment Chitotriosidase Colourimetric test	Cystine or functional test in cells, Genetic	Cystine or functional test in CVS and cultured cells, Genetic	AR *CTNS* 17p13.2
Sialic acid storage disease Infantile (ISSD) (269920) Salla, adult form (604369)	Sialin (sialic acid transporter)	Sialic and uronic acids	Urinary free sialic acid	Free sialic acid in fibros, Genetic	Free sialic acid in CVS & cells. Genetic	AR *SLC17A5* 6q13
Cobalamin F disease (Methylmalonic aciduria and homocystinuria, cblF type) (277380)	Cobalamin transporter	Cobalamin	Urine & blood methylmalonic acid and homocysteine	Functional test in fibros Genetic	Not tested?	AR *LMBRD1* 6q13
Danon (300257)	Lysosome-associated membrane protein 2 (LAMP-2)	Cytoplasmic debris and glycogen	–	Detection of LAMP-2 in WBC/ tissue Genetic	Not tested?	X-LD *LAMP2* Xq24
LIMP-2 deficiency /Action myoclonus renal failure syndrome (254900)	LIMP-2 (Lysosomal integral membrane protein 2 or SCARB2 Scavenger Receptor Class B)	Not characterised	–	β-gluco-cerebrosidase in fibros, protein detection	Not tested?	AR *SCARB2* 4q21.1
Malignant infantile osteopetrosis (607649)	Mucolipin-1 (TRPML, transient receptor potential mucolipin)	Lipids	Blood gastrin	EM fibros. Genetic	EM of cells and genetic	AR *MCOLN1* 19p13.2
(602727) **Mucolipidosis IV** (252650)	CLCN7, chloride channel 7	–	–	Radiology genetic	Genetic	AR *CLCN7* 16p13.3
	OSTM-1, osteopetrosis-associated transmembrane protein	–	–	Radiology genetic	Genetic	AR *OSTM1* 6q21
Niemann–Pick type C1 Chapter 11 (257220)	Niemann–Pick type C1 protein (proton-driven transporter)	Cholesterol & other lipids	Serum chitotriosidase, cholesterol oxidation products	Filipin staining of fibros Functional test Genetic	Genetic	AR *NPC1* 18q11–q12
Niemann–Pick type C2 Chapter 11 (607625)	Niemann–Pick type C2 Protein (soluble lysosomal protein)	Cholesterol & other lipids	Serum chitotriosidase	Filipin staining of fibros Functional test Genetic	Genetic	AR *NPC2* 14q24.3

Neuronal ceroid lipofuscinoses (CLNs) (Chapter 18)

Disease (OMIM)	Enzyme/Protein deficiency	Storage material	Preliminary test	Diagnostic test ‡§	Prenatal diagnosis*	Inheritance, Gene symbol and location
CLN1 disease (Infantile NCL, INCL)# (256730)	Palmitoyl protein thioesterase 1 (PPT1)	Lipofuscin, Saposins		Enzyme in WBC/DBS Genetic	Enzyme, Genetic histology in CVS	AR *PPT1* 1p34.2
CLN2 disease (Late infantile NCL, LINCL)# (204500)	Tripeptidyl peptidase 1 (TPP1)	Lipofuscin, subunit c of ATPase		Enzyme in WBC/DBS Genetic	Enzyme, Genetic histology in CVS	AR *TPP1* 11p15.4
CLN3 disease (Juvenile NCL, JNCL Batten disease) (204200)	CLN3, lysosomal and/or Golgi transmembrane protein	Lipofuscin, subunit c of ATPase	Vacuolated lymphocytes	Histology and genetic	Histology in CVS. Genetic	AR *CLN3* 16p11.2
Recessive Adult NCL (ANCL Kufs) (204300)	CLN6 transmembrane protein in ER	Lipofuscin, subunit c of ATPase	Histology	Genetic	–	AR *CLN6* 15q23
CLN4 disease (Dominant Adult NCL, Parry disease) (162350)	CSPα	Lipofuscin, subunit c of ATPase	Histology	Genetic	–	D *DNAJC5* 20q13.33
CLN5 disease (variant late infantile, vLINCL) (256731)	CLN5, soluble lysosomal protein	Lipofuscin, subunit c of ATPase	Histology	Histology and genetic	Histology in CVS. Genetics	AR *CLN5* 13q22.3
CLN6 disease (variant late infantile, vLINCL) (601780)	CLN6 transmembrane protein in ER	Lipofuscin, subunit c of ATPase	Histology	Histology and genetic	Histology in CVS. Genetic	AR *CLN6* 15q23
CLN7 disease (variant late infantile, vLINCL) (610951)	CLN7/MFSD8 (major facilitator superfamily domain-containing protein 8), transporter	Lipofuscin, subunit c of ATPase	Histology	Histology and genetic	Histology in CVS. Genetic	AR *MFSD8* 4q28.2
CLN8 disease (variant late infantile, vLINCL) (600143)	CLN8 transmembrane protein in ER	Lipofuscin, subunit c of ATPase	Histology	Histology and genetic	Histology in CVS. Genetic	AR *CLN8* 8p23.3
CLN9 disease (609055)	Unknown	Lipofuscin, subunit c of ATPase	Histology	Histology	–	–
CLN10 disease (congenital/late infantile) (610127)	Cathepsin D	Lipofuscin Saposins A&D	Histology	Enzyme in WBC/fibros Genetic	Enzyme histology in CVS. Genetic	AR *CTSD* 11p15.5

(Continued)

Table 5.1 (*Cont'd*)

Defects in lysosome and lysosome-related organelle biogenesis (Chapter 19)

Disease (OMIM)	Enzyme/Protein deficiency	Storage material	Preliminary test	Diagnostic test [‡§]	Prenatal diagnosis[*]	Inheritance, Gene symbol and location
Chediak-Higashi syndrome (214500)	LYST		Bone Marrow examination and blood film including electron microscopy of leucocytes and platelets	Genetic	Microscopy and Genetic	AR *CHS1/LYST* 1q42.3
Griscelli syndrome type 1 (214450)	Myosin 5A	Melanin granules	Decreased pigmentation	Genetic	Microscopy and Genetic	AR *MYO5A* 15q21.2
Griscelli syndrome type 2 (607624)	Rab27A (soluble GTPase)	Melanin granules	Decreased pigmentation	Genetic	Microscopy and Genetic	AR *RAB27A* 15q21.3
Griscellli syndrome type 3 (609227)	Melanophilin	Melanin granules	Decreased pigmentation	Genetic	Microscopy and Genetic	AR *MLPH* 2q37.3
Hermansky-Pudlak syndrome (203300) **Types 1–9** See Chapter 19 and references therein for details of deficient protein, diagnosis and genetics of subtypes		Lipofuscin/ ceroid	Platelet function and bone marrow examination for pigment – containing macrophages	EM of platelets Genetic	Genetic	AR

Abbreviations: AF, amniotic fluid; AR, autosomal recessive; CS, chondroitin sulfate; CSF, cerebrospinal fluid; CVS, chorionic villi biopsy; D, dominant; DBS, dried blood spot; DS, dermatan sulfate; fibros, cultured fibroblasts; Glc-Cer, glucosylceramide; GM1, GM1-ganglioside; GM2, GM2-ganglioside; HS, heparan sulfate; KS, keratan sulfate; oligos, oligosaccharides; WBC, white blood cells; X-LD, X-linked dominant; X-LR, X-linked recessive.

§ Pseudodeficiency of enzyme

‡ Mass spectrometric assay published

Can be early or later onset, name refers to predominant phenotype

* CVS is used in preference but most tests can be performed on cultivated amniotic fluid cells and some metabolites can be determined in amniotic fluid. Molecular genetic testing can be performed for all pregnancies where the underlying molecular defect in the family is well established. For some very rare disorders prenatal diagnosis has not been reported but the techniques have been assessed.

† As unaffected females may have low activity foetal sex testing must be carried out

§ Genetic association to be confirmed

PART 2

The Individual Diseases

CHAPTER 6

Gaucher Disease

Deborah Elstein and Ari Zimran

Gaucher Clinic, Shaare Zedek Medical Center, Jerusalem, Israel

A representative case history

In June 1994, a 20-year-old woman was seen in our clinic with complaints of overt and progressive increase in abdominal girth as well as unremitting fatigue. She had been diagnosed at her induction for (compulsory) army service 2 years previously because of hepatosplenomegaly. Subsequent enzyme analysis showed low levels of β-glucocerebrosidase activity but (unfortunately) a sternal bone marrow aspiration was nevertheless performed elsewhere for "confirmation". She had always suffered from intermittent epistaxis and bruising after mild trauma. She had undergone several hospitalizations as a teenager because of unexplained bone pains in her knees and back, accompanied by a pronounced limp and fevers (typical for bone crises which many times are mistaken for osteomyelitis or other misdiagnoses). She has an older brother, who also has Gaucher disease but who had already suffered avascular necrosis of the left hip, but only minimal organomegaly: both siblings have the same genotype N370S/V394L. ERT with imiglucerase was initiated at 15units/kg body weight/infusion (the "low-dose" regimen, which we use in Israel for adult patients) in October, 1994. Within three years, there was dramatic reduction in hepatosplenomegaly, an increase in hemoglobin and platelet counts and bone pains (and hence the limp) had disappeared. At her most recent clinic evaluation, after approximately 16 years of ERT, she is totally asymptomatic with normalization of blood counts and near-normalization of organ volumes.

Gaucher disease

Gaucher disease was first described by Philippe Gaucher in 1882. He was able to detect the abnormally enlarged cells in the spleen but he erroneously identified the condition as a primary neoplasm. In 1965, the primary defect was recognized as the inability of the mutated enzyme β-glucocerebrosidase to degrade glucocerebroside adequately. The activated macrophages, or "Gaucher" cells, harbour the accumulated undegraded substrate. Purification of the enzyme with subsequent cloning of the gene in 1985 led not only to identification of the many mutations that cause the disease but also to the concept of management. Enzyme replacement therapy (ERT) was successfully tested in a clinical trial in 1991 [1] leading to a revolution in the management of the disease. A decade later, substrate reduction therapy (SRT) was evaluated with potential to also impact the neurological manifestations of Gaucher disease [2].

Epidemiology

Gaucher disease is inherited as an autosomal recessive disorder. It is a panethnic disorder like the other lysosomal storage disorders but has a predilection among Ashkenazi Jews with a carrier frequency of 1: 17 and an expected birth frequency of 1: 850. Two distinct neuronopathic forms of Gaucher disease are common in Northern Sweden and in the area of the Palestinian town of Jenin, respectively. The estimated global frequency of Gaucher disease is 1: 50,000 to 1: 100,000.

Lysosomal Storage Disorders: A Practical Guide, First Edition. Edited by Atul Mehta and Bryan Winchester.
© 2012 John Wiley & Sons, Ltd. Published 2012 by John Wiley & Sons, Ltd.

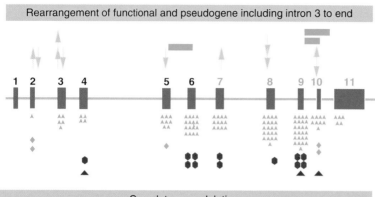

Over 300 mutations in Gaucher disease

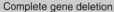

Figure 6.1 Most common Gaucher disease mutations in the β-glucocerebrosidase gene. (Courtesy of Prof. Gregory A. Garbowski, MD, Cincinnati Children's Hospital Medical Center.)

Etiology and pathogenesis: genetic basis

The glucocerebrosidase gene is located on chromosome 1q21. More than 300 mutations have been described (Figure 6.1) with an updated list published in 2008 [3]. The most common mutation, N370S, accounts for approximately 75% of the mutant alleles among Ashkenazi Jewish patients and approximately 30% among non-Jewish patients. Patients homozygous for N370S tend to have relatively mild phenotype; N370S is generally considered "protective" of development of neuronopathic features [4].

Mutations causing protein misfolding may induce endoplasmic reticulum (ER) associated degradation (ERAD) by the ER quality control system. In order to also avoid the proteotoxic effect of the mutated protein, and to circumvent ERAD, the new therapeutic modality of pharmacological chaperones (PC) [5] has been evaluated, facilitating trafficking from ER to Golgi to lysosome, and ultimately reducing storage of glucocerebroside in the lysosome.

Clinical forms

Three clinical forms have been defined, based on absence (type 1) or presence (types 2 and 3) of neurological signs.;

Such classification is useful when talking about management options and genetic counselling.

Type 1

Type 1, the putatively non-neuronopathic form, is the most prevalent. The phenotypic spectrum ranges from virtually asymptomatic (these patients typically are diagnosed incidentally) to severe life-threatening disease. Age of onset of signs and symptoms and disease course are accordingly variable; the younger the age at presentation the more severe the clinical course. Anaemia and/or thrombocytopenia are common presenting findings, as is hepatosplenomegaly (Figure 6.2), which even in children may be massive. In children, too, height retardation may be noted [6] although there is catch-up growth in most cases irrespective of intervention. Erlenmeyer flask deformity of the distal femur (Figure 6.3), osteopenia (Figure 6.4), and varying degrees of bone pain are common.

Symptomatic skeletal features, including "bone crises", osteonecrosis of joints, and pathological fractures of long bones (Figure 6.5) and vertebrae with collapse (Figure 6.6), although less prevalent, are, however, the leading causes of morbidity [6, 7]. Various imaging modalities assess/quantify bone involvement, but presymptomatic prediction of onset and rate of progression

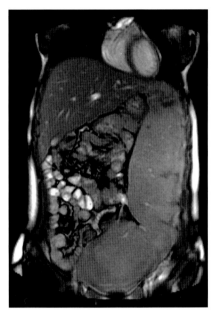

Figure 6.2 Massive splenomegaly reaching into the true pelvis in a 20-year-old female with a slightly erratic history of imiglucerase therapy since age 4 years.

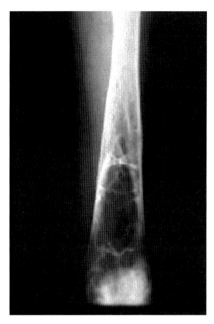

Figure 6.4 Osteopenia in the femur.

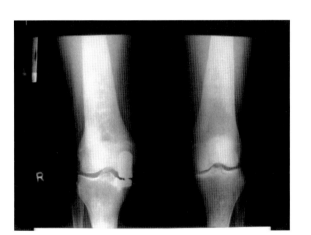

Figure 6.3 Ehrlenmayer Flask deformity.

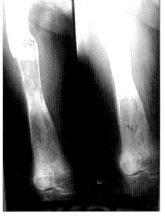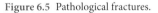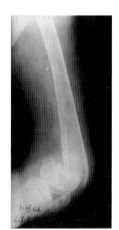

Figure 6.5 Pathological fractures.

of bone disease has not yet been achieved. Lung involvement, especially infiltrative disease (i.e. of "Gaucher" cells), is an uncommon but serious complication usually in young children with severe genotype (including type 3) or in splenectomized adult patients with severe liver involvement. "Gaucher" cell infiltration can also be seen in other tissues and organs, notably the lymph nodes in various locations (Figure 6.7). Patients with type 1, despite being "non-neuronopathic", may be at some increased risk for Parkinsonism and/or may develop peripheral neuropathies [6, 7].

Type 2

Type 2 is a lethal neuronopathic form associated with homozygosity or compound heterozygosity for severe and/or null mutations and is characterized by hypertonic posturing, strabismus, trismus and retroflexion of the head shortly after birth; death following aspiration

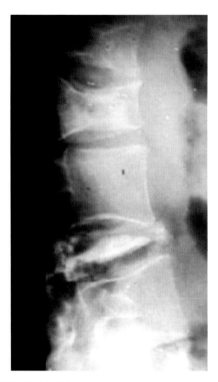

Figure 6.6 Vertebral fractures.

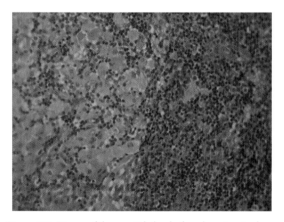

Figure 6.7 Biopsy of the parotid gland of a splenectomized 45-year-old male patient with a parotid gland adenoma also showing "Gaucher" cell infiltration despite 18 years of treatment with imiglucerase.

pneumonia and/or apnea/laryngospasm usually occurs by 2 years. Massive hepatosplenomegaly and lung involvement are common [6, 7].

Type 3

Type 3 is both a more heterogeneous and a more attenuated neuronopathic form [6, 7], presenting in childhood and characterized by the pathognomonic sign of supranuclear horizontal gaze palsy (SHGP). Most patients have at least one L444P mutation or other missense/null mutation. There is a subset of patients who are homozygous for the D409H mutation and develop progressive calcification of heart valves.

Table 6.1 presents all the subtypes of Gaucher disease and their characteristics.

Diagnosis

The gold standard for diagnosing Gaucher disease is the detection of reduced β-glucocerebrosidase activity in peripheral blood cells compared to same-day normal controls. The recently-introduced methodology to assess the enzymatic activity on a dry blood spot could be used for large-scale screening (e.g. research purposes) but it is commonly associated with both false-positive and false-negative results and hence cannot replace the gold-standard assay [7]. The enzymatic diagnosis should be combined with the identification of mutations at the DNA level, and here too, in order to avoid pitfalls, it should be performed by complete gene sequencing. Although still commonly performed, bone marrow aspiration and biopsies for the identification of Gaucher cells is not the appropriate diagnostic test.

Biomarkers

Biomarkers add quality assurance to biochemical diagnoses, but are more importantly used to quantify dynamic changes in the clinical course over time, reflecting disease progression (usually in the untreated patient) or clinical improvement with specific therapy. Chitotriosidase activity, which is elevated hundreds-fold in Gaucher disease, has been used in the past decade as the preferred surrogate marker [8], but, because of a genetic deficiency of chitotriosidase in ~6% of the population, CCL18 (PARC) levels are additionally evaluated. There is an ongoing search for new biomarkers (such as MIP-1alfa, MIP-1beta and others) to better predict future complications.

Routine follow-up of patients

At minimum, monitoring disease expression and the effect of ERT include serial evaluation of haematological

Table 6.1 Subtypes of Gaucher disease and their characteristics.

Subtype	Type 1		Type 2		Type 3		
	Symptomatic	Asymptomatic	Infantile	Neonatal	3a	3b	3c
Common genotype	N370S/other or 2 mild mutations	N370S/N370S or 2 mild mutations	1 null and 1 severe mutations	2 null or recombinant mutations	D409H/D409H	L444P/L444P	None
Common presenting features	Hepatosplenomegaly hypersplenism bleeding bone pains	None	*SNGP; strabismus opsithotonus, trismus	Hydrops foetalis; congenital ichthyosis	SNGP; cardiac valves' calcifications	SNGP; hepatosplenomegaly growth retardation	SNGP; myoclonic seizures
CNS involvement	None	Parkinsonism?	Severe	Lethal	SNGP; brachycephalus	SNGP; gradual cognitive deterioration	SNGP; slowly progressive neurologic deterioration
Bone involvement	Mild to severe (variable)	None	None	None	Minimal	Moderate to severe; kyphosis (gibbus)	Mild
Lung involvement	None to (rarely) severe	None	Severe	Severe	Minimal	Moderate to severe	Mild–moderate
Life expectancy	Normal / near-normal	Normal	Death before 2 years	Neonatal death	Death in early adulthood	Death in mid-adulthood	Death during childhood
Treatment options	ERT	None	Plliative	None	Valve replacement	ERT	ERT

*SNGP = supranuclear gaze palsy; ERT = enzyme replacement therapy.

parameters and reduction in hepatosplenomegaly. Although ultrasonography may be recommended for repeat assessments as the least invasive and having no risk of radiation, especially in children, it is the least used because of issues of reliability and reproducibility and the importance of observer experience. Computed tomography (CT) was employed in the past, but today, magnetic resonance imaging (MRI), especially because of justifiable concerns about radiation with periodic assessments, is preferred. Similarly, scintography is rarely justified. The most sensitive tool for the follow-up of bone involvement is probably Quantitative Chemical Shift Imaging (QCSI) but is the least available.

MRI is also frequently used to monitor bone disease, using various assessment scores in addition to skeletal X-rays and bone densitometry (DEXA). The value of plasma and urine bone markers has not been confirmed. There are also specific tools for quality of life assessment, used mainly in clinical trials.

Enzyme replacement therapy (ERT) for Gaucher disease: alglucerase and imiglucerase

The first ERT for Gaucher disease, alglucerase (Ceredase®, Genzyme Corp., Cambridge MA, USA), was a human placental derivative, tested in a seminal 9-month clinical trial of 12 patients with type 1 disease [1]. Within the first years of the availability of alglucerase, its safety and efficacy in improving haemoglobin levels and platelet counts, in reducing splenic and hepatic enlargement, and in ameliorating bone pains were confirmed.

In 1994, the human recombinant form of β-glucocerebrosidase, imiglucerase (Cerezyme®, also from Genzyme Corp.), was approved on the basis of two clinical trials: the first compared the safety and efficacy of imiglucerase with alglucerase, at (high-dose) regimen of 60 units/kg body weight/2 weeks [9] and the second compared the frequency of administration of imiglucerase, every 2 weeks *versus* 3 times a week, at (low-dose) 15 units/kg body weight/every-other-week [10]. There were no significant differences between and among the groups.

With 20 years of experience with ERT, the important conclusion seems to be that, at the advent of ERT, most patients suffer from several clinically relevant signs and symptoms of Gaucher disease, and that these gradually (2–5 years) improve with continuation of ERT so that near-normalization of many parameters is possible with most dosing regimens above 15 units/kg/ every-other-week [7]. The greater the deviation of many of the clinical parameters from normal values (but not platelet counts) the more dramatic the initial response. Platelet counts (particularly, but not only, in patients with massively enlarged spleens) may require longer periods to respond. In other cases, there may be no response of the platelets at all, even to high-dose, prolonged ERT; some of these patients may additionally have immune thrombocytopenia.

After 2–5 years, regardless of dosages, the responsiveness of the major disease-specific features and biomarkers tends to plateau and most patients achieve stabilization. Some symptomatic patients do not respond well or perhaps not even adequately, so that these are now considered to be "poor responders" or even "non-responders".

Attempts have been made to define "therapeutic goals" of disease-specific treatments, which are based on the cumulative patient experience with imiglucerase in a (Genzyme-sponsored) international Gaucher (ICGG) registry [11]. These goals are also applied when evaluating the efficacy of new Gaucher-specific therapies [12].

Neurological signs and symptoms

Because the enzyme is too large to traverse the blood–brain barrier, patients with neurological features only benefit from the effect of ERT on visceral, haematological and skeletal features.

Bone disease

Skeletal involvement often appears randomly both in asymptomatic patients and in patients on ERT for long periods of time. Among patients from the seminal alglucerase trial, radiological evidence of skeletal improvement was noted only 42 months after advent of therapy, so ERT may only slowly affect bone [7, 11]. However, pathological damage such as osteonecrosis, bone infarcts, fractures, etc., is apparently not reversible. Splenectomy is the most predictable trigger of bony damage, but with the introduction of ERT, splenectomy is less often indicated and, hence, early ERT may be seen as the best way of preventing bony damage. ERT may also improve BMD and osteopenia/osteoporosis [11]. Nonetheless, for patients with irreversible osteonecrosis of the large joints, total joint replacement relieves the pain and restores functionality (Figure 6.8).

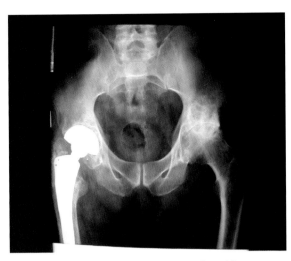

Figure 6.8 Avascular necrosis of the hip with total hip replacement in the contralateral hip.

Dosing regimens

The dosage controversy has never been adequately resolved. The first concern was the cost per unit, but beyond this was the question of whether higher doses actually translate into clinically significant more effective therapy [7]. More recently concerns were raised regarding untoward impact of ERT on associated diseases including diabetes, hyperlipidemia, malignancies and Parkinsonism [13].

Malignancies

Although, in general, patients with Gaucher disease are equally at risk for cancers as the population-at-large, there are some concerns in the literature about increased risks among those with mild Gaucher disease for malignancies, cardiovascular and cerebrovascular events, and decreased life expectancy [7, 13]. Because many of these statistics were culled from the International Collaborative Gaucher Group (ICGG) registry data, larger and unbiased studies are mandatory for verification. Most groups have shown an increased incidence of monoclonal gammopathies and multiple myeloma, neither of which is responsive to ERT. Conversely, there is a putatively low incidence of breast, ovarian and prostate cancers.

Global shortage of imiglucerase (June 2009)

In June 2009 the Genzyme Corporation announced a viral contamination at its manufacturing site. The reduction in

enzyme availability to 20% of expected supplies, with many patients required to stop or significantly reduce dosage, has led to re-evaluation of the clinical impact of withdrawal from ERT [7]. Early access programs of two new forms of the enzyme for ERT, which were at the pre-licence stage, were initiated at the request of regulatory agencies in both the USA and Europe.

Velaglucerase alfa

Velaglucerase alfa (VPRIV™, Shire HGT, MA, USA) is a human recombinant glucocerebrosidase with an amino acid sequence identical to that of the wild-type enzyme. It is produced by Gene-Activation™ technology in a human cell line [14], and has been commercially available since 2010. It was originally tested in a 9-month Phase 1/2 open-label, single centre trial and ongoing extension study [14]. Three Phase 3 clinical trials (involving nearly 100 patients, including children aged >2 years) were successfully completed: a two-dose study in treatment-naive patients, a switch-over study addressing the safety of the switch from imiglucerase to velaglucerase alfa, and a head-to-head comparison between imiglucerase and velaglucerase, which demonstrated a lack of inferiority of the new enzyme. Velaglucerase alfa seems to be the least immunogenic of the four enzymes developed to date and currently more than 1,200 patients worldwide receive this ERT.

Taliglucerase alfa

Taliglucerase alfa (Elelyso™, Protalix Biotherapeutics, Carmiel, Israel) is a human recombinant glucocerebrosidase produced from transduced carrot cells in a high-yield plant-cell system, which is easily scaled up in disposable bioreactors and is free from exposure to mammalian tissues [15]. It has completed a Phase 3 clinical trial and there are currently 2 additional ongoing clinical trials: one in naïve-to-treatment children and another among both adults and pediatric patients switching from imiglucerase. Taliglucrase alfa became commercially available in 2012.

Comparison of ERTs

While velaglucerase alfa seems to be the least immunogenic enzyme preparation, the evaluation of comparative efficacy of these ERTs requires the follow-up of larger cohorts of patients over time in order to assess whether the initial impressions based on short-term trial cohorts can be verified. In the discrete clinical trials of the four ERT options using the regimen of 60 units/kg body weight every-other-week, all showed good efficacy in all disease-specific parameters.

Other treatment options: substrate reduction therapy (SRT)

Substrate reduction therapy (SRT) was first tested in 1998 [2] using the orally-delivered, glucose analogue imino-sugar, N-butyldeoxynojirimycin (miglustat; Zavesca™, Actelion Pharmaceuticals Ltd; Allschwil Switzerland). Miglustat is a reversible inhibitor of the ceramide-specific glucosyltransferase that induces reduction in substrate biosynthesis. Because of its more problematic safety profile, miglustat was approved by the EMA (2002) only for adult patients with mild to moderate disease unsuitable for standard enzyme therapy and by the FDA (2003) with a similar caveat. Efficacy in treating Gaucher-specific parameters with miglustat is less good than ERTs but in a surveillance study, BMD as well as hematological parameters and organ reduction improved within 6 months. An important potential advantage of this agent is its ability to traverse the blood-brain-barrier and therefore to impact neuronopathic disease features; however, clinical trials failed to show any benefits. However, traversing the blood-brain barrier is also relevant for other lysosomal disorders on the glucosyltransferase pathway.

Genzyme Corporation (Cambridge, MA USA) has three ongoing Phase 3 clinical trials of SRT with eliglustat, a ceramide analogue. Preliminary results from Phase 1/2 trials of disease-specific efficacy are very encouraging, including improvement in BMD. Unlike miglustat, this compound is incapable of traversing the blood-brain barrier.

Summary

Gaucher disease is the most common autosomal recessive lipid storage disorder. Deficiency of β-glucocerebrosidase results in accumulation of glucocerebroside in lysosomes. Type 1 patients have no primary neuronopathic symptoms, but there is tremendous phenotypic variability even among patients with the same genotype. There is involvement of the central nervous system in type 2, an infantile lethal form, and type 3 disease, a subacute form with greater phenotypic heterogeneity. Diagnosis of Gaucher disease depends on demonstration of a deficiency of β-glucocerebrosidase activity with identification of mutations as an adjunct to prediction of type, to some extent, disease severity and for accurate identification of carriers. Disease manifestations include hepatosplenomegaly, thrombocytopenia, anemia, osteoporosis with risk of pathological fractures and osteonecrosis, and less commonly, pulmonary involvement. For symptomatic patients, safe and effective enzyme replacement therapy with imiglucerase has been available since 1994 and since 2002, substrate reduction therapy with miglustat, with less optimal efficacy and a problematic safety profile. In 2009, two new enzymatic options, velaglucerase alfa and taliglucerase alfa, became available at the pre-licensing stage because of a shortage of imiglucerase; both new ERTs now commercially available. Chaperone therapy is also being tested for type 1 disease and may ultimately be most valuable for neuronopathic patients.

References

1 Barton NW, Brady RO, Dambrosia JM, *et al.* Replacement therapy for inherited enzyme deficiency. Macrophage targeted glucocerebrosidase for Gaucher's disease. *N Engl J Med* 1991; **324**: 1464–1470.

2 Cox T, Lachmann R, Hollak C, *et al.* Novel oral treatment of Gaucher's disease with N-butyldeoxynojirimycin (OGT 918) to decrease substrate biosynthesis. *Lancet* 2000; **355**: 1481–1485.

3 Hruska KS, LaMarca ME, Scott CR, Sidransky E. Gaucher disease: mutations and polymorphism spectrum in the glucocerebrosidase gene (GBA). *Hum Mutat* 2008; **29**: 567–583.

4 Fairley C, Zimran A, Phillips M, *et al.* Phenotypic heterogeneity of N370S homozygotes with type I Gaucher disease: an analysis of 798 patients from the ICGG Gaucher Registry. *J Inherit Metab Dis* 2008; **31(6)**: 738–744.

5 Ron I, Horowitz M: ER retention and degradation as the molecular basis underlying Gaucher disease heterogeneity. *Hum Mol Genet* 2005; **14(16)**: 2387–2398.

6 Zimran A, Elstein D. Lipid storage diseases. In: Lichtman MA, *et al.* (eds.), *Williams Hematology* (8th edition). New York: McGraw-Hill, 2010; pp. 1065–1071.

7 Zimran A. How I treat Gaucher disease. *Blood* 2011; **118(6)**: 1463–1471.

8 Hollak CEM, van Weely S, van Oers MHJ, Aerts JMFG. Marked elevation of plasma chitotriosidase activity. A novel hallmark of Gaucher disease. *J Clin Invest* 1994; **98**: 1288–1292.

9 Grabowski GA, Barton NM, Pastores G, *et al.* Enzyme therapy in Gaucher disease type 1: comparative efficacy of mannose-terminated glucocerebrosidase from natural and recombinant sources. *Ann Int Med* 1995; **122**: 33–39.

10 Zimran A, Elstein D, Levy-Lahad E, *et al.* Replacement therapy with imiglucerase for type 1 Gaucher's disease. *Lancet* 1995; **345**: 1479–1480.

11 Pastores GM, Weinreb NJ, Aerts H, *et al.* Therapeutic goals in the treatment of Gaucher disease. *Semin Hematol* 2004; **41**: 4–14.

12 Weinreb N, Taylor J, Cox T, *et al.* A benchmark analysis of the achievement of therapeutic goals for type 1 Gaucher

disease patients treated with imiglucerase. *Am J Hematol* 2008; **83**: 890–895.

13 Zimran A, Ilan Y, Elstein D. Enzyme replacement therapy for mild patients with Gaucher disease. *Am J Hematol* 2009; **84**(**4**): 202–204.

14 Zimran A, Altarescu G, Phillips M, *et al*. Phase I/II and extension study of velaglucerase alfa (Gene-Activated[TM] Human Glucocerebrosidase) replacement therapy in adults with type 1 Gaucher disease: 48 month experience. *Blood* 2010; **115**(**23**): 4651–4656.

15 Aviezer D, Brill-Almon E, Shaaltiel Y, *et al*. A plant-derived recombinant human glucocerebrosidase enzyme – a preclinical and phase I investigation. *PLoS ONE* 2009; **4**(**3**): e4792.

CHAPTER 7

Fabry Disease

Atul Mehta[1] and Uma Ramaswami[2]

[1]Lysosomal Storage Disorders Unit, Department of Haematology, University College London Royal Free Hospital, London, UK
[2]The Willink Biochemical Genetics Unit, Genetic Medicine, St Mary's Hospital, Manchester, UK

Fabry disease (Online Mendelian Inheritance in Man #301500) is a rare X-linked metabolic disorder caused by the partial or complete deficiency of the lysosomal enzyme, α-galactosidase A.

Case history

A 16-year-old boy presents with a skin rash. Raised red spots have been noted around his upper lip for a few months. Similar spots are present around the umbilicus and at the tops of the thighs. He has a long history of pain in the hands and feet, typically occurring after exercise and described as 'burning'. He has noticed difficulty in sweating. He is intolerant of heat and exercise, which induce and aggravate his limb pains. He complains of increasing swelling of his lower limbs. He also has a long history of cramping abdominal pain with diarrhoea; as a child, these abdominal pains were associated with headache and often caused him to miss school. He suffered an episode of sudden deafness at the age of 11 years. His mother's brother died of renal failure, aged 42 years; and his grandmother died of a stroke, aged 61 years. Examination confirms the skin rash. He has bilateral high tone deafness. Cardiac examination, ECG and echocardiogram are normal, but his left ventricular size is at the upper limit of normal. He has 2+ proteinuria but renal function is normal. He undergoes a skin biopsy and renal biopsy and the diagnosis of Fabry disease is made.

Epidemiology

Fabry disease is generally considered to be the second most prevalent lysosomal storage disorder, after Gaucher disease, with an estimated incidence ranging between 1:40,000 and 1:170,000 persons. It may be much more common, and a recent study showed that 1:3,200 neonates in northern Italy have missense mutations in the alpha-galactosidase A gene, but many of these may be clinically silent. The diagnosis is often missed in childhood. All ethnic groups are affected. Although it is sex linked, heterozygous females are frequently symptomatic. The mechanisms underlying this are unknown, but may relate to skewed X inactivation. Up to 3–4% of adult male patients with cryptogenic stroke or unexplained left ventricular hypertrophy may have atypical Fabry disease.

Genetic basis

The AGAL A (*GLA*) gene is located at Xq22.1 and approximately 600 mutations have been identified (mainly missense mutations but also nonsense mutations and single amino acid deletions and insertions). Most of these mutations are 'private', having been identified only in individual families, while others, located at CpG dinucleotides (e.g. R227X), have been found as independent mutational events.

Lysosomal Storage Disorders: A Practical Guide, First Edition. Edited by Atul Mehta and Bryan Winchester.
© 2012 John Wiley & Sons, Ltd. Published 2012 by John Wiley & Sons, Ltd.

Pathophysiology

Neutral sphingolipids with terminal α-galactosyl residues (predominantly globotriaosylceramide (Gb3)) accumulate in the lysosomes of cells in a range of different organs and tissues. This includes endothelial, perithelial and smooth muscle cells of blood vessels, epithelial cells of glomeruli and tubules of the kidneys, cardiac myocytes, ganglion cells of the autonomic system, cornea and histiocytic and reticular cells of connective tissue. An accumulation of lysosphingolipids (i.e. glycosphingolipids that do not have N-acylated fatty acids) may be of particular significance in Fabry diseases and may lead to biochemical and structural changes which damage the cells. Abnormal proliferation of cells, e.g. of the intimal musculature of blood vessels, may be a part of the vascular pathology of Fabry disease.

Clinical presentation

Fabry disease is a progressive, multisystem disorder which typically results in a global reduction in quality of life of affected individuals (see Box 7.1). Symptoms in

---

Box 7.1 **Typical signs and symptoms of Fabry disease according to age.**

Childhood and adolescence (≤16 years)
- Neuropathic pain
- Ophthalmological abnormalities (cornea verticillata and tortuous retinal blood vessels)
- Hearing impairment
- Dyshidrosis (hypohidrosis and hyperhidrosis)
- Hypersensitivity to heat and cold
- Gastrointestinal disturbances and abdominal pain
- Lethargy and tiredness
- Angiokeratomas
- Onset of renal and cardiac signs, e.g. microalbuminuria, proteinuria, abnormal heart rate variability

Early adulthood (17–30 years)
- Extension of any of the above
- Proteinuria and progressive renal failure
- Cardiomyopathy
- Transient ischaemic attacks, strokes
- Facial dysmorphism

Later adulthood (age >30 years)
- Worsening of any of the above
- Heart disease (e.g. left ventricular hypertrophy, angina, arrhythmia and dyspnoea)
- Stroke and transient ischaemic attacks
- Osteopenia and osteoporosis

---

childhood typically relate to lethargy, tiredness, pain, cutaneous abnormalities (Figure 7.1), changes to sensory organs and often gastrointestinal disturbances. In early adulthood patients may suffer extension of any of the above symptoms and often develop lymphodema, proteinuria and the first signs of renal, cardiac or central nervous system/cerebrovascular disease. A characteristic facial appearance has been noted (Figure 7.2). In late adulthood (age >30 years) symptoms include worsening of the above and more severe organ dysfunction (cardiac disease, renal disease and cerebrovascular disease). The

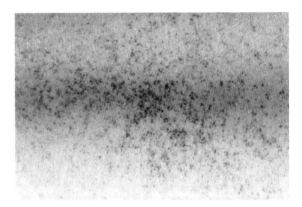

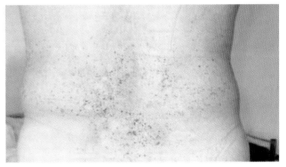

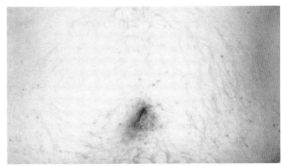

Figure 7.1 Typical angiokeratomas. (Courtesy of Dominique P. Germain, University of Versailles, France.)

late onset forms of Fabry disease may present as stroke/ TIA, left ventricular hypertrophy or renal failure.

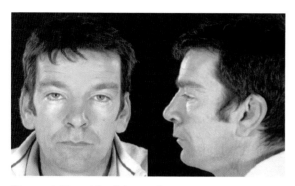

Figure 7.2 Typical facial dysmorphism in a patient with Fabry disease. Male patient treated with ERT for 10 years, showing prominent supra orbital ridges, bushy eyebrows, periorbital puffiness, mild ptosis, prominent jaw line. Facial features seem to normalize to a degree in patients on ERT.

Natural history

The life expectancy for males with Fabry disease is reduced by about 15 years; for females the reductions are less, about 10 years. The commonest cause of death in males and females is cardiovascular disease. There is some preliminary evidence that ERT is having an impact by extending life expectancy and reducing the impact of renal disease on mortality. As Fabry patients live longer, cognitive disturbances, mood disorders and vascular disease are becoming more apparent.

Laboratory diagnosis

Diagnosis (see Figure 7.3) in males is confirmed by the demonstration of deficient α-galactosidase A activity in plasma, serum, or leukocytes and the identification of the pathogenic mutation. The disease is X-linked and therefore females have variable, occasionally even normal, levels of enzyme activity. DNA confirmation of the

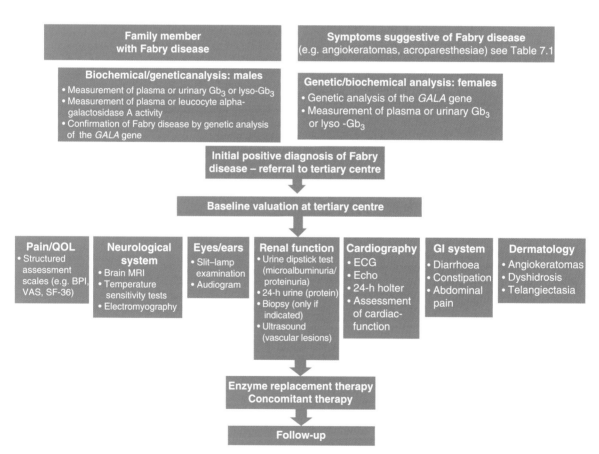

Figure 7.3 Diagnostic pathway in Fabry disease.

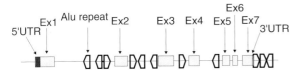

Figure 7.4 The Fabry (*GLA*) gene.

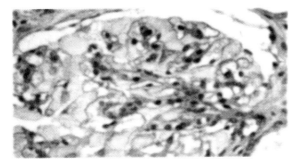

Figure 7.5 Kidney biopsy: accumulation of globotriaosyl-ceramide within the lysosomes of glomerular podocytes. (Courtesy of Dominique P. Germain, University of Versailles, France.)

diagnosis is essential. Enzyme activity in plasma and leucocytes in heterozygote females can be at the lower end of the normal range, and DNA confirmation is required. The gene is illustrated in Figure 7.4.

Biopsy of tissues, such as skin and kidney (Figure 7.5), demonstrates the presence of lipid deposition and multilamellated myelin bodies in electron micrographs. As Gb3 deposition starts *in utero*, prenatal diagnosis can be performed from chorionic villi or culture of amniotic cells, where low α-galactosidase A activity can be demonstrated.

Treatment

Two products, agalsidase alfa (Replagal, Shire HGT) and agalsidase beta (Fabrazyme, Genzyme Corporation), are licensed as enzyme replacement treatments for Fabry disease. Both have a broad evidence base from data in randomized trials, observational registry studies and case series. ERT is generally advocated in all males with Fabry disease with signs or symptoms referable to the disease, and in all females who have demonstrable signs of the disease. The two products are broadly equivalent. ERT has made a substantial impact in males, females and children. It is likely that life expectancy is improved as ERT improves the function of critical organs (e.g. kidney, heart). ERT does not reverse severe organ damage,

however, and there are questions over the time to start treatment, dose and impact of antibodies. Small molecule therapy in the form of orally administered chaperone drugs are in trial and show promise in patients with selected mutations which have residual activity.

Adjuvant therapies are very important. Pain must be adequately controlled, and blood pressure control is important in maintaining renal/cardiac function and reducing the risk of stroke. Proteinuria can be controlled by the use of angiotensin converting enzyme (ACE) inhibitors or angiotensin receptor blockade. Aspirin may be used to reduce the risk of thrombosis, heart rhythm should be monitored, and social support is valuable. Patients have an increased risk of depression.

Treatment guidelines

Formal guidelines recommend that all adults – males and females – who have evidence of organ damage should receive ERT. Adults with severe pain, or reduced quality of life, but without organ damage, should also receive ERT. ERT has been shown to be safe in children. As ERT does not reverse established organ damage and does not prevent cerebrovascular disease, it should therefore be instituted early in the course of the disease. In June 2009, Genzyme Corporation reported a reduced capacity to manufacture agalsidase beta and the majority of Fabry patients have subsequently either been treated with reduced doses of agalsidase beta or switched to agalsidase alfa. The impact of this 'shortage' and 'switching' is currently the subject of intense scruniny and no firm conclusions can be drawn. At the time of writing, however, supplies of agalsidase beta appear to be recovering.

Further reading

1 Mehta A, Beck M, Eyskens F, *et al.* Fabry disease: a review of current management strategies. *Qly J Med* 2010; **103**: 641–659.

2 Meikle PJ, Hopwood JJ, Clague AE, Carey WF. Prevalence of lysosomal storage disorders. *J Am Med Assoc* 1999; **281**: 249–245.

3 Spada M, Pagliardini S, Yasuda M, *et al.* High incidence of later-onset Fabry disease revealed by newborn screening. *Am J Hum Genet* 2006; **79**: 31–40.

4 Garman SC, Garboczi DN. The molecular defect leading to Fabry disease: structure of human alpha- galactosidase. *J Mol Biol* 2004; **337**: 319–335.

5 Deegan PB, Baehner AF, Barba Romero MA, *et al.* Natural history of Fabry disease in females in the Fabry Outcome Survey. *J Med Genet*, 2006; **43**: 347–352.

6 Hughes DA, Ramaswami U, Elliott P, *et al.* Guidelines for the diagnosis and anagement of Anderson Fabry disease. http://www.dh.gov.uk/prod_consum_dh/groups/dh_di-gitalassets/@dh/@en/documents/digitalasset/dh_4118408 2005.

7 Germain DP, Waldek S, Banikazemi M, *et al.* Sustained long term renal stabilization after 54 months of agalasidase beta therapy in patients with Fabry disease. *J Am Soc Nephrol* 2007; **18**: 1547–1557.

8 Replagal summary of product characteristics, 2010. http://emc.medicines.org.uk/medicine/19760/SPC/Replagal+1mg+ml+concentrate+for+solution+for+infusion/

9 Fabrazyme summary of product characteristics, 2010. http://emc.medicines.org.uk/medicine/18404/SPC/Fabrazyme+35+mg%2c+powder+f or+concentrate+for+solution+for+inf usion/

10 Mehta A, Beck M, Giugliani R, *et al.* Enzyme replacement therapy with agalasidase alfa in patients with Fabry's disease: an analysis of registry data. *Lancet* 2009; **374**: 1986–1996.

11 Linthorst GE, Germain DP, Hollak CEM, *et al.* Expert opinion on temporary treatment recommendations for Fabry disease during the shortage of enzyme replacement therapy (ERT). In: Molecular genetics and metabolism. 2011. p. 99–102.

CHAPTER 8

The Gangliosidoses

Joe T.R. Clarke

Centre Hospitalier Universitaire, Sherbrooke, and University of Toronto, Toronto, Canada

The gangliosidoses are a clinically heterogeneous group of disorders resulting from hereditary defects of the metabolism of sialic acid-containing glycoconjugates caused by primary deficiencies of the lysosomal hydrolases, β-galactosidase or β-*N*-acetylgalactosaminidase (β-hexosaminidase), or proteins necessary for the stabilization or hydrolytic activity of the enzymes *in vivo*. All are neurodegenerative disorders in which non-neurological manifestations of the primary genetic defects are often clinically trivial. The most common variants of the diseases generally present in early infancy and progress rapidly to death; late-onset variants pursue a more protracted course, varying from years to decades, before death. All are very rare, autosomal recessive disorders. All are panethnic, although Tay–Sachs disease occurred with a frequency approaching 1 in 2,500 births among Ashkenazi Jews prior to the establishment of screening programmes for carriers of the disease.

GM1-gangliosidosis (OMIM #230500)

The first cousin Brazilian parents of a 7-month-old infant boy reported that he had not made any developmental progress since 3-4 months of age, no longer fixed and followed objects or faces with his eyes, was floppy and irritable. On physical examination, the infant was found to have subtle facial dysmorphism (frontal bossing, depressed bridge of the nose, long philtrum, macroglossia and gingival hypertrophy), an enlarged liver and spleen, and a fundoscopic examination revealed the presence of macular cherry-red spots. Over the ensuing several weeks, he developed complex partial seizures and regressed to a neurovegetative state. Radiographs showed dysplastic changes of the long bones and vertebrae similar to those seen in Hurler disease. Examination of a bone marrow aspirate showed the presence of storage cells with ultrastructural features typical of ganglioside accumulation (Figure 8.1). Urinary screening tests for mucopolysaccharides were negative or only weakly positive. By contrast, thin-layer chromatographic analysis of urinary oligosaccharides show marked abnormalities consistent with GM1-gangliosidosis (Figure 8.2). The diagnosis is confirmed by demonstrating a marked and specific deficiency of β-galactosidase in peripheral blood leukocytes. The child died at age 22 months of inanition and pneumonia. The clinical course and biochemical abnormalities are characteristic of generalized GM1-gangliosidosis, type I.

Classification

The most common variant of generalized GM1-gangliosidosis, type I, presents in early infancy and progresses rapidly to death, usually by 2–3 years of age [1]. Death in the first few months of life from severe cardiomyopathy occurs in some cases, before the development of severe neurodegenerative manifestations of the disease. Severe GM1-gangliosidosis may present as non-immune foetal hydrops.

Generalized GM1-gangliosidosis, type II, is characterized by the onset between 6 and 36 months of age of developmental arrest, then regression with seizures and spasticity, in the absence of the prominent hepatosplenomegaly, skeletal abnormalities or macular cherry-red spots seen in infants with type I disease. The course of the

Lysosomal Storage Disorders: A Practical Guide, First Edition. Edited by Atul Mehta and Bryan Winchester.
© 2012 John Wiley & Sons, Ltd. Published 2012 by John Wiley & Sons, Ltd.

(a)

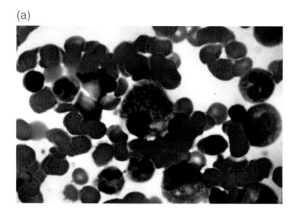

(b)

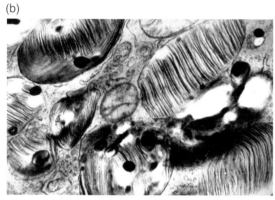

Figure 8.1 Storage histiocytes in bone marrow. Panel (a): Light microscopic appearance, Wright stain. Panel (b): Electron microscopic appearance of lamellar membranous inclusions.

disease is more protracted, generally culminating in death late in the first decade of life.

Type III disease is a late-onset variant presenting as generalized dystonia with dysarthria and ataxia. Parkinsonism and other signs of extrapyramidal involvement are common. Cognitive impairment develops later in the course of the disease. Survival is generally measured in decades after the initial onset of symptoms.

Galactosialidosis is a very rare disorder of ganglioside metabolism caused by deficiency of protective protein (cathepsin A) resulting in combined deficiency of lysosomal β-galactosidase and α-neuraminidase [2, 3]. This disease is covered more completely in Chapter 15.

Epidemiology

The global incidence of GM1-gangliosidosis is estimated to be 1 in 300,000 to 100,000 births; however, the incidence is much higher in some genetic isolates, such as in the Canary Islands, southern Brazil, and among Roma gypsies.

Classification

By far the most common variant of GM2-gangliosidosis is late-infantile Tay–Sachs disease, caused by *HEXA* mutations. The disease generally presents towards the middle of the first year of life with developmental arrest, loss of visual fixation, abnormalities of tone, macrocephaly, and an exaggerated startle reflex ("hyperacusis"). It pursues a stereotypic clinical course, with rapid neurological deterioration, the appearance of classical

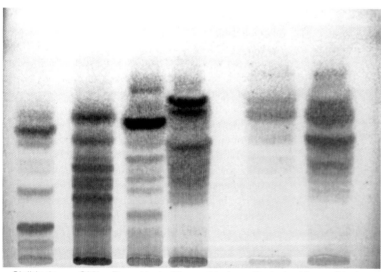

Sialidosis   GM1   Fucosidosis   Mannosidosis   Control   Mannosidosis

Figure 8.2 Thin-layer chromatogram of urinary oligosaccharides. The pattern of oligosaccharides characteristic of various lysosomal storage diseases is revealed by staining the oligosaccharides separated by TLC with orcinol/sulfuric acid.

GM2-gangliosidosis (OMIM #272800, #272750, #268800)

The 7-year-old son of unrelated Caucasian parents presented with a history of incoordination and progressive speech difficulty beginning at age 4–5 years. His development was otherwise unremarkable. However, over the subsequent few months, his gait became slower and more uncoordinated, with frequent falls. Physical examination was unremarkable apart from marked dysarthria and moderately severe ataxia of his gait. Apart from his speech difficulty, he showed no cranial nerve deficits, and muscle bulk, power and tone were normal; deep tendon reflexes were symmetrical and brisk, but judged to be within normal limits. There was no dysmorphism or organomegaly. CNS imaging by MRI was reported to be within normal limits. Skeletal radiographs were also normal. Electrophysiological testing showed a normal EEG and nerve conductions. Urinary screening tests for MPS and oligosaccharides were normal. A lumbar puncture was also normal. However, although total serum β-hexosaminidase activity was normal, β-hexosaminidase A activity was only 2% of normal; β-hexosaminidase B activity was increased. The results were consistent with a diagnosis of juvenile-onset GM2-gangliosidosis, Tay–Sachs variant.

The clinical course of the condition was characterized by further progressive deterioration of speech and gait, marked muscle wasting, and evidence of cognitive impairment. By age 10 years, he was wheelchair bound, with no intelligible speech and marked cognitive impairment. He died at age 13 years of pneumonia.

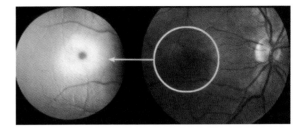

Figure 8.3 Macular cherry-red spot. The accumulation of ganglioside in ganglion cells creates a ring of pallor resulting in abnormal prominence of the centre of the macula which is devoid of ganglion cell bodies in the normal retina. (Courtesy of Dr. Alex Levin.)

Adult-onset Tay–Sachs disease is much more common than adult-onset Sandhoff disease, but the onset, clinical course and outcome are the same. It is more common in Ashkenazi Jews than among other populations because of the frequency of heterozygosity for severe *HEXA* mutations in that population. Adult-onset Tay–Sachs disease is often the result of compound heterozygosity for one of the two common severe *HEXA* mutations (1278insTATC; IVS12 + 1 G > C), along with a mild mutation, such as G269S. This variant may present at any age as an atypical cerebellar ataxia, atypical motor neurone disease or psychosis. Cognitive impairment only occurs late in the course of the disease.

Tay–Sachs disease caused by deficiency of the GM2 activator protein (*GM2A* mutations) is clinically indistinguishable from classical variants of Tay–Sachs disease. Diagnosis is complicated owing to the fact that measurements of β-hexosaminidase activity using synthetic substrates are invariably normal.

Epidemiology

The overall incidence of GM2-gangliosidosis is of the same order as GM1-gangliosidosis. However, approximately 1 in 25–30 Ashkenazi Jews is a carrier of the disease, and prior to the introduction of screening for carriers of the disease, Tay–Sachs disease (late-infantile GM2-gangliosidosis, TSD variant) was 100 times more common in Ashkenazi Jews than in other populations. Large-scale screening programmes to identify carriers and provide genetic counselling, including prenatal diagnosis, have led to a marked decrease in the incidence of the disease [5]. Sandhoff disease (late-infantile GM2-gangliosidosis, Sandhoff variant) is very rare, except in some relatively isolated, inbred communities. Although carrier detection of Tay–Sachs disease also identifies carriers of Sandhoff disease, carrier detection programmes

cherry-red spots of the macula (Figure 8.3), blindness and seizures, culminating in death at 3–4 years of age.

Late-infantile Sandhoff disease is clinically almost indistinguishable from Tay–Sachs disease. However, mild enlargement of the liver and radiographic evidence of skeletal involvement may be found. The clinical course is the same as for Tay–Sachs disease.

The juvenile variants of Tay–Sachs disease and Sandhoff disease are indistiguishable [4]. The onset is often heralded by the development of dysarthria and incoordination progressing to frank ataxia. Cognitive impairment is highly variable; some patients presenting in later childhood show very little or no intellectual impairment until late in the course of the disease. Acute psychoses are very common in patients with the juvenile variants of the diseases. The psychoses are characteristically resistant to treatment with conventional antipsychotic medications.

Table 8.1 Genetics of the gangliosidoses.

Disease	Gene	Chromosomal locus	Gene product	Function
GM1-gangliosidosis	*GLB1*	3p21.33	β-Galactosidase Elastin-binding protein	1. Lysosomal hydrolase cleaves the non-reducing terminal galactose from gangliosides and other glycoconjugates 2. Occurs in a complex with α-neuraminidase and lysosomal protective protein/cathepsin A (see Chapter 15)
GM2-gangliosidosis (Tay-Sachs or B variant)	*HEXA*	15q23-q24	Alpha subunit of β-hexosaminidase	Subunit of heterodimeric enzyme that is necessary for the enzymic cleavage of non-reducing terminal N-acetylgalactosaminide from GM2-ganglioside
GM2-gangliosidosis (Sandhoff or O variant)	*HEXB*	5q13	Beta subunit of β-hexosaminidase	1. Subunit of heterodimeric β-hexosaminidase necessary for stability of the enzyme 2. Cleaves the non-reducing terminal N-acetylgalactosaminide from neutral glycosphingolipids
GM2-gangliosidosis (AB variant)	*GM2A*	5q31.3-q33.1	GM2 activator protein	Solubilizes GM2-ganglioside, necessary for the enzymic hydrolysis of GM2-ganglioside by β-hexosaminidase

have not had a significant impact on the frequency of the disease because of the focus on Ashkenazi Jews and the fact that the disease is very rare and the frequency of the condition is not increased in that population.

Genetics

The genetics of the gangliosidoses is summarized in Table 8.1. The genetic basis of the different variants of GM2-gangliosidosis is shown in Figure 8.4. All are autosomal recessive disorders. Carrier detection and prenatal diagnosis of all of them are possible by appropriate mutation analysis of the relevant gene.

Pathophysiology

The higher molecular weight gangliosides, including GM1-ganglioside, occur in highest concentration in cerebral gray matter. GM2-ganglioside, which represents the first product of the enzymic degradation of GM1, also occurs almost exclusively in the brain. Accumulation of these acidic glycosphingolipids in neurones would appear to account for the progressive neurodegenerative course of the three disorders, GM1-gangliosidosis, galactosialidosis,

and GM2-gangliosidosis. The observation that some patients with galactosialidosis exhibit no primary neurological abnormalities suggests that the β-galactosidase deficiency does not cause cerebral GM1-ganglioside storage, just as patients with Morquio disease, type B, a disease that is also caused by β-galactosidase deficiency, do not exhibit significant primary neurological involvement, though the skeletal manifestations of the enzyme deficiency may be very severe. The details of the mechanism of the neuronal cell death and secondary demyelination are unknown, although various observations suggest they may include disruptions of endoplasmic reticulum stress responses, axoplasmic transport and neuronal–glial interactions, as well as secondary inflammatory reactions and activation of autophagy [1, 6].

The non-neurological manifestations of GM1-gangliosidosis (dysmorphic facies, dysostosis multiplex, hepatosplenomegaly) are the result, in part at least, of accumulation of other glycoconjugates, such as oligosaccharides derived from the incomplete degradation of glycoproteins, which are excreted in the urine. In the case of Sandhoff disease, the central neurological

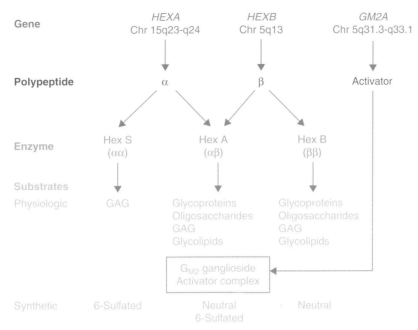

Figure 8.4 Genetics of GM2-gangliosidosis. Abbreviations: GAG, glycosaminoglycans. (Adapted from Winchester [14], with permission from Oxford University Press.)

abnormalities are likely attributable entirely to GM2-ganglioside accumulation in brain resulting from deficiency of Hex A. Gangliosides, as well as acidic synthetic substrates, such as 4MU-β-Gal sulfate (4MUGS), are not substrates for Hex B. However, deficiency of Hex B does slow the normal degradation of neutral glycosphingolipids, such as asialo-GM1-ganglioside, which is thought to be the cause of the subtle hepatosplenomegaly and skeletal abnormalities occurring in some cases of the severe, late-infantile variant of the disease.

Laboratory diagnosis

In the case of GM1-gangliosidosis and galactosialidosis, vacuolated lymphocytes are seen in the peripheral blood smear and foamy storage cells occur in the bone marrow. The urinary oligosaccharide profile is almost always obviously abnormal as a result of the excretion of large amounts of non-ganglioside glycoconjugates (oligosaccharides derived from the incomplete degradation of glycoproteins) (Figure 8.2). The demonstration of accumulation of GM1-ganglioside or GM2-ganglioside, as a way to make the diagnosis of GM1 or GM2-gangliosidosis, is not practical: accumulation of the lipids is generally only easily demonstrable in brain tissue obtained by biopsy, which is generally not necessary for diagnostic purposes. Confirmation of the diagnosis rests

in each case on the demonstration of primary deficiency of the gene product, by measurement of enzyme activity or by physical quantitification of non-catalytic proteins, or by mutation analysis. The enzyme activities are measureable in serum or in any cells containing lysosomes, including in platelets. The activities of β-galactosidase (GM1-gangliosidosis and galactosialidosis) and β-hexosaminidase (GM2-gangliosidosis) are easily measured fluorometrically with the use of synthetic substrates: 4-methylumbelliferyl-β-D-galactoside (4MU-β-Gal) and 4-methylumbelliferyl-β-D-*N*-acetylglucosaminide (4MU-β-Hex), respectively. Confirmation by the demonstration of mutations in the relevant genes, *GMB1*, *HEXA* or *HEXB*, may be necessary in some cases to rule out the possibility of pseudo-deficiency. Pseudo-deficiency is a phenomenon in which deficiency of enzyme activity towards a synthetic substrate, such as 4MU-β-Gal, is found though activity towards the natural substrate is sufficient to prevent clinical disease. This is a rare phenomenon which generally comes to attention when a clinically healthy individual is found incidentally or in the course of high-risk screening to have marked deficiency of the relevant enzyme activity as generally measured using a synthetic substrate. Mutation analysis is one way to rule out a clinically significant enzyme deficiency in an individual who might be thought to be pre-symptomatic.

The diagnosis of Tay–Sachs disease (B variant of GM2-gangliosidosis) relies on the ability to demonstrate deficiency of β-hexosaminidase A (Hex A) in the presence of a large excess of β-hexosaminidase B (Hex B). The isozymes can be separated by a variety of physical manipulations; however, the most common is to take advantage of the marked difference in the heat stability of the isoenzymes: Hex A is heat-labile, while Hex B is relatively heat-stable.

The B1 variant of GM2-gangliosidosis is clinically indistinguishable from other variants of GM2-gangliosidosis. It is caused by mutations a the catalytic site of the α-subunit of Hex A. It represents a diagnostic challenge because Hex A and Hex B enzyme activities are normal when measured using 4MU-β-Hex as substrate. However, enzyme activity towards the sulfated substrate, MUGS, is markedly deficient. The apparent paradox is caused by the fact that the neutral substrate, 4MU-β-Hex, is hydrolyzed by the active site of the β-subunit of Hex A, which does not hydrolyze the sulfated substrate or GM2-ganglioside. Hence, the apparently "normal" Hex A activity obtained with the conventional 4MU-β-Hex substrate is actually the result of hydrolysis of the substrate by the β-subunit of mutant Hex A. The diagnosis is also possible by demonstrating the presence of an active site mutation, such as Arg178His, in the α-subunit of the enzyme [8].

In the case of deficiency of GM2 activator (AB variant of GM2-gangliosidosis), the diagnosis may be difficult. The activity of β-hexosaminidase measured with the use of synthetic substrates is invariably normal, and measurement of enzyme activity using suitably labelled natural substrate, GM2-ganglioside, is exceedingly cumbersome, even if a supply of labelled substrate is available. Confirmation of the diagnosis is only practically possible by immuno-quantification of the GM2 activator protein or by the demonstration of mutations in the *GM2A* gene.

Treatment

Current treatment of all the gangliosidoses is still entirely supportive and symptomatic; no primary treatment, by replacement or enhancement of the gene product, has been developed so far. Despite normalization of relevant enzyme activity, the results of treatment of the gangliosidoses by bone marrow transplantation have been disappointing; however, experience is very limited, and whether it might be more effective if undertaken pre-symptomatically is not clear. Studies done in mutant mice suggest that haematopoietic stem cell transplantation might alter the course of the diseases if done before the development of neurological symptoms. Because the clinical manifestations are predominantly, if not exclu-sively, limited to the central nervous system (CNS), treatment by enzyme replacement therapy (ERT) has not been considered to be feasible. However, research is currently underway to develop variants of the normal enzyme capable of crossing the blood–brain barrier, which might make treatment by ERT feasible in the future. The results of attempts to modify the otherwise disastrous course of GM2-gangliosidosis by substrate reduction therapy, with miglustat, have been disappointing [9].

Research is currently focused more on efforts to stabilize mutant enzyme proteins by chaperone treatment. Unlike exogenous enzyme administered intravenously, chaperone molecules are more likely to cross the blood–brain barrier. Moreover, relatively small increases in enzyme activity would appear to be sufficient to modify the clinical course of diseases such as GM2-gangliosidosis dramatically [10]. Mutant β-galactosidase enzyme activity in fibroblasts from a patient with adult-onset GM1-gangliosidosis is increased 2–3 fold by exposure to galactose *in vitro* [11]. The preliminary results of the treatment of late-onset GM2-gangliosidosis with the anti-parasitic drug, pyrimethamine, are promising [12, 13]. Chaperone therapy is only effective in cases where the decreased enzyme activity is the result of instability of the mutant polypeptide; mutations of the active site, such as in the B1 variant of GM2-gangliosidosis, or those resulting in no gene product being formed, such as occurs in classical late-infantile Tay–Sachs disease, would not be expected to respond to this approach to therapy.

Experiments on neural stem cell transplantation and on gene transfer therapy of GM2-gangliosidosis in animals have produced some encouraging preliminary results which have not yet been explored in humans.

References

1 Brunetti-Pierri N, Scaglia F. GM1-gangliosidosis: review of clinical, molecular, and therapeutic aspects. *Mol Genet Metab* 2008 Aug; **94**(4): 391–396.

2 Strisciuglio P, Sly WS, Dodson WE, *et al.* Combined deficiency of beta-galactosidase and neuraminidase: natural history of the disease in the first 18 years of an American patient with late infantile onset form. *Am J Med Genet* 1990 Dec; **37**(4): 573–577.

3 Kleijer WJ, Geilen GC, Janse HC, *et al.* Cathepsin A deficiency in galactosialidosis: studies of patients and carriers in 16 families. *Pediatr Res* 1996 Jun; **3B9**(6): 1067–1071.

4 Maegawa GH, Stockley T, Tropak M, *et al.* The natural history of juvenile or subacute GM2-gangliosidosis: 21 new cases and literature review of 134 previously reported. *Pediatrics* 2006 Nov; **118**(5): e1550–1562.

5 Natowicz MR, Prence EM. Heterozygote screening for Tay–Sachs disease: past successes and future challenges. *Curr Opin Pediatr* 1996 Dec; **8**(6): 625–629.

6 Walkley SU, Zervas M, Wiseman S. Gangliosides as modulators of dendritogenesis in normal and storage disease-affected pyramidal neurons. *Cereb Cortex* 2000 Oct; **10**(10): 1028–1037.

7 Galjart NJ, Morreau H, Willemsen R, *et al.* Human lysosomal protective protein has cathepsin A-like activity distinct from its protective function. *J Biol Chem* 1991 Aug 5; **266**(22): 14754–14762.

8 Tanaka A, Ohno K, Sandhoff K, *et al.* GM2-gangliosidosis B1 variant: analysis of beta-hexosaminidase alpha gene abnormalities in seven patients. *Am J Hum Genet* 1990 Feb; **46**(2): 329–339.

9 Maegawa GH, Banwell BL, Blaser S, *et al.* Substrate reduction therapy in juvenile GM2-gangliosidosis. *Mol Genet Metab* 2009 Sep–Oct; **98**(1–2): 215–224.

10 Conzelmann E, Sandhoff K. Partial enzyme deficiencies: residual activities and the development of neurological disorders. *Dev Neurosci* 1983; **6**(1): 58–71.

11 Caciotti A, Donati MA, d'Azzo A, *et al.* The potential action of galactose as a "chemical chaperone": increase of beta galactosidase activity in fibroblasts from an adult GM1-gangliosidosis patient. *Eur J Paediatr Neurol* 2009 Mar; **13**(2): 160–164.

12 Clarke JT, Mahuran DJ, Sathe S, *et al.* An open-label Phase I/II clinical trial of pyrimethamine for the treatment of patients affected with chronic GM2-gangliosidosis (Tay–Sachs or Sandhoff variants). *Mol Genet Metab* 2011 Jan; **102**(1): 6–12.

13 Maegawa GH, Tropak M, Buttner J, *et al.* Pyrimethamine as a potential pharmacological chaperone for late-onset forms of GM2-gangliosidosis. *J Biol Chem* 2007 Mar 23; **282**(12): 9150–9161.

14 Winchester B. Primary defects in lysosomal enzymes. In: *Lysosomal Disorders of the Brain: Recent Advances in Molecular and Cellular Pathogenesis and Treatment*. Platt FM, Walkley SU (eds). Oxford: Oxford University Press, 2004.

CHAPTER 9

Metachromatic Leukodystrophy and Globoid Cell Leukodystrophy

Volkmar Gieselmann,[1] David A. Wenger[2] and Ingeborg Krägeloh-Mann[3]

[1] Institut fuer Biochemie und Molekularbiologie, Rheinische-Friedrich-Wilhelms Universität, Bonn, Germany
[2] Department of Neurology, Thomas Jefferson University, and Jefferson Medical College, Philadelphia, PA, USA
[3] Department of Pediatric Neurology and Developmental Medicine, University Children's Hospital, Tübingen, Germany

MLD and GLD

Metachromatic leukodystrophy (MLD) and globoid cell leukodystrophy (Krabbe disease, GLD) are autosomal recessively inherited disorders caused by the deficiency of arylsulfatase A (ASA) and galactosylceramidase (GALC), respectively. Since both enzymes depend on the assistance of activator proteins saposin B (ASA) and A (GALC), respectively, clinically indistinguishable diseases can also be caused by the deficiencies of these activator proteins (Figure 9.1). The pathological hallmark of both diseases is a loss of oligodendrocytes and thus myelin leading to multiple progressive and finally lethal neurologic symptoms [1, 2].

Case studies

Late-infantile MLD

A 3-year-old girl had an unrevealing family history, pregnancy and birth; her early development also was normal – she learned to sit within 7 months, crawled at 8 months, stood up with help at 10 months. Thereafter, however, motor development stagnated. At 18 months she learned to walk but was unstable. Language development was normal until then (first words at 12 months, two word combinations at 18 months). Eight months later, LD was diagnosed after demonstration of ASA deficiency.

At 27 months she had a febrile infection and deteriorated thereafter, lost walking 1 month later, developed swallowing problems; she could no longer sit at 33 months and her speech became dysarthric; at 35 months she could no longer grasp, and also stopped speaking ; at 3 years, head control was lost as well as interest in her surroundings. She survived several years in this severely impaired condition. Her gross motor course is illustrated in Figure 9.2.

Adult MLD

A woman presented with clumsiness, dysfunctional and bizarre behaviour, memory deficits, and apathy at the age of 37 years. She had been working as a housewife and was described as well-organized and intelligent. At the age of 32 years she showed progressive apathy and loss of interest in daily living routines, including care of her three children. Memory functions deteriorated dramatically. She could recall neither the names nor birthdays of her relatives. She developed bladder incontinence. At the age of 37 she fell down stairs and developed a subdural haematoma. In the course of diagnostic procedures in a neurosurgery department she underwent MRI which revealed typical leukodystrophic alterations. Biochemical and molecular studies confirmed the diagnosis of MLD. Upon neurologic examination at that time she revealed no abnormalities, especially no clinical signs of neuropathy. Muscle tone and gait were normal. Cognitive and mental functions were severely

Lysosomal Storage Disorders: A Practical Guide, First Edition. Edited by Atul Mehta and Bryan Winchester.
© 2012 John Wiley & Sons, Ltd. Published 2012 by John Wiley & Sons, Ltd.

impaired, with fluctuating vigilance and loss of concentration. Immediate and delayed verbal recall was impaired. She showed frontal signs with grasping and perseveration. Follow-up examinations at the age of 38 and 40 years revealed further cognitive decline but still no motor impairment.

Infantile GLD

At 4½ months of age a female infant came to our attention because of a 2-month history of apathy and poor motor development. At this time the infant was very irritable, crying almost 24 hours a day. The child was experiencing generalized twitching of the extremities and was hyper-extending the head. The hands were kept tightly clenched. She had unexplained elevations in her body temperature. By 6 months of age she had no purposeful movement and appeared to be blind. At 8 months of age seizures became frequent. She died at 9 months of age after a high fever that could not be controlled. This case is typical of many patients with the infantile form of GLD. The diagnosis of GLD was confirmed by the finding of very low GALC activity. While some live longer due to improved symptomatic care, the clinical regression in untreated infantile-onset GLD patients is rather typical.

Adult GLD

A woman, currently 48 years of age, was considered normal until about 28 years of age when she suffered the onset of lower extremity paresis with episodes of tripping and clumsiness on walking. Magnetic resonance imaging done at this time showed symmetrical white matter lesions affecting the posterior limb of the internal capsules, thalami, corona radiate, centrum semiovale and subependymal white matter (especially about the occipital horns). She underwent physiotherapy to help her legs but continued to experience spastic paresis with a clumsy gait and difficulty on rising from a squatting or sitting position. There was no obvious intellectual impairment. She is married, continues to work part time and is the mother of a healthy daughter born when she was 43 years old. Her sister, who is 1½ years younger, was considered normal until 4 to 5 years of age when she developed progressive weakness in all extremities. She experienced rapid mental deterioration and onset of seizures. She is currently wheelchair-bound and significantly mentally disabled. EMG studies performed when the younger sister was 37 years of age showed severe sensorimotor peripheral polyneuropathy with axonal and demyelinating features including median motor distal latency prolongation, median motor conduction velocity slowing, and prolongation of the median F-response. Similar studies performed at the same time in the older sister showed that the abnormalities were far less severe than in the more symptomatic younger sister. These sisters have the same low GALC activity and the same mutations in the GALC gene. Clearly other genetic and/ or environmental factors play a role in modifying disease onset and progression in the later-onset forms of Krabbe disease.

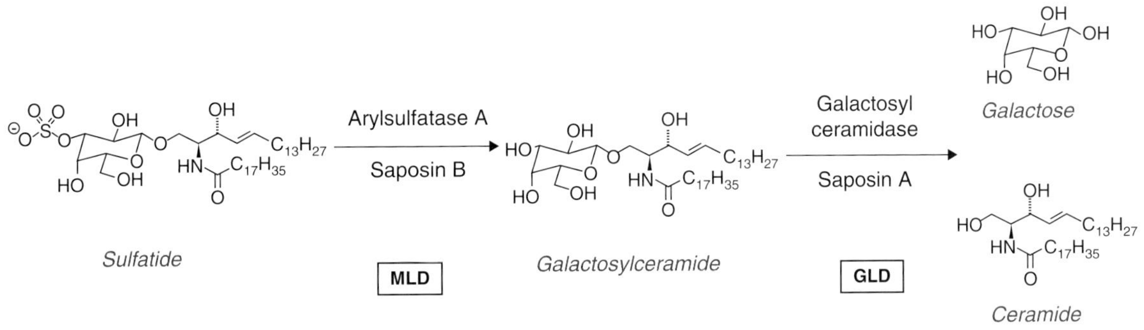

Figure 9.1 Enzymes and activator proteins involved in degradation of sulfatide and galactosylceramide. Sulfatide is hydrolyzed by arylsulfatase A (ASA) to yield galactosylceramide and sulfate. The activator protein saposin B solubilizes sulfatide and presents it to the enzyme. Sulfatide accumulates in the absence of either protein. This step is defective in metachromatic leukodystrophy (MLD). Galactosylceramide is cleaved into galactose and ceramide by galactosylceramidase (GALC). This enzyme depends on the assistance of saposin A. A deficiency of either of these proteins causes globoid cell leukodystrophy (GLD) (Krabbe disease).

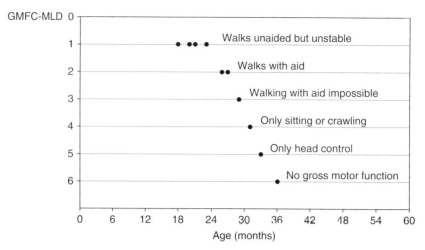

Figure 9.2 Natural course of MLD. Typical course of gross motor function in a child with late-infantile MLD (see case history of late-infantile MLD) described by a gross motor function classification, the GMFC-MLD [9]: first abnormalities at 18 months (walks unstable); once level 2 (walking only with aids) is attained, gross motor function rapidly deteriorates and at the age of 3 years, there is no gross motor function anymore.

Epidemiology

In the European population the incidence of MLD and GLD is estimated to be about 0.6 in 100,000 live newborns for each disorder [3]. Activator protein deficiencies are much rarer. Their incidence has not been exactly determined. In general, the diseases occur in all ethnicities. Higher incidences of MLD are found in Habbanite Jews (1:75), Christian Arabs (1:8,000), Eskimos and Navajo Indians. A higher frequency of GLD has been described in certain Druze and Arab villages in Israel (1:170) [4]. To initiate therapy before symptoms are obvious, New York State instituted a newborn screening test for Krabbe disease using dried blood spots in August 2006. Since that time over 1.2 million newborns have been tested, and 4 were found to have infantile Krabbe disease based on a combination of mutation analysis and follow-up enzyme testing.

Genetics

The genes for ASA and GALC are located on 22q13.31-qter (ASA) and 14q31 (GALC), respectively. Whereas the ASA is a small gene in which the 8 exons encompass only about 3 kb of genomic sequence, the 17 exons of the GALC gene span 56 kb.

More than 150 mutations are known in the ASA gene. Among Caucasians, only a few of them are frequent (c.459 + 1 g > a, p.426P > L, p.179I > S) accounting for ~ 60%

of all alleles, whereas many of the other mutations were only found in a few, mostly single, families (Table 9.1). More than 110 mutations in the GALC gene are known. One mutation (p.57 G > S) in the GALC gene is common in southern Italy. Japanese patients display a different spectrum of genetic defects in both disorders. In the ASA gene this is a p.99 G > R substitution and for the GALC gene it is a deletion/insertion mutation c.683_694del12insCTC. Table 9.1 summarizes the most common disease-causing mutations found in patients with MLD and GLD.

In both diseases there is a limited genotype/phenotype correlation. In MLD, homozygosity for mutations which do not allow the synthesis of any functional enzyme, always cause the severe late infantile form of disease. The presence of one allele associated with residual enzyme activity mitigates the disease to the juvenile form, whereas homozygosity for two alleles with residual ASA activity in most cases will result in a late juvenile or even adult form of MLD (Figure 9.3). Thus, residual enzyme activity which, in late-onset patients, is in the range of 2–4% of normal, is one determinant of clinical severity. However, clinical variability in late-onset patients – even in siblings with identical ASA genotype – is considerable, showing that other genetic or epigenetic factors influence the disease course substantially. Therefore, a precise prediction of the individual course of disease based on genotype analysis is impossible.

Data on genotype/phenotype correlations in GLD are more limited than in MLD, but the data available suggests

Table 9.1 Most common mutations and polymorphisms found in patients with MLD and GLD.

Location	cDNA position (based on GALC original numbering system)[1]	Base change	Effect (for GALC original numbering system)	Comments[2,3]
Frequent mutations causing MLD				
Ex 2	c. 296G > A	GGC > GAC	p.99G > D	Late-infantile Japanese
In 2	c. 459 + 1 g > a	CAGgta > CAGata	Loss of splice donor site	Late-infantile
Ex 3	c. 536T > G	ATC > AGC	p.179I > S	Late-onset
Ex 8	c. 1277C > T	CCG > CTG	p.426P > L	Late-onset
Polymorphisms in the ASA pseudodeficiency allele				
Ex 6	c. 1049A > C	AAT > ACT	p.350N > S	Polymorphism
Ex 8	c. 1620A > G	aataac > agtaac	Loss of polyadenylylation signal	Polymorphism
Frequent mutations causing GLD				
Ex 1	c. 169G > A (c. 121G > A)	GGC > AGC	p.57G > S (p.41G > S)	Late-onset, southern Italy
Ex 4	c. 332G > A (c. 284G > A)	GGC > GAC	p.111G > D (p.95G > D)	Infantile
Ex 4	c. 334A > G (c. 286A > G)	ACT > GCT	p.112T > A (p.96T > A)	Late-onset
Ex 7	c. 683 del + ins (c. 635 del + ins)	del 12, ins 3	del 5 aa + ins 2 aa	Infantile, Japanese, Korean
Ex 8	c. 857G > A (c. 809G > A)	GGC > GAC	p.286G > D (p.270G > D)	Late-onset
Ex 8	c. 908C > T (c. 860C > T)	TCC > TTC	p.303S > F (p.287S > F)	Infantile
In 10-end	30 kb deletion	30 kb del	Short mRNA	Infantile
Ex 11	c. 1186C > T (c. 1138C > T)	CGG > TGG	p.396R > W (p.380R > W)	Infantile
Ex 13	c. 1472 delA (c. 1424delA)	TAAGG > TAGG	FS, PS	Infantile
Ex 14	c. 1586C > T (c. 1538C > T)	ACG > ATG	p.529T > M (p.513T > M)	Infantile
Ex 15	c. 1700A > C (c. 1652A > C)	TAC > TCC	p.567Y > S (p.551Y > S)	Infantile
Ex 16	c. 1901T > C) (c. 1853T > C)	TTA > TCA	p.634L > S (p.618L > S)	Infantile
Polymorphisms in the GALC gene				
Ex 4	c. 550C > T (c. 502C > T)	CGT > TGT	p.184R > C (p.168R > C)	Always with 30 kb deletion
Ex 6	c. 742G > A (c. 694G > A)	GAT > AAT	p.248D > N (p.232D > N)	
Ex 8	c. 913A > G (c. 865A > G)	ATC > GTC	p.305I > V (p.289I > V)	Japanese
Ex 14	c. 1685T > C (c. 1637T > C)	ATA > ACA	p.562I > T (p.546I > T)	Very common

[1] The original numbering system of the GALC cDNA was based on the use of a start codon 48 nucleotides shorter than another start codon identified later.
[2] The comments reflect the best information available from published and unpublished data.
[3] Designation as infantile or later-onset is based on the identification of multiple patients with these mutations either homozygous or heterozygous with other known mutations.
Note: Almost all of the disease-causing mutations in the GALC gene also contain known polymorphisms in the same copy of the gene.
Abbreviations: aa = amino acids; del = deletion; ins = insertion; FS = frame shift; PS = premature stop.

that correlations in GLD and MLD follow similar rules. The finding of certain mutations in the GALC gene, either homozygous or heterozygous with known mutations, can predict a severe phenotype in a newborn individual. The presence of other known mutations in the GALC gene will predict a later-onset form of GLD. Late-onset MLD patients frequently present initially with psychiatric symptoms rather than motor problems. This phenotype correlates with a certain genotype. Patients presenting psychiatrically are frequently heterozygous for a null allele and the p.179I > S amino acid substitution [5]. The molecular basis for this peculiar genotype/phenotype correlation remains unclear.

For diagnostic reasons it is important to realize that for both genes polymorphisms are known, which lead to substantial but harmless enzyme deficiencies (termed pseudodeficiencies – see Chapter 3). There is no convincing evidence that these pseudodeficiencies are linked to any

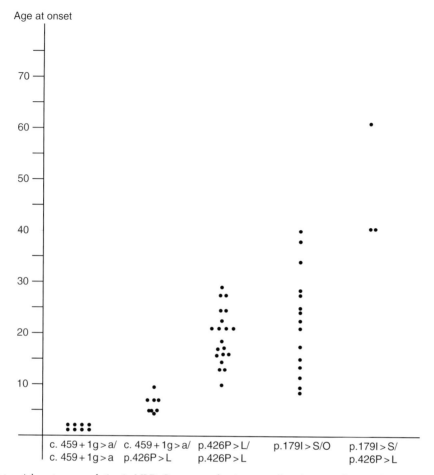

Figure 9.3 Genotype/phenotype correlation in MLD. Genotypes of patients are plotted against the age of diagnosis. c.429 + 1 g > a is the most frequent null allele of the ASA locus, p.426P > L and p.179I > S are frequent alleles with residual enzyme activity. 0 represents any null allele. (Reproduced from Gieselmann V. *Acta Paediatr Suppl* 2008; **97**: 15–21, with permission from Wiley).

other disease, but they must be excluded before the diagnosis of MLD or GLD is made. The pseudodeficiency allele of the ASA gene is frequent occurring in about 15% of Europeans. The frequent allele contains two polymorphisms, one leads to the loss of one oligosaccharide side chain (p.350N > S) and the other to the loss of a polyadenylation signal, which is important for a proper termination of the transcription of the gene (Table 9.1). Whereas the first has only minor effects on enzyme stability, the latter causes the loss of 90% of mRNA, leading to a substantially reduced synthesis of an otherwise fully functional enzyme.

There are several common polymorphisms in the GALC gene that have an effect on the measured GALC activity (Table 9.1) [2]. These include p.184R > C, p.248D > N, p.305I > V and p.562I > T, using the new numbering system.

Expression studies have shown that the very common polymorphism p.562I > T significantly lowers the measured GALC activity. While even the inheritance of multiple copies of these polymorphisms on both GALC alleles does not result in true pseudodeficiency, their presence does result in a very wide "normal" range for GALC activity. In addition, their presence on the same allele as a disease-causing mutation may play a significant role in determining whether that mutation is disease-causing.

Pathophysiology

ASA and GALC are involved in the degradation of two major myelin sphingolipids, 3-O sulfogalactosylceramide (sulfatide) and galactosylceramide, respectively

(Figure 9.1). Whereas sulfatide accumulates in MLD, the overall level of galactosylceramide is not increased in brain from patients with GLD. At the cellular level, however, in GLD there is substantial storage of galactosylceramide in macrophages. An inability to degrade these myelin sphingolipids results in loss of oligodendrocytes and myelin. In Krabbe disease (GLD) this is accompanied by infiltration of frequently multinucleated macrophages, which were termed globoid cells. These cells are so characteristic that they gave the disease its name. In both diseases, the lysolipids of sulfatide and galactosylceramide, lysosulfatide and psychosine, respectively, also accumulate. They have potent biological activities such as inhibition of protein kinase C, interference with IGF-1 signalling and phospholipase A2 activation [6, 7]. For these reasons they are considered to play an essential role in the pathogenesis although their exact mode of action *in vivo* remains to be elucidated. As far as MLD is concerned, substantial storage of sulfatide also occurs in a number of neurons. In a mouse model of this disease the early symptoms correlate with the increase of sulfatide in neurons in the absence of demyelination. Therefore, this disease should not be considered as affecting oligodendrocytes only. Furthermore, in humans, symptoms – at least in the early stages – may also be caused by neuronal storage before symptoms due to demyelination dominate the clinical picture.

Clinical presentation

The clinical phenotype of MLD and GLD is due to the global and progressive loss of myelin. Therefore, in both disorders, clinically relevant pathology is limited to both the central and peripheral nervous systems. Demyelination causes various neurologic symptoms which are finally lethal. Both diseases are clinically heterogeneous with respect to the age of onset, progression of symptoms and initial symptoms. In the typical late-infantile form of MLD (defined as onset before 2½ years of age), children develop symptoms usually in the second year of life after an initially normal development. Symptoms involve gait problems due to neuropathy and spasticity, ataxia, abnormal movement patterns and mental regression. The disease is progressive and patients mostly die before the age of 5 years in a decerebrated state. In the juvenile (onset 2½ to 16 years) and more so in adult forms (onset after 16 years) concentration, behavioural and psychiatric symptoms resulting in, for example, school problems may prevail in the early stages before the neuromotor problems become

dominant. In the past this has occasionally led to the misdiagnosis of schizophrenia or bipolar disease. In adults, MLD may start as late as 60 years of age [8]. Progression in adults is slower and patients have a mean survival time of about 12 years after diagnosis. Decline in intellectual capabilities, bizarre behaviour, emotional instability and memory deficits are frequent initial signs. Mostly the disease affects both the peripheral and the central nervous system. Whereas early involvement of the peripheral nervous system has been noted in a number of patients, there are patients in which there is marked demyelination in central nervous system while the peripheral nervous system is preserved. A detailed description of the natural course of MLD revealed that in late-infantile and juvenile patients the disease progression, as measured with a gross motor function classification (GMFC-MLD [9]), is not linear as might have been expected [10]. Patients maintain their motor functions in early stages of the disease over several months. This initial phase is followed by a rapid decline, during which the patients lose most of their motor function in a narrow time window of about 6 months, and this is not only seen in late-infantile but also juvenile patients (Figure 9.4).

In contrast, the infantile form of GLD is more aggressive than late-infantile MLD. Children develop rapidly-progressing symptoms already during the first 6 months of life. Characteristic is an initial general hyper-irritability to various stimuli, hyperesthesia and limb stiffness. A severe and motor deterioration rapidly develops with marked hypertonicity, spastically extended and crossed legs and hyperactive reflexes. Patients lose vision and mostly die before the age of 24 months. There are also attenuated juvenile and adult forms of GLD in which the clinical phenotype is more variable. Disease may start with loss of vision, spastic paraparesis, ataxia and slow psychomotoric deterioration.

Diagnosis by MRI

MRI shows characteristic abnormalities in these two leukodystrophies (Figures 9.5 and 9.6). Central white matter is affected early (with a characteristic tigroid pattern in MLD) whereas U-fibres are spared until rather late in the disease course; atrophy is also a late sign. Whereas, in MLD, the corpus callosum shows early abnormalities regardless of type of onset, this is seen in GLD mainly in the infantile form. Cerebellar abnormalities, especially signal hyperintensity on T2w in the N. dentatus, are a rather early sign in GLD, whereas cerebellar white matter is affected late in MLD.

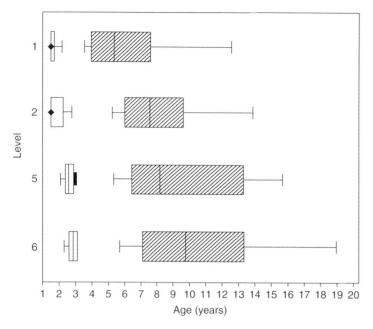

Figure 9.4 Natural course of MLD. Natural course of gross motor function in late late-infantile (left, white) and juvenile (right, hatched) MLD described with a gross motor function classification, the GMFC-MLD. Age at entry into a specific level of the motor score is illustrated and shows a very rapidly declining course in late infantile MLD, whereas juvenile MLD is more variable, but level 2 (loss of independent walking) and level 5 (only head control) are also very close, illustrating a rapid homogeneous decline in that specific disease period. The whiskers of the box plots indicate 10%-percentiles and 90%-percentiles. (Adapted from Kehrer [10], with permission from Wiley.)

Especially for MLD there are systematic data on the development of MRI abnormalities during the disease course, indicating that in late-infantile MLD changes develop rapidly with disease progression, whereas in the juvenile form patients already show clear white matter changes at disease onset [11].

MR spectroscopy (MRS) is abnormal early and shows an increase of choline-containing compounds and a decrease in N-acetylaspartate (NAA), indicating demyelination; lactate is often elevated (Figures 9.5 and 9.6).

Laboratory diagnosis

In general, the laboratory diagnosis depends on the demonstration of an enzyme deficiency in leukocytes. Prenatal diagnosis is possible for both disorders. It must be emphasized, however, that for both disorders, especially MLD, the biochemical diagnosis is complicated by the existence of pseudodeficiency alleles and the activator protein deficiencies. Thus, there are individuals, with or without neurologic symptoms, who have low ASA or GALC activities measured in the laboratory but (it is important to realize) do not have MLD or GLD. Therefore, a pseudodeficiency must always be excluded when low ASA or GALC activities are found in a patient with neurologic symptoms of unknown origin. The polymorphisms determining pseudodeficiencies can be identified by gene sequencing. The

diagnostic situation, however, is complicated by the fact that disease-causing mutations can occur on the background of the pseudodeficiency allele. Thus, the proof of pseudodeficiency depends on the complete sequencing of the ASA and GALC gene: sequencing should identify the polymorphisms and exclude disease-causing mutations [12, 13].

Moreover laboratory diagnosis has to take in to account that normal ASA or GALC activity does not exclude the diagnosis of MLD or GLD since the diseases may be due to saposin B or A deficiency, respectively. However, it should be noted that the activator deficiency forms of MLD and GLD diseases are very rare and other more common causes for white matter disease should also be considered. When the activator proteins are deficient, the enzymatic activities measured in the laboratory using activator protein-independent substrates will not be low. Thus, when the clinical picture strongly suggests MLD or GLD in the presence of normal enzyme activities, activator protein deficiencies must be excluded. In MLD the determination of sulfatide excretion in urine is of high diagnostic relevance when the diagnosis is questionable. Pseudodeficient individuals do not excrete sulfatide, whereas saposin B-deficient patients do. Thus, high amounts of sulfatide in urine when ASA activity is normal is almost a proof of saposin B deficiency. The definitive diagnosis, however, of saposin A or B deficiency depends on gene sequencing or direct demonstration of

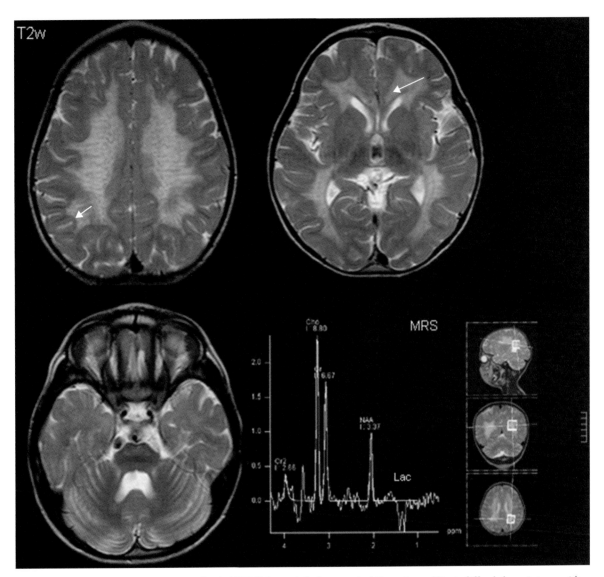

Figure 9.5 MRI of a MLD patient. Late-infantile MLD (37 months): the central white matter on T2w is diffusely hyperintense with typical patchy appearance (tigroid pattern), the U-fibres are in part affected (small arrow) and the corpus callosum is hyperintense (long arrow); the projection fibres also show signal abnormalities (anterior limb isointense, post limb hyperintense); the third ventricle is mildly enlarged, but otherwise no supratentorial atrophy; whereas the cerebellum is mildly atrophic and the central cerebellar white matter slightly hyperintense. MR-spectroscopy (MRS) in the posterior white matter shows an elevated choline peak and a massively reduced NAA, as well as pathological lactate (negative double peak).

saposin deficiency via Western Blots. Given the complications of laboratory diagnosis due to pseudodeficiencies and saposin deficiencies, a specialized laboratory should be consulted to ensure proper prenatal and postnatal diagnostic procedures.

Treatment

Hitherto, there is no truly satisfying treatment, other than symptomatic, for either disease. Haematopoietic stem cell transplantation (HSCT) has been tried in both diseases.

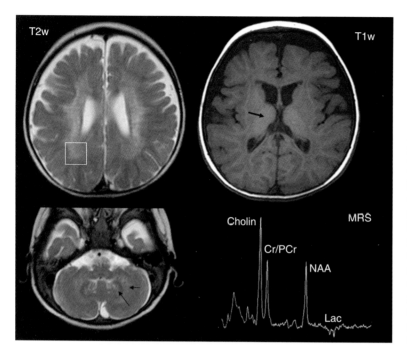

Figure 9.6 MRI of a GLD patient. Infantile Krabbe (13 months): the central white matter on T2w is diffusely hyperintense, U-fibres are spared and the corpus callosum is not affected; the central cerebellar white matter slightly hyperintense (small arrow) and also the N. dentatus is in part hyperintense (long arrow). On T1w, the thalamus is mildly hyperintense (thick arrow). MR-spectroscopy in the posterior white matter shows an elevated choline peak and a massively reduced NAA, as well as a small pathological lactate (negative double peak).

For MLD a definite conclusion has so far not been drawn. Clinical data, however, indicates that HSCT may be beneficial in the early stages of disease in late-onset patients, whereas it is not indicated in late-infantile patients in whom symptoms have already developed. Umbilical cord blood transplantation has been shown to retard the disease progression in infantile GLD patients when transplantation is done at a pre-clinical stage. For this reason newborn screening for GLD has been introduced in New York State. Three infants diagnosed by newborn screening received haematopoietic stem cell transplantation by 1 month of age; one died of transplant complications, and two have significant graft-versus-host disease and other developmental issues but are doing better than if they had received no treatment. Other newborns were found to have low GALC activity and mutations previously found in later-onset patients. These individuals are being monitored by neurodiagnostic testing to see if, in fact, they will develop a later-onset form of Krabbe disease and when to start therapy. These individuals present a serious dilemma for both the parents and physicians taking care of them. Apart from stem cell transplantation, a number of clinical studies are currently ongoing or planned for near future to evaluate other therapeutic approaches for GLD.

Intravenous enzyme replacement therapy for MLD was examined in a phase I/II clinical trial in a limited number of patients. The results have not yet been published but, overall, there was no apparent clinical improvement in the patients. This may not be surprising since the enzyme would have to pass the blood–brain barrier in order to be therapeutically active. Several other therapeutic approaches are being evaluated for MLD, including intrathecal replacement of recombinant ASA, HSCT-based gene therapy in pre-clinical late-infantile patients and AAV-mediated gene therapy based on the direct multiple injection of ASA expressing viral vectors into the brain of patients. Clearly better treatments, probably involving combined therapies, will be needed to arrive at a more satisfactory outcome for newly diagnosed individuals [14].

Natural history studies

Especially with regard to the developments in therapy, but also with respect to patients' counselling, standardized information on the natural history of the diseases is of high interest. As indicated above, there are studies available especially for the late-infantile and juvenile forms of MLD with respect to a standardized description of the deterioration of gross motor function and also of white matter changes and atrophy on MRI [9–11]. As several studies are ongoing on a national and international level, more systematic data is to be expected which will give more insight into the natural disease course of MLD and GLD. This information will be very useful for evaluating the success of treatments under investigation.

References

1 von Figura K, Gieselmann V, Jaeken J. Metachromatic leuko-dystrophy. In: Scriver CR, *et al.* (eds.), *The Metabolic and Molecular Bases of Inherited Disease* (8th edn.). New York: McGraw-Hill, 2001; pp. 3695–3724.

2 Wenger DA, Suzuki K, Suzuki Y, *et al.* Galactosylceramide lipidosis. Globoid cell leukodystrophy (Krabbe disease). In:, Scriver CR, *et al.* (eds.), *The Metabolic and Molecular Bases of Inherited Disease* (8th edn). New York: McGraw-Hill, 2001; pp. 3669–3694.

3 Heim P, Claussen M, Hoffmann B, *et al.* Leukodystrophy incidence in Germany. *AmJ Med Genet* 1997; **71**(4): 475–478.

4 Rafi MA, Luzi P, Zlotogora J, *et al.* Two different mutations are responsible for Krabbe disease in the Druze and Moslem Arab populations in Israel. *Hum Genet* 1996; **97**(3): 304–308.

5 Rauschka H, Colsch B, Baumann N, *et al.* Late-onset metachromatic leukodystrophy: genotype strongly influences phenotype. *Neurology* 2006; **67**(5): 859–863.

6 Ballabio A, Gieselmann V. Lysosomal disorders: from storage to cellular damage. *Biochim Biophys Acta* 2009; **1793**(4): 684–696.

7 Zaka M, Rafi MA, Rao HZ, *et al.* Insulin-like growth factor-1 provides protection against psychosine-induced apoptosis in cultured mouse oligodendrocyte progenitor cells using primarily the PI3K/Akt pathway. *Mol Cell Neurosci* 2005; **30**(3): 398–407.

8 Perusi C, Lira MG, Duyff RF, *et al.* Mutations associated with very late-onset metachromatic leukodystrophy. *Clin Genet* 1999; **55**(2): 130.

9 Kehrer C, Blumenstock G, Raabe C, *et al.* Development and reliability of a classification system for gross motor function in children with metachromatic leucodystrophy. *Dev Med Child Neurol* 2011; **53**: 156–160.

10 Kehrer C, Blumenstock G, Gieselmann V, *et al.* The natural course of gross motor deterioration in metachromatic leukodystrophy. *Dev Med Child Neurol* 2011 Sep; **53**(9): 850–855.

11 Groeschel S, Kehrer C, Engel C, *et al.* Metachromatic leuko-dystrophy: natural course of cerebral MRI changes in relation to clinical course. *J Inherit Metab Dis* 2011 Oct; **34**(5): 1095–1102.

12 Rafi MA, Coppola S, Liu SL, *et al.* Disease-causing mutations in cis with the common arylsulfatase A pseudodeficiency allele compound the difficulties in accurately identifying patients and carriers of metachromatic leukodystrophy. *Mol Genet Metab* 2003; **79**(2): 83–90.

13 Wenger DA, Rafi MA, Luzi P. Molecular genetics of Krabbe disease (globoid cell leukodystrophy): diagnostic and clinical implications. *Hum Mutat* 1997; **10**(4): 268–279.

14 Sevin C, Aubourg P, Cartier N. Enzyme, cell and gene-based therapies for metachromatic leukodystrophy. *J Inherit Metab Dis* 2007; **30**(2): 175–183.

CHAPTER 10

Types A and B Niemann–Pick Disease

Melissa P. Wasserstein, Robert J. Desnick, and Edward H. Schuchman

Department of Genetics and Genomic Sciences, Mount Sinai School of Medicine, New York, NY, USA

Representative case histories

Types A and B Niemann–Pick disease (NPD, OMIM 257200 & 607616) are two distinct forms of a lysosomal storage disorder due to the inherited deficiency of acid sphingomyelinase (ASM, EC 3.1.4.12) activity. They are representative of a wide spectrum of disease caused by mutations in the ASM gene (*SMPD1*, OMIM 607608). Type A NPD is the infantile, neurodegenerative form of the disorder, while patients with type B NPD generally have little or no neurological involvement and may survive into adolescence or adulthood. Intermediate cases have also been described.

Type A

A 3-month-old previously well boy was noted to have hepatosplenomegaly during a routine pediatric visit. Over the next several months, the infant acquired developmental milestones appropriately and learned how to roll over, vocalize, and sit with support. By 10 months of age his abdomen was markedly enlarged, and the extremities appeared thin. Over the next few months, the baby developed gastrointestinal reflux and had difficulty feeding. His liver and spleen weree massively enlarged, and he developed ascites and liver dysfunction. He never learned how to crawl, stand, or walk, and over time lost the abilities to sit, roll over, and vocalize. At 23 months of age, he acquired pneumonia and died from respiratory failure. He had absent ASM activity and was compound heterozygous for the p.R496L and p.fsP330 mutations in the *SMPD1* gene (see below).

Type B

A 15-year-old girl presented with short stature and delayed onset of puberty. She had a history of hepatosplenomegaly which was first noted at 4 years of age, and reported a shortness of breath with prolonged exercise. She reached her developmental milestones appropriately, and is an intellectually normal teenager. A chest radiograph reveals diffuse reticulonodular interstitial changes. Her pulmonary function shows a restrictive pattern of lung involvement with abnormal diffusing capacity. Blood analysis reveals a mixed dyslipidemia, thrombocytopenia, and elevated transaminases. She is found to have low ASM activity and is compound heterozygous for the p.deltaR608 and p.R600H mutations in the *SMPD1* gene.

Epidemiology

ASM deficiency is a rare genetic disorder, and limited information is available regarding its demographics and incidence. Several studies have estimated the birth rate of this disorder at ~0.5 to 1 per 100,000 [1, 2]. However, these estimates relied on data from biochemical testing laboratories where suspected cases were referred by clinicians for enzymatic confirmation, rather than on population screening. Thus, they are only approximations, and probably under-represent the true disease frequency. This is particularly true for the late-onset (type B) cases, where the clinical diagnosis may not be readily apparent.

The only population where DNA-based screening has taken place for ASM-deficient NPD is the Ashkenazi

Lysosomal Storage Disorders: A Practical Guide, First Edition. Edited by Atul Mehta and Bryan Winchester.
© 2012 John Wiley & Sons, Ltd. Published 2012 by John Wiley & Sons, Ltd.

Jewish community, where the carrier frequency of three common mutations causing the type A form of the disorder has been estimated to be between ~1:90 and 1:120 [3, 4]. This suggests an estimated birth rate of ~2–3 per 100,000 for this form of the disorder among Ashkenazi Jewish individuals.

Demographic data is currently available at the Mount Sinai School of Medicine for ~1,000 individuals referred for mutational analysis over a 20-year period (Schuchman *et al.,* unpublished information). About 300 of these patients were referred with an infantile, neurological phenotype ("type A" NPD), and of these, ~60% were Ashkenazi Jewish. The remaining patients derived from over 40 countries, and in contrast to the type A patients, very few of these individuals had Ashkenazi Jewish ancestry. The majority of these individuals were from North America and western Europe, although this may be reflective of enhanced awareness and diagnosis of lysosomal storage disorders in these regions, rather than a higher disease frequency. A significant number also were from North Africa and the Middle East, suggesting that ASM deficiency may be more common in these regions than was previously thought. In fact, over 40% of the NPD patients referred to Mount Sinai from Europe were of North African, Turkish or Arab ancestry. A significant number also were referred from South America, particularly Chile and Brazil. Asia had the fewest number of ASM-deficient NPD cases referred to our centre.

Genetics

The *SMPD1* gene is located on the short arm of chromosome 11 (11p15.4) [5]. The gene spans ~6 kb and consists of 6 exons encoding the 629 amino acids of the full-length ASM polypeptide [6]. Notably, *SMPD1* is the only gene encoding a lysosomal protein for which genomic imprinting has been demonstrated; i.e. it is preferentially expressed from the maternal chromosome (paternally imprinted) [7].

The clinical presentation of ASM-deficient NPD is largely dependent on the type of mutation(s) the patient inherits, and the resultant effect(s) of these mutations on the residual ASM polypeptide. However, because the *SMPD1* gene is imprinted, the phenotypic variability may also be due, at least in part, to the inheritance of specific mutations on the maternal vs. paternal alleles. In addition, abnormal clinical and laboratory findings have been reported in heterozygous individuals carrying only one *SMPD1* mutation [8]. This could similarly be due to the inheritance of a single, "severe" *SMPD1* mutation on the preferentially expressed maternal chromosome.

To date, over 100 mutations have been found within the *SMPD1* gene causing ASM-deficient NPD (http://www.hgmd.org/). These include point mutations, small deletions, and splicing abnormalities. No "hot-spots" exist for these mutations, although since ~40% of the ASM polypeptide is encoded by exon 2 of the *SMPD1* gene, a preponderance of mutations can be found within this region. Several polymorphisms also have been found within this gene, including a varying number of repeated nucleotides within the ASM signal peptide region [9, 10]. In addition, there are two in-frame ATG initiation codons within the *SMPD1* gene, and mutation analysis has revealed that both may be functional [11]. Because the *SMPD1* cDNA and gene may vary in length, the nomenclature for the same mutation may differ between reports based on the reference sequence that is used. For example, the p.deltaR608 mutation originally described by Levran *et al* [12] may also be referred to as p.deltaR610.

Identification of mutations in ASM-deficient NPD patients has permitted the first genotype/phenotype correlations for this disorder, and the first genetic screening efforts. Several mutations have been found within specific populations leading to severe, intermediate, or less severe phenotypes. For example, three mutations account for over 90% of Ashkenazi Jewish type A NPD infants [13–15], and homozygosity for these mutations (or the presence of one of these mutations in combination with another) is predictive of the severe NPD form. Another mutation, p.deltaR608, only occurs in non-neurological ASM-deficient NPD patients, and is found in ~15–20% of such individuals in western Europe and North America [12]. This mutation is considered "neuroprotective" since, even when found together with one of the severe type A mutations, the patients lack neurological involvement. The deltaR608 mutation is also prevalent in NPD patients from North Africa [16]. Yet another mutation, p.Q292K, is associated with an intermediate, neurological phenotype [17]. These and other findings have assisted physicians, genetic counselors and families in predicting the phenotypic outcome in individual ASM-deficient NPD patients, and in the future may lead to large-scale screening for this disorder in other populations.

Pathophysiology

The primary accumulating lipid in ASM-deficient NPD is sphingomyelin, a major structural component of all cell membranes. Thus, unlike several of the other sphingolipid storage disorders (e.g. Gaucher, Fabry, Tay–Sachs, etc.), the primary lipid affected in ASM-deficient NPD is an abundant component of all cells. Sphingomyelin accumulation in cells from ASM-deficient patients may first be detected within the lysosomal/endosomal compartments, but is also found in the plasma membrane and other cellular membranes. These membrane abnormalities, in turn, may result in many downstream cellular changes, including abnormalities in cell signalling pathways, receptor function, transport mechanisms, etc. Moreover, as in all lysosomal disorders, , many other lipid (and non-lipid) molecules may accumulate in ASM-deficient NPD cells, secondary to the primary metabolic abnormality, including cholesterol, ceramide, sphingosine and others, contributing to the cellular dysfunction. Indeed, the early detection of cholesterol accumulation in ASM-deficient cells led to the misclassification of types A and B NPD, and type C NPD, as allelic forms of the same disorder. It is now known that type C NPD is a distinct disorder due to mutations in one of two genes encoding proteins involved in cholesterol transport (see Chapter 11).

Many of the secondary lipids accumulating in ASM-deficient NPD cells have important biological effects on cell survival and proliferation, which likely contributes to the disease pathogenesis (for a review, see [18]). For example, ceramide and sphingosine are important cell-signalling lipids that are abnormally expressed following cellular stress or in response to many common disease pathologies (e.g. diabetes, fibrosis, sepsis, cancer, etc.). The activity of ASM is a major source of ceramide in cells, and although the primary "housekeeping" function of the enzyme appears to be within the lysosome, it is also subject to rapid and specific translocation to the cell surface when cells are stressed, and can be readily detected in the circulation. The pathogenic consequence of the deficiency of cell surface and secreted ASM in NPD patients remains unknown, as is the direct effect of the secondary lipid abnormalities on the disease pathology.

The primary organ systems affected in all ASM-deficient patients are the spleen, liver and lung. Lipid-filled foam cells can be readily detected in the parenchymal tissues of the spleen and liver, as well as in the pulmonary airways. The onset and severity of pulmonary disease in ASM-deficient NPD is highly variable, and is primarily due to the infiltration of inflammatory cells into the airways. In ASM-deficient mice (see below), the infiltration of inflammatory cells can be correlated with the elevated release of lung chemokines, including MIP1alpha [19]. Once present, these inflammatory cells can be very long-lived, and in the case of ASM deficiency also exhibit defective phagocytosis and other biological properties (Figure 10.1).

Foam cells (often referred to as "NPD" cells) are readily detected in the bone marrow of ASM-deficient patients, although the effect of this enzyme deficiency on bone and cartilage disease has not been studied in much detail. It is notable that many adult ASM-deficient NPD patients exhibit joint and bone pain, and there may be a higher incidence of fractures in these patients as well. In addition, there is a growing literature showing the importance of sphingolipid metabolism, and sphingomyelin/ceramide in particular, on normal cartilage and bone homeostasis.

Due to the cellular abnormalities in the liver and spleen, ASM-deficient NPD patients often present with abnormal haematological and plasma lipid findings. For example, low platelets are a common finding in the disease, as is the combination of very low HDL, high LDL and high triglycerides. The consequences of these lipid abnormalities on cardiac disease in ASM deficiency is not clearly understood, although there is evidence for early cardiac calcifications in some patients and early cardiovascular disease. Growth abnormalities also are frequently found in children with ASM deficiency, and may be due to abnormalities in the IGF-1 signalling pathway [20].

Finally, in patients with type A NPD, the brain is severely affected. Although little is known about brain pathology in ASM-deficient NPD patients, a series of recent studies in the ASM knockout mice (see below) revealed numerous abnormalities, including Purkinje cell death in the cerebellum, as well as abnormal synaptic vesicle release and uptake, calcium homeostasis, neuronal polarization, myelin production and immune responses (for a review, see [21]).

Clinical presentation

Type A Niemann–Pick disease

Most patients with type A NPD present with hepatosplenomegaly at a median age of 3 months. Early development and attainment of developmental milestones are typically normal. Absence of deep tendon reflexes and hypotonia are the most common, early abnormalities on neurologic examination. At approximately 9 months of age, development plateaus and then regresses. Retinal cherry-red spots are apparent by 12 months of age. Many patients develop significant gastroesophageal reflux, which makes feeding difficult. The liver and spleen continue to enlarge until they occupy most of the abdominal and pelvic cavity, and some patients develop significant ascites. Chest radiographs reveal diffuse interstitial disease. Laboratory abnormalities include elevated levels of SGOT, SGPT, total cholesterol and triglycerides, low HDL-C and platelets, and elevated chitotriosidase levels.

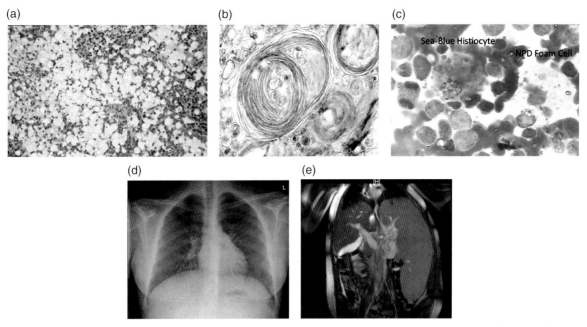

Figure 10.1 (a) Typical H & E staining of a liver section from an ASM-deficient NPD patient. Note the massive infiltration of lipid filled macrophages (foam cells). (b) Electron micrograph showing membrane-like inclusions in the brain of a type A NPD patient. (c) Bone marrow from a type B NPD patient showing an NPD foam cell and sea-blue histiocyte, both characteristic of ASM-deficient NPD. (d) Chest radiograph of a type B NPD patient showing the diffuse, reticulonodular interstitial changes. (e) High resolution CT showing hepatosplenomegaly in a type B NPD patient.

Type B Niemann–Pick disease

Type B NPD is clinically heterogenous, and the age of clinical onset, disease manifestations, and severity varies considerably. Hepatosplenomegaly is the most common initial presentation of type B NPD, often presenting in childhood. Pulmonary disease is apparent on chest radiograph and high resolution chest CT, and many patients have low FEV1, FVC and DLCO on pulmonary function testing consistent with restrictive lung disease. Although children with type B NPD typically have bone age delay, delayed onset of puberty and short stature, most patients eventually reach a normal adult height. Many patients have early satiety due to gastric compression by the enlarged spleen. Decreased bone mineral density and osteopenia occur in the majority of patients, and pathologic fractures are not uncommon (McGovern *et al.* in preparation). Bleeding episodes, especially recurrent epistaxis, are common in younger patients. Hepatic manifestations can include elevated transaminases, hepatic fibrosis, cirrhosis, and ascites. Most patients have an abnormally low concentration of HDL-cholesterol, high total and LDL-cholesterol, and high plasma triglycerides. They are also at risk to develop coronary artery disease [22]. Although ophthalmic examination in about 25% of all type B patients will reveal cherry-red spots, most do not have abnormal neurological symptoms.

Natural history

Infants with type A NPD typically develop failure to thrive by 15 months of age as their neurologic disease begins its rapid progression. They become weaker, less interactive, and most die before 3 years of age. The cause of death is often respiratory failure following pulmonary infection.

Patients with more severe phenotypes of type B NPD can develop significant life-threatening complications of their disease, including liver failure, oxygen dependency, pulmonary infections and splenic rupture. The most common causes of disease-related morbidity and mortality are respiratory and liver failure (Wasserstein *et al.* unpublished information). A detailed description of the natural history of type B NPD has been published [23].

Table 10.1 Typical clinical and laboratory findings of ASM-deficient NPD.

Feature	Type A	Type B
Age at onset/diagnosis	Early infancy	Childhood/adolescence
Neurodegenerative course	+	–
Cherry-red macula	+	+/–
Dyslipidemia	+	+
Hepatosplenomegaly	+	+
Marrow NPD cells	+	+
Pulmonary disease	+	+
Liver disease	+	+/–
Age at death	2 3 years	Childhood/adulthood
Autosomal recessive inheritance	+	+
Ashkenazic Jewish predilection	+	–
Acid sphingomyelinase activity	<5%	<10%

Laboratory diagnosis

Suspect cases of ASM deficiency can be readily confirmed by determining ASM activity in white blood cells, cultured EBV-transformed lymphoblasts and/or primary skin fibroblasts. In general, skin fibroblasts have the highest level of normal ASM activity, and are the most consistent and reliable source for enzymatic confirmation of ASM-deficient NPD. Numerous assay methods exist to detect ASM activity in cell extracts, and residual ASM activities in ASM-deficient NPD patients are usually below 10%. However, the residual activities may appear higher in white blood cells, and there is no reliable correlation of residual ASM activity and clinical presentation. Whenever possible, *SMPD1* mutation analysis should be used to confirm the enzymatic diagnosis, and may provide some additional utility in terms of phenotype prediction. However, mutation analysis alone should not be used for the diagnosis of ASM-deficient NPD since many of the DNA changes that may be found have not been expressed, and therefore could be polymorphisms and lead to normal or near normal levels of ASM activity. ASM activity and mutation analysis also can be performed on amniotic or chorionic villi cells for the prenatal diagnosis of ASM-deficient NPD (see Table 10.1).

Treatment

No specific treatment is available for ASM-deficient NPD, and patients are therefore managed symptomatically. Infants with type A disease initially benefit from feeding and physical therapies with the goal of maintaining muscle mass and minimizing aspiration risk. Typically they consume concentrated, high calorie formula food, and many require either nasogastric or gastrostomy tubes as the disease progresses. Children with type B disease are encouraged to consume frequent, nutritionally dense smaller meals throughout the day. Supplementation with calcium, maintenance of therapeutic vitamin D levels and weight-bearing exercises are required to reduce the risk of osteopenia. Some children with type B disease have successfully taken growth hormone with resultant increased growth velocity and no evident deleterious side effects. Patients are told to avoid contact sports and other activities that could potentially damage the enlarged spleen. Many adult patients are treated for dyslipidemia, but liver function must be closely monitored, as some type B patients have worsening of elevated transaminases while on statins and other antilipidemic medications.

Bone marrow, cord blood, and liver transplantation have been carried out in ASM-deficient NPD patients, but long-term follow-up has only been reported in a very small number of cases. In general, these procedures can potentially slow or even reverse some aspects of the non-neurological phenotype, but will have little or no effect on the central nervous system (CNS) disease. In addition, they are often associated with high morbidity or mortality, and should only be considered after careful consultation with physicians experienced with the disease and procedure.

Several potential therapies also have been evaluated in the mouse models of ASM-deficient NPD [24, 25], including stem cell transplantation, gene therapies, and enzyme replacement therapy (ERT). For example, ERT was evaluated in the complete "knockout" (ASMKO) mouse using a recombinant human ASM isolated from the media of overexpressing Chinese hamster ovary cells [26]. The reticuloendothelial organ pathology could be effectively prevented or reversed in these mice using enzyme doses as low as 0.3 mg/kg, but there was no effect on the CNS, even when doses as high as 10 mg/kg were administered. The liver and spleen were particularly responsive to ERT, followed by the lung, which exhibited a slower response due to the slow clearance of alveolar macrophages from the airways.

Based on these preclinical studies, an FDA-approved phase I clinical trial of ERT was undertaken in adult patients with non-neurological ASM-deficient NPD. Several safety biomarkers were identified, and the lowest safe initiating dose was determined. Based on these results, a phase II (repeat dosing) trial has been designed and will be initiated following the receipt of regulatory approval.

Acknowledgements and conflicts of interest

The authors wish to thank the many patients and physicians who have contributed to the type A and B NPD research programme at Mount Sinai. EHS also acknowledges the many colleagues who have worked in his laboratory over the past 25 years on ASM and NPD. This research has been funded by grants from the National Institutes of Health, the National Niemann–Pick Disease Foundation (NNPDF), and the Genzyme Corporation. EHS and RJD are also inventors on patents that have been licensed to Genzyme for the diagnosis and treatment of NPD.

References

1 Meikle PJ, Hopwood JJ, Clague AE, Carey WF. Prevalence of lysosomal storagedisorders. *JAMA* 1999; **281**(3): 249–254.

2 Poorthuis BJ, Wevers RA, Kleijer WJ, *et al.* The frequency of lysosomal storage diseases in The Netherlands. *Hum Genet* 1999; **105**(1–2): 151–156.

3 ACOG Committee on Genetics. ACOG Committee Opinion No. 442: Preconception and prenatal carrier screening for genetic diseases in individuals of Eastern European Jewish descent. *Obstet Gynecol* 2009; **114**(4): 950–953.

4 Schuchman EH, Miranda SR. Niemann–Pick disease: mutation update, genotype/phenotype correlations, and prospects for genetic testing. *Genet Test* 1997; **1**(1): 13–19. Review.

5 da Veiga Pereira L, Desnick RJ, Adler DA, *et al.* Regional assignment of the human acid sphingomyelinase gene (SMPD1) by PCR analysis of somatic cell hybrids and in situ hybridization to 11p15.1-p15.4. *Genomics* 1991; **9**(2): 229–234.

6 Schuchman EH, Levran O, Pereira LV, Desnick RJ. Structural organization and complete nucleotide sequence of the gene encoding human acid sphingomyelinase (SMPD1). *Genomics* 1992; **12**(2): 197–205.

7 Simonaro CM, Park JH, Eliyahu E, *et al.* Imprinting at the SMPD1 locus: implications for acid sphingomyelinase-deficient Niemann–Pick disease. *Am J Hum Genet* 2006; **78**(5): 865–870.

8 Lee CY, Krimbou L, Vincent J, *et al.* Compound heterozygosity at the sphingomyelin phosphodiesterase-1 (SMPD1) gene is associated with low HDL cholesterol. *Hum Genet* 2003 May; **112**(5–6): 552–562.

9 Schuchman EH, Levran O, Suchi M, Desnick RJ. An MspI polymorphism in the human acid sphingomyelinase gene (SMPD1). *Nucleic Acids Res* 1991; **19**(11): 3160.

10 Wan Q, Schuchman EH. A novel polymorphism in the human acid sphingomyelinase gene due to size variation of the signal peptide region. *Biochim Biophys Acta* 1995; **1270**(2–3): 207–210.

11 Pittis MG, Ricci V, Guerci VI, *et al.* Acid sphingomyelinse: identification of nine novel mutations among Italian Niemann–Pick type B patients and characterization of in vivo functional in-frame start codon. *Hum Mutat* 1994; **24**(2): 186–187.

12 Levran O, Desnick RJ, Schuchman EH. Niemann–Pick type B disease. Identification of a single codon deletion in the acid sphingomyelinase gene and genotype/phenotype correlations in type A and B patients. *J Clin Invest* 1991; **88**(3): 806–810.

13 Levran O, Desnick RJ, Schuchman EH. Identification and expression of a common missense mutation (L302P) in the acid sphingomyelinase gene of Ashkenazi Jewish type A Niemann–Pick disease patients. *Blood* 1992; **80**(8): 2081–2087.

14 Levran O, Desnick RJ, Schuchman EH. Type A Niemann–Pick disease: a frameshift occurs in the acid sphingomyelinase gene (fsP330) from Ashkenazi Jewish patients. *Hum Mutat* 1993; **2**(4): 317–319.

15 Levran O, Desnick RJ, Schuchman EH. Niemann–Pick disease: a frequent missense mutation in the acid sphingomyelinase gene of Ashkenazi Jewish type A and B patients. *Proc Natl Acad Sci USA* 1991; **88**(9): 3748–3752.

16 Vanier MT, Ferlinz K, Rousson R, *et al.* Deletion of arginine (608) in acid sphingomyelinase is the prevalent mutation among Niemann–Pick disease type B patients from northern Africa. *Hum Genet* 1993; **92**(4): 325–330.

17 Wasserstein MP, Aron A, Brodie SE, *et al.* Acid sphingomyelinase deficiency. Prevalence and characterization of an intermediate phenotype of Niemann–Pick disease. *J Pediatr* 2006; **149**(4): 554–559.

18 Gault CR, Obeid LM, Hannun YA. An overview of sphingolipid metabolism: from synthesis to breakdown. *Adv Exp Med Biol* 2010; **688**: 1–23. Review.

19 Dhami R, Passini MA, Schuchman EH. Identification of novel biomarkers for Niemann–Pick disease using gene expression analysis of acid sphingomyelinase knockout mice. *Mol Ther* 2006; **13**(3): 556–564.

20 Wasserstein MP, Larkin AE, Glass RB, *et al.* Growth restriction in children with type B Niemann–Pick disease. *J Pediatr* 2003; **142**(4): 424–428.

21 Ledesma MD, Prinetti A, Sonnino S, Schuchman EH. Brain pathology in Niemann–Pick disease type A: insights from the acid sphingomyelinase knockout mice. *J Neurochem* 2011; **116**(5): 779–788. Review

22 McGovern MM, Pohl-Worgall T, Deckelbaum RJ, *et al.* Lipid abnormalities in children with types A and B Niemann–Pick disease. *J Pediatr* 2004; **145**(1): 77–81.

23 McGovern MM, Wasserstein MP, Giugliani R, *et al.* A prospective, cross-sectional survey study of the natural history of Niemann–Pick disease type B. *Pediatrics* 2008; **122**(2): e341–349.

24 Horinouchi K, Erlich S, Perl DP, *et al.* Acid sphingomyelinase deficient mice: a model of types A and B Niemann–Pick disease. *Nat Genet* 1995; **10**(3): 288–293.

25 Jones I, He X, Katouzian F, *et al.* Characterization of common SMPD1 mutations causing types A and B Niemann–Pick disease and generation of mutation-specific mouse models. *Mol Genet Metab* 2008; **95**(3): 152–162.

26 Miranda SR, He X, Simonaro CM, *et al.* Infusion of recombinant human acid sphingomyelinase into Niemann–Pick disease mice leads to visceral, but not neurological, correction of the pathophysiology. *FASEB J* 2000; **14**(13): 1988–1995.

CHAPTER 11

Niemann–Pick Disease Type C

Marie T. Vanier[1] *and Marc C. Patterson*[2]

[1] Institut National de la Santé et de la Recherche Médicale, and Hospices Civils de Lyon, Lyon, France
[2] Department of Neurology, Pediatrics and Medical Genetics, Mayo Clinic, Rochester, MN, USA

Niemann–Pick disease type C [NPC] (Online Mendelian Inheritance in Man (OMIM)# 257220 – NPC1, OMIM# 607625 – NPC2) is a rare autosomal recessive metabolic disorder caused by the deficient function of either of two proteins, named NPC1 and NPC2, which act cooperatively to facilitate the egress of free cholesterol and other compounds from the endolysosomal system. The impaired activity of these proteins is associated with the accumulation of free cholesterol and a variety of sphingolipids in the lysosomes but their precise function(s) have not yet been fully elucidated [1–3].

Case histories

Case history 1

An 8-year-old girl presented with progressive school failure. She had experienced increasing difficulty attending in class and in learning and retaining new material over the past year. Her parents reported that she became clumsy from 4 or 5 years of age, and that she had become overtly ataxic in the last year, with frequent falls. She also experienced sudden falls associated with loss of muscle tone that were provoked by laughter. The examination is noteworthy for gait and appendicular ataxia, dystonic posturing of the feet and fingers with stressed gait, mild cerebellar dysarthria and dysphagia, and vertical supranuclear gaze palsy. The deep tendon reflexes are increased in the lower extremities, with flexor plantar responses. The spleen is palpable 10 cm below the left costal margin, and is firm and non-tender. The general examination is otherwise unremarkable.

The child was the product of an uncomplicated first pregnancy to unrelated parents of northern European ancestry; she experienced prolonged jaundice as a neonate, and had hepatosplenomegaly. The liver was not palpably enlarged after 3 months, but the splenomegaly persisted.

The diagnosis of Niemann–Pick disease type C was confirmed after a skin biopsy showed a characteristic pattern of staining with filipin, and the presence of polymorphous cytoplasmic bodies on electron microscopic examination. Molecular analysis demonstrated two mutations *in trans* in the *NPC1* gene.

Case history 2

Twin sisters from a consanguineous marriage showed pronounced cholestatic jaundice from birth. One of them died at 15 days of age and the diagnosis of NPC was rapidly confirmed by quantitating liver and spleen lipids post mortem. In the other twin, the diagnosis was confirmed on a skin biopsy, which showed a classic filipin staining pattern. Icterus resolved at 3 months of age. Hepatosplenomegaly was present from day 8. She sat up at 10 months of age, but could not stand at 12 months of age. Motor regression and a progressive intention tremor began at 15 months. At 28 months, she could no longer maintain a sitting position or hold her head up. She developed swallowing problems, then severe pyramidal tract involvement from the age of 33 months. The child died at 38 months. This patient was found to be homoallelic for a p.Q775P *NPC1* mutation.

Lysosomal Storage Disorders: A Practical Guide, First Edition. Edited by Atul Mehta and Bryan Winchester.
© 2012 John Wiley & Sons, Ltd. Published 2012 by John Wiley & Sons, Ltd.

Case history 3

This girl attended secondary school without problems but was reported to have "speech problems" (dysarthria) from the age of 12 and mild gait problems beginning at 14 years. At 17.5 years, the neurologic examination showed dysarthria, gait and limb cerebellar ataxia, minor pyramidal signs, and slow horizontal and downward saccades. Her spleen was not palpable, but abdominal ultrasound showed slight splenomegaly. She had started to have learning problems at school. Testing showed memory difficulties. A skin biopsy was made and the diagnosis of NPC was confirmed after studies showed a "variant" filipin pattern and a rate of LDL-induced cholesterol esterification at the lower end of the normal range. One of her *NPC1* alleles carries a new missense mutation, and the other a frameshift mutation.

Epidemiology

Niemann–Pick disease type C has a calculated incidence of 1:100,000–120,000 live births [3, 4]. It is likely more common than this number suggests, as adult onset cases are being recognized more often, and as awareness of the wide range of presentations of this disease grows among physicians. All ethnic groups are affected; genetic isolates with an increased carrier frequency and incidence have been described in the Acadian descendants of Jean Amirault in Nova Scotia, in a Hispanic group in New Mexico and Colorado and in a Bedouin group [1].

Genetic basis

Mutations in the *NPC1* gene, which is located at 18q11-q12, are present in about 95% of patients with NPC. More than 300 disease-causing mutations (and numerous polymorphisms) have now been identified (about one-third of which are missense mutations; the remainder comprise frameshift and nonsense mutations, single amino acid deletions and insertions, splice mutations and large deletions) [5]. Only the p.I1061T and p.P1007A mutations are globally frequent and account together for close to 20% of mutated alleles in several countries. An increasing number of recurrent mutant alleles are being described, but a majority of mutations are "private". Twenty different mutations in the *NPC2* gene (located at 14q24.3) have been described in about 40 families. *NPC1* and *NPC2* mutations correlate with the neurological form of the disease, not with the systemic manifestations.

Pathophysiology

The pathophysiology of NPC is incompletely understood. The microscopic and macroscopic consequences of NPC1 and NPC2 mutations are well documented: variable enlargement of the liver and spleen, with foam cell infiltrates and sea blue histiocytes there and in the bone marrow. In the brain, neurons are ballooned with stored lipids, and ectopic dendritogenesis, meganeurite formation and neuroaxonal dystrophy are characteristic. A major feature is progressive neuronal death, particularly of Purkinje cells. Neurofibrillary tangles are seen in the cortex [1]. Biochemical analysis shows marked storage of unesterified cholesterol, sphingomyelin, bis(monoacylglycero)phosphate, free sphingoid bases (sphingosine and sphinganine) and several glycosphingolipids in peripheral tissues (especially spleen), with mostly increased glycosphingolipids in the brain [1, 3].

The sequence of events that leads to these tissue changes is not known, but current theories centre around cholesterol, free sphingoid bases and glycosphingolipid accumulation as the initiating events. The "classical" model stresses the central role of NPC1 and NPC2 proteins in the trafficking of cholesterol in the late endosomal/lysosomal system [6], and infers that cholesterol accumulation further impairs trafficking and leads to the accumulation of other lipid species as a secondary event. Based on *in vitro* studies indicating that free sphingosine is the first species to accumulate in NPC1 fibroblasts, a challenging model has been proposed, where sphingosine accumulation leads to abnormal intracellular distribution of calcium that in turn triggers accumulation of cholesterol and sphingolipids [7]. That NPC2 and NPC1 are able to bind and transfer free cholesterol in a sequential fashion seems fairly well established [6]; secondary effects of the lysosomal storage of cholesterol on trafficking of sphingolipids have also been described. Similarly, the potential deleterious effects of abnormally high levels of free sphingoid bases or lysosphingolipids have been documented. Considering the severity of NPC in the nervous system, an apparently intriguing point is the limited accumulation of cholesterol seen in neurons, although this can probably be explained by the specifics of cholesterol metabolism in the brain [8]. Of note is the fact that the increase in free sphingosine is also small in the brain, where the most conspicuous accumulation is that of ganglioside GM2. Interestingly, early and repeated intrathecal administration of cyclodextrin to the cat model normalized the levels of all three lipids. Thus, whatever the mechanism, increases of cholesterol,

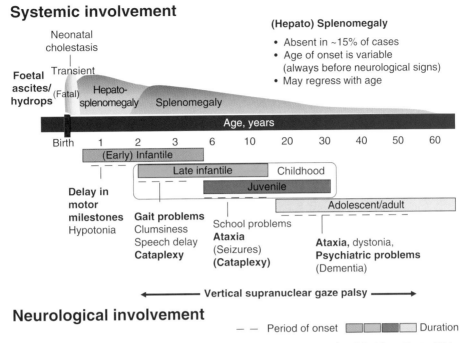

Figure 11.1 Schematic representation of the clinical aspects of Niemann–Pick C disease. (Modified from Vanier [3].)

sphingosine and ganglioside appear to be closely linked. More work is needed to better understand the brain dysfunction in NPC, particularly to identify the trigger (or triggers) for patterned neuronal loss.

Clinical presentation

In the perinatal period and early infancy, NPC presents with visceral manifestations; beyond that, NPC is a progressive neurodegenerative disease (Figure 11.1). The earliest (rare) presentation of NPC is with foetal hydrops and/or foetal ascites; these babies commonly have hepatic failure, plus or minus respiratory failure, and as many as 50% die in early infancy. In the neonatal period, prolonged cholestatic jaundice of varying severity with hepatosplenomegaly occurs in up to 40–50% of children with NPC, but in most cases resolves without sequelae. Isolated hepatosplenomegaly or splenomegaly can also be detected in the first months of life. Some infants have hypotonia and motor delay that becomes evident in the latter part of infancy; they usually have hepatosplenomegaly. Vertical supranuclear gaze palsy (VSGP) has generally not been reported, but may be easily overlooked, as it is often detected on careful examination. Other children are found to have incidental splenomegaly in

childhood; the onset of neurologic symptoms in such cases may be delayed by many years. In the authors' experience, the first sign of neurologic involvement is increased latency and slowing of vertical saccades. These findings slowly evolve to complete vertical supranuclear gaze paralysis; horizontal supranuclear gaze palsy also occurs, but its onset is later. NPC patients who survive long enough will have complete vertical and horizontal saccadic paralysis.

NPC presents insidiously in childhood and later. Children commonly experience difficulty concentrating and learning new material, and may have dyspraxia. There is often a history of preceding clumsiness, that eventually declares itself as frank ataxia of gait. The ataxia reflects the loss of cerebellar Purkinje cells, which also causes progressive dysarthria and dysphagia. About one-third of patients have gelastic cataplexy, and as many as one-half of children with NPC have epileptic seizures, which may be medically intractable. Dystonia is common, often beginning as action dystonia in one limb, spreading to involve the limbs and axial muscles in some patients. Increased deep tendon reflexes are frequent, particularly in the lower limbs. The disease is relentlessly progressive, and patients who do not succumb to uncontrolled seizures or intercurrent infection will eventually lose the

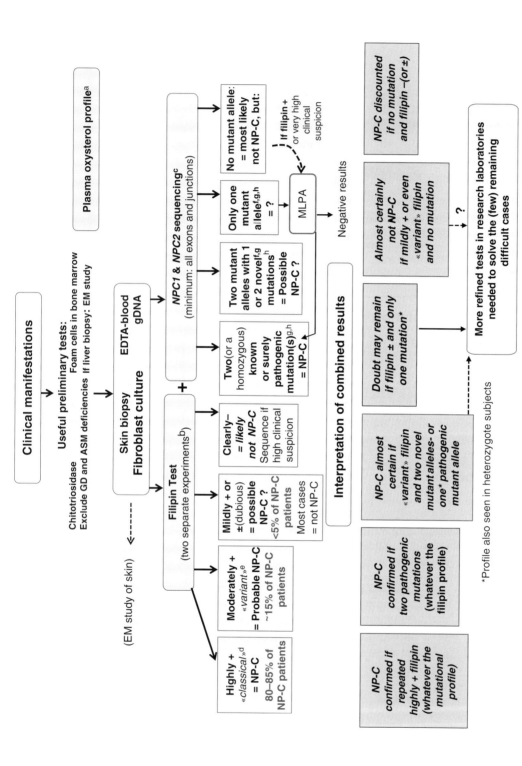

Figure 11.2 Algorithm for the laboratory diagnosis of Niemann–Pick C disease.

Abbreviations: GD: Gaucher disease; ASM: acid sphingomyelinase; EM: electron microscopy; MLPA: Multiplex Ligation-dependent Probe Amplification. This technique evaluates copy number changes, and has allowed detection of large deletions, so far only in the *NPC1* gene. It has also been useful to detect a false homozygous status with a deletion on the other allele. [a] New test under clinical development, see text. [b] Two sequential filipin tests (not duplicates). [c] Wherever possible. Conclude quickly on *NPC2* in children <10 months. [d] I-cell disease (ML II and III) gives a false positive result (but very different clinical features). [e] ASM deficiency and some heterozygotes can give a similar filipin pattern. [f] Not certainly pathogenic [g] cDNA is usually needed to study the effect of splice mutations [h] Check alle e segregation by parental study ability to walk, speak, feed and care for themselves before death from respiratory failure.

Adolescents and adults are more likely to present with fragmentary phenotypes, particularly with psychiatric syndromes, including major depression, bipolar disorder and schizophreniform disorder, or with atypical early-onset dementia. Recent experience suggests that adult forms without psychiatric symptoms are more frequent than previously reported. Some authors have suggested that VSGP may be absent in later-onset patients, but that has not been the experience of the authors. Siblings with NPC most often have similar neurological courses, particularly in severe, early-onset disease, but patients with a perinatal fatal form can have siblings with a neurological form. The authors have also experienced several kindreds in which affected siblings, usually with juvenile or adult onset, have discordant clinical courses, perhaps reflecting the influence of so far unidentified modifier genes.

Natural history

In the few babies presenting with foetal ascites or neonatal hepatic failure, with or without pulmonary infiltrates, mortality from systemic disease in early infancy is high. Otherwise, the life expectancy tends to be reduced in proportion to the age of onset of neurological symptoms. Children presenting in infancy usually die before the age of 6–7 years, those with a neurological onset around 3–5 years of age rarely survive the age of 12–15, while children presenting later commonly survive into the third or fourth decades. Patients with adolescent or adult neurological onset may survive into the seventh decade. Patients with medically intractable seizures have a worse prognosis for function and survival, and once the abilities to walk, swallow and speak have been lost, the prognosis for survival is much worse.

The commonest cause of death is respiratory failure, related to a combination of brainstem failure and pulmonary infection, as discussed above.

Laboratory diagnosis

Foam cells and sea-blue histiocytes are often present in bone marrow, but these findings are not specific for NPC. In particular, similar cells are found in sphingomyelinase deficiencies (Niemann–Pick A and B).

Currently, the diagnosis of NPC is confirmed by demonstrating impaired trafficking of endocytosed cholesterol in living cells, completed whenever possible by molecular study of the *NPC1* and *NPC2* genes

(Figure 11.2). A skin biopsy is used to obtain a fibroblast culture. The cells are conditioned in a cholesterol-free medium to upregulate LDL-receptors, and exposed to a pulse of LDL-enriched medium. In NPC cells, cholesterol formed from LDL hydrolysis cannot exit lysosomes, and is therefore unable to evoke the expected cellular homeostatic responses; those are all impaired, cholesterol re-esterification (catalyzed by ACAT in the endoplasmic reticulum) being the most affected one [1]. The lysosomal accumulation of cholesterol can be visualized by fluorescence microscopy using filipin, a fluorescent polyene macrolide antibiotic derived from *Streptomyces filipensis*, which binds strongly to unesterified cholesterol. Staining fixed cells with filipin has proved to be the most sensitive assay for NPC [1, 3, 4, 9] The measurement of the early rate of LDL-induced cholesterol esterification in fibroblasts, long used as a secondary test, is so variable in clinical practice that it should now be replaced by mutation analysis. NPC cells stained by filipin classically show intense fluorescent vesicles in a perinuclear distribution, However in 10–15% of cases, a less intense staining pattern is observed, which may overlap with that seen in some heterozygotes (Figure 11.3). In this so-called "variant" biochemical form [9], determined by specific mutations [2], final diagnosis may be difficult and require mutation analysis (esterification may be normal in these cells). Molecular analysis of the *NPC1* and *NPC2* genes would seem preferable to an invasive skin biopsy as a primary test. However, in about 10–15% of the cases, the test may also be inconclusive, owing to the significant percentage of unidentified mutations found in laboratories that perform such analyses and difficulties in determining if new missense or splice mutations are really disease-causing. The filipin test and molecular studies are therefore complementary for optimal diagnosis of an index case. Provided two mutations *in trans* have been identified, molecular analysis is the preferred means of diagnosis in siblings and above all for prenatal diagnosis (where it may be the only possible approach; it is always safer and faster).

Where appropriate expertise is available, a portion of the skin biopsy (or of the liver biopsy in specific cases) should be appropriately fixed for electron microscopic examination. The demonstration of characteristic polymorphous cytoplasmic bodies is essentially diagnostic. Expert biochemical lipid studies in a liver biopsy have also proved useful in the past, but such expertise is rarely available today.

Recent investigations have found that two oxysterols (7-OH cholesterol and a triol) are significantly elevated in

Normal   NPC *classic*   NPC *variant*

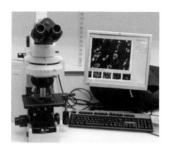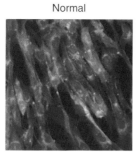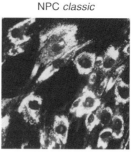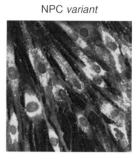

Figure 11.3 Filipin staining of cultured skin fibroblasts in normal and Niemann–Pick C disease cell lines. (Modified from Vanier and Millat [2] with permission from Wiley-Blackwell.)

plasma of children and adults with NPC [10]. It seems likely that this investigation will shortly become available clinically, and will constitute a new screening test for NPC.

Treatment

Miglustat is an iminosugar that acts as a competitive inhibitor of glucosylceramide synthase, the administration of which delays the onset of symptoms and signs and prolongs survival in murine and feline models of NPC [11]. The drug has been approved for the management of neurologic manifestations of NPC in several countries, including the European Union, Brazil, Canada and Australia. Published data suggests that it may stabilize established disease for a period of time, and that it is most beneficial in patients with later-onset, more slowly progressive disease [12–15]. The most common adverse effects of miglustat are gastrointestinal; guidelines for their management are available [16].

Treatment guidelines

Diagnostic and management guidelines based on expert opinion and the limited treatment literature for NPC have been published [4,17,18]. All patients are likely to benefit from multimodality treatment aimed at managing the symptoms and signs of NPC, including epilepsy, dystonia, gelastic cataplexy, dysphagia and dysarthria. Intercurrent infections must be diagnosed and treated early and aggressively, and children and adults should receive appropriate physical, occupational and speech therapy.

References

1 Patterson MC, Vanier MT, Suzuki K, *et al*. Niemann–Pick disease type C: a lipid trafficking disorder. In: Scriver CR, *et al*. (eds.), *The Metabolic and Molecular Bases of Inherited Disease*. New York: McGraw-Hill, 2001; pp. 3611–3634.

2 Vanier MT, Millat G. Niemann–Pick disease type C. *Clin Genet* 2003; **64**: 269–281.

3 Vanier MT. Niemann–Pick disease type C. *Orphanet J Rare Dis* 2010; **5**: 16.

4 Wraith JE, Baumgartner MR, Bembi B, *et al*. Recommendations on the diagnosis and management of Niemann–Pick disease type C. *Mol Genet Metab* 2009; **98**: 152–65.

5 Runz H, Dolle D, Schlitter AM, Zschocke J. NPC-db, a Niemann–Pick type C disease gene variation database. *Hum Mutat* 2008; **29**: 345–350. http://www.npc.fzk.de

6 Kwon HJ, Abi-Mosleh L, Wang ML, *et al*. Structure of N-terminal domain of NPC1 reveals distinct subdomains for binding and transfer of cholesterol. *Cell* 2009; **137**: 1213–1224.

7 Lloyd-Evans E, Morgan AJ, He X, *et al*. Niemann–Pick disease type C1 is a sphingosine storage disease that causes deregulation of lysosomal calcium. *Nat Med* 2008; **14**: 1247–1255.

8 Aqul A, Liu B, Ramirez CM, *et al*. Unesterified cholesterol accumulation in late endosomes/lysosomes causes neurodegeneration and is prevented by driving cholesterol export from this compartment. *J Neurosci* 2011; **31**: 9404–9413.

9 Vanier MT, Rodriguez-Lafrasse C, Rousson R, *et al*. Type C Niemann–Pick disease: spectrum of phenotypic variation in disruption of intracellular LDL-derived cholesterol processing. *Biochim Biophys Acta* 1991; **1096**: 328–337.

10 Porter FD, Scherrer DE, Lanier MH, *et al*. Cholesterol oxidation products are sensitive and specific blood-based biomarkers for Niemann–Pick C1 disease. *Sci Transl Med* 2010; **2**: 56ra81.

11 Zervas M, Somers KL, Thrall MA, Walkley SU. Critical role for glycosphingolipids in Niemann–Pick disease type C. *Curr Biol* 2001; **11**: 1283–1287.

12 Patterson MC, Vecchio D, Prady H, *et al*. Miglustat for tre:tment of Niemann–Pick C disease: a randomised controlled study. *Lancet Neurol* 2007; **6**: 765–772.

13 Pineda M, Wraith JE, Mengel E, *et al*. Miglustat in patients with Niemann–Pick disease Type C (NP-C): a multicenter observational retrospective cohort study. *Mol Genet Metab* 2009; **98**: 243–249.

14 Patterson MC, Vecchio D, Jacklin E, *et al.* Long-term miglustat therapy in children with Niemann–Pick disease type C. *J Child Neurol* 2010; **25**: 300–305.

15 Wraith JE, Vecchio D, Jacklin E, *et al.* Miglustat in adult and juvenile patients with Niemann–Pick disease type C: Long-term data from a clinical trial. *Mol Genet Metab* 2010; **99**: 351–357.

16 Belmatoug N, Burlina A, Giraldo P, *et al.* Gastrointestinal disturbances and their management in miglustat-treated patients. *J Inher Metab Dis* 2011; **34**: 991–1001.

17 Patterson MC, Hendriksz CJ, Walterfang M *et al.* Recommendations for the diagnosis and management of Niemann-Pick disease type C: An update. *Mol Genet Metab* 2012; **106**: 330–344.

18 Wijburg FA, Sedel F, Pineda M *et al.* Development of a suspicion index to aid diagnosis of Niemann-Pick disease type C. *Neurology* 2012; **78**: 1560–1567. www.npc-si.com

CHAPTER 12

The Mucopolysaccharidoses

Roberto Giugliani

Department of Genetics, Federal University of Rio Grande do Sul, and Medical Genetics Service, Hospital de Clinicas, Porto Alegre, Brazil

The mucopolysaccharidoses (MPSs) are a group of 11 disorders, each one characterized by an enzyme deficiency – caused by a gene defect – which affects one of the steps of the degradation pathway of glycosaminoglycans (GAGs) (Table 12.1), leading to progressive storage of these compounds in tissues and organs. This storage, along with other pathogenic mechanisms, leads to several clinical consequences, with wide phenotypic variability.

Case history

A 6-year-old boy was taken to the doctor to review the skeletal X-rays, requested on the previous consultation. The mother reported that pregnancy and birth were uneventful. The boy was born with Mongolian spots and early development was normal. Surgery for umbilical hernia and shortly thereafter for inguinal hernia was performed during the second year of life, and bilateral tympanostomy was made during the third year of life due to recurrent otitis. Upper respiratory infections and nasal secretion became frequent and tonsillectomy and adenoidectomy were performed, resulting in transient improvement. When the patient was 4 years old the mother noticed that the joints were becoming "swollen". In a consultation at that age the paediatrician observed an abnormal curvature of the spine and a slightly increased liver size, and recommended that the patient should come every 6 months for follow-up. When the family's neighbours noticed that the child's face was becoming "coarse", the mother took the boy again to the doctor, who asked for an eye and ear examination. These evaluations disclosed slight corneal clouding and some degree of hearing loss. The doctor also noticed some degree of regression on motor and intellectual skills, and requested skeletal x-rays as the joints were becoming stiff and the growth rate seemed to be decreasing. After a biochemical investigation, the diagnosis of MPS II (Hunter syndrome) was established.

Epidemiology

Data about the epidemiology of MPSs is available only for few countries and regions. Although MPSs, as a group, are estimated to occur in one in every 22,000 individuals, individual prevalence of each MPS is much lower. The relative frequency of different MPS types also differs from region to region, but MPS II seems to be the most common in most places, followed by MPS III (A and B), MPS I and MPS IV A. MPS VI is rare in Europe and North America, but relatively frequent in some countries as Brazil and Turkey. MPS VII, MPS IV B and MPS III (C and D) are much rarer, and MPS IX has been described in only two families so far. Although it is believed that the majority of the severe cases of MPS are identified, usually after a long diagnostic "odyssey", it is probable that the diagnosis of MPS in some attenuated patients is missed. It is noteworthy that many children with MPS are submitted to surgery before a diagnosis is confirmed.

Genetic basis

With the exception of MPS II, which is X-linked, all of these diseases are inherited as autosomal recessive traits (Table 12.1). These diseases are genetically very

Lysosomal Storage Disorders: A Practical Guide, First Edition. Edited by Atul Mehta and Bryan Winchester.
© 2012 John Wiley & Sons, Ltd. Published 2012 by John Wiley & Sons, Ltd.

Table 12.1 The classification of the mucopolysaccharidoses.

MPS	Name	Increased GAGs	Inheritance	Enzyme deficiency	Gene location
I	Hurler (IH), Hurler-Scheie (IHS) or Scheie (IS)	HS + DS	Autosomal Recessive	α-Iduronidase	4p16.3
II	Hunter	HS + DS	X-linked recessive	Iduronate sulfatase	Xq28
III A	Sanfilippo A	HS	Autosomal recessive	Heparan-N-sulfatase	17q25.3
III B	Sanfilippo B	HS	Autosomal recessive	α-N-acetylglucosaminidase	17q21.2
III C	Sanfilippo C	HS	Autosomal recessive	AcetylCoA α- glucosamine acetyltransferase	8p11.21
III D	Sanfilippo D	HS	Autosomal recessive	N-acetylglucosamine 6-sulfatase	12q14.3
IV A	Morquio A	KS	Autosomal recessive	Galactosamine-6-sulfate sulfatase	16q24.3
IV B	Morquio B	KS	Autosomal recessive	β-Galactosidase	3p22.3
VI	Maroteaux-Lamy	DS	Autosomal recessive	N-acetylgalactosamine 4-sulfatase	5q14.1
VII	Sly	HS + DS	Autosomal recessive	β-Glucuronidase	7q11.21
IX	Natowicz	Hyaluronan	Autosomal recessive	Hyaluronidase 1	3p21.31

Notes:

(1) Scheie syndrome was initially classified as MPS V, but when the enzyme defect was identified it was recognized as the attenuated end of the MPS I spectrum; to avoid confusion, MPS V was no loger used.

(2) An enzyme defect was found and proposed as MPS VIII, but shortly thereafter this was recognized as a laboratory mistake, and the new type of MPS was withdrawn; also, to avoid confusion, MPS VIII was no longer used.

heterogeneous, with many mutations described for each MPS type. In general, there is a trend that nonsense and frameshift mutations lead to more severe disease, while missense mutations are associated with more attenuated pictures, but it is usually difficult to predict phenotype from the genotype on an individual basis. All the MPS types, including MPS II, are true recessive diseases, with no detectable manifestations in carriers. A few females with MPS II were reported, these being extremely rare occurrences not related to carrier status but to major rearrangements and/or skewed inactivation.

Pathophysiology

Although MPS storage plays an important role in the pathophysiology of MPSs, it is now known that it is not the only pathogenic mechanism involved in these diseases. While some clinical signs, such as hepatosplenomegaly, are caused directly by the storage of partially degraded GAGs within the lysosomes, these molecules are also located outside of the acidic organelle. Therefore they can activate inflammatory pathways and an innate immune response via the toll-like receptor 4 and the complement system, which might contribute to some

aspects of these diseases, including neuroinflammation, short bones and aortic fragmentation. The undegraded GAGs can also upregulate the expression of destructive proteases and induce apoptosis in tissues such as the joints and the bones.

Clinical presentation

The MPSs are a group of heterogeneous and multisystem disorders, with broad heterogeneity across types. Most cases have disease manifestations which bring major impairment to lifespan and quality of life. Within the same type there are severe and attenuated patients with intermediate cases confirming a continuum of disease severity between the two extremes. From the clinical point of view, MPS cases can be classified into three main groups: patients with predominant "visceral phenotype", those with predominant "neurodegenerative phenotype" and those with predominant "skeletal phenotype". The group with predominant "visceral phenotype" includes patients with MPS I, MPS II, MPS VI and MPS VII, who present with the main manifestations of coarse facies, visceromegaly (hepatosplenomegaly), hernia, joint stiffness, upper airway obstruction and heart disease

(a)

(b)

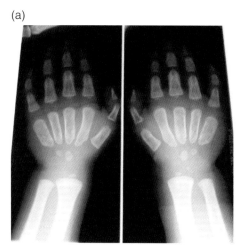
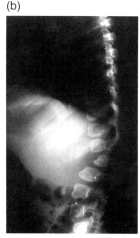

Figure 12.1 Dysostosis multiplex observed in X-rays of (a) hands and (b) spine of a MPS I patient. The broad and short metacarpals are typical, as are the shape of the vertebral bodies.

(Figure 12.1). Bone dysplasia, known as "dysostosis multiplex", and other skeletal deformities are present (Figure 12.2). Although growth may be normal and even increased in the first years, short stature is eventually established, and mental deterioration starting in childhood occurs in the severe cases of MPS I and MPS II and also in MPS VII. Corneal clouding is frequent (except in MPS II), and also hearing loss (marked in MPS II). The group with the "neurodegenerative phenotype" is formed by patients with MPS III. In these patients, the visceromegaly, coarse facies, joint disease and bone dysplasia (dysostosis multiplex) are relatively mild, and the clinical picture is marked by neurodegeneration, which usually starts between 3 and 5 years of age and progresses steadily. Behavioural disturbances and hyperactivity are often reported in the early stages of the disease (Figure 12.3). The group with the "skeletal phenotype" is formed by patients with MPS IV, who show a skeletal dysplasia (different from dysostosis multiplex) with genu valgum, pectus carinatum, kyphoscoliosis, hypoplasia of odontoid with atlanto-axial instability, among other bone problems. Patients are mentally normal and have very short stature, presenting corneal opacity and valve disease. They do not have visceromegaly or coarse facies, and usually show joint laxity instead of joint stiffness (Figure 12.4). MPS IX was not included in any of these 3 phenotypes since in the cases reported the main clinical finding is the presence of joint swellings and synovial masses.

Natural history

The MPSs are progressive diseases which lead to a shortened life span in most cases. Affected patients are usually normal at birth. Rare cases, especially of MPS VII, may

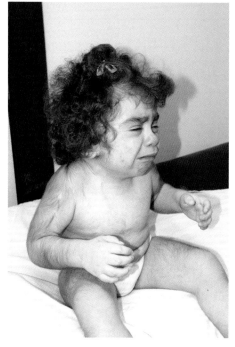

Figure 12.2 Patient with MPS I, presenting the "visceral phenotype". Noteworthy are the coarse facies, protruded abdomen due to hepatosplenomegaly, umbilical hernia, swollen and stiff joints. Patient also presented with heart murmur, corneal clouding and short stature.

present with foetal hydrops. The clinical picture usually becomes apparent between 2 and 4 years of age in the severe cases. The majority of these severe cases die before the end of the second decade of life, usually from cardiopulmonary complications. Attenuated cases usually live to adulthood,

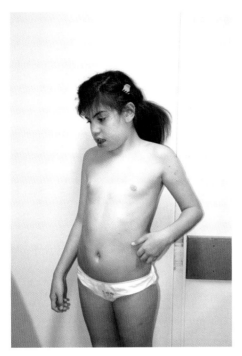

Figure 12.3 Patient with MPS III B presenting the "neurodegenerative phenotype". The physical changes are hardly noticeable and, the behavioural changes, hyperactivity and neurological regression are more important.

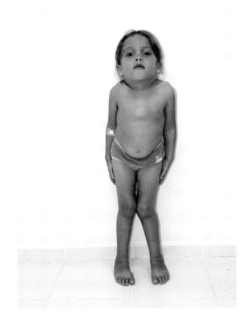

Figure 12.4 Patient with MPS IV A presenting the "skeletal phenotype". Coarse facies and stiff joints are not present, and skeletal changes marked by genu valgum, pectus carinatum and kyphoscoliosis are prominent.

but with important disabilities due mainly to the skeletal, visual, respiratory and cardiac manifestations of the disease. Only patients at the milder end of the spectrum have a normal life span, despite presenting disease manifestations in several organs.

Laboratory diagnosis

A suggested algorithm for the laboratory diagnosis of the MPS types is displayed in Figure 12.5 When a MPS is suspected (due to clinical findings or family history) a urine and blood sample should be obtained to perform a diagnostic work-up. The suspicion could be initially checked by a screening test for GAGs in a urine sample, as in all MPS types (except in MPS IX), there is abnormal urinary GAG excretion. If the test is positive, the same sample could be used for a quantitative assay of urinary GAGs and a qualitative evaluation of the GAG species (usually by electrophoresis or thin-layer chromatography). Cases with a negative screening but with a high clinical suspicion of MPS should be considered carefully and checked again, especially if the types suspected are MPS III or MPS IV (which occasionally present with urinary GAGs

within normal levels). The qualitative pattern of urinary GAGs, taken along with the clinical presentation, provides a helpful insight to the MPS diagnosis. Patients with predominant excretion of heparan sulfate most probably have MPS III; patients with predominant excretion of dermatan sulfate most probably have MPS VI; patients with predominant excretion of keratan sulfate most probably have MPS IV; and patients with predominant excretion of both dermatan and heparan sulfate most probably have MPS I, MPS II or MPS VII. According to this pattern (Figure 12.6), the blood sample is retrieved and could now be used to perform specific enzyme assays to confirm the diagnosis and assign the specific MPS type. The blood sample could be also used for the identification of the genetic defect, which is seldom needed for diagnosis as it can be established by the enzyme assay. However, genotyping is important for carrier detection, especially in MPS II, the X-linked type of MPS, genetic counselling and could help with the prenatal diagnosis, which could also be performed by enzyme assay. The genotype could also help to predict the phenotype, which is especially important for treatment decisions in young MPS I patients. Despite its usefulness in diagnosis and evaluation of immediate response to ERT (its level is usually very high in untreated patients, with a sharp decrease

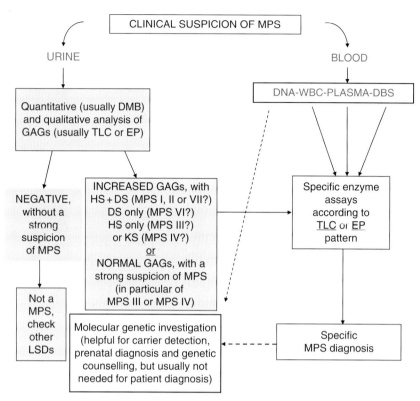

Figure 12.5 Proposed flowchart for the laboratory diagnosis of MPS from samples of urine and blood (dashed line indicates that test is optional for diagnosis). All enzymes could be assayed in blood, some in plasma and WBC and some only in WBC. This flowchart does not detect MPS IX as the increased urinary GAG excretion is not seen in this extremely rare type of MPS. (Abbreviations: MPS – mucopolysaccharidosis; GAGs – glycosaminoglycans; LSDs – lysosomal storage diseases; DMB – dimethylene blue; TLC – thin-layer chromatography; EP – electrophoresis; WBC – white blood cells; DBS – dried blood spots.)

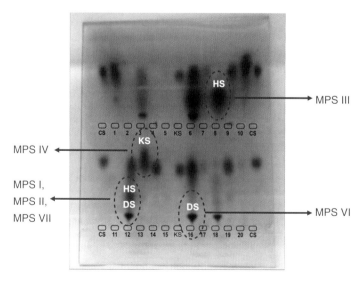

Figure 12.6 Electrophoretic separation of urinary GAGs in agarose with toluidine blue staining. Four different pathological patterns are observed, which is helpful to select the diagnostic enzyme assays to be performed in blood. (Abbreviations: DS – dermatan sulfate; HS – heparan sulfate; KS – keratan sulfate.)

Table 12.2 Present status of the specific therapies for the mucopolysaccharidoses (situation in October 2011).

MPS type	BMT/HSCT	Intravenous ERT	Intrathechal ERT	Other
I	Indicated for children with the severe form (MPS IH)? below 2½ years	Approved	In clinical development (cognitive deficit); Case report (spinal cord compression)	Gene therapy in pre-clinical development
II	Case reports, no conclusive evidence	Approved	In clinical development (cognitive deficit)	Substrate inhibition with genistein in clinical trials; gene therapy in pre-clinical development.
III A	Not usually recommended	–	In clinical development (cognitive déficit)	Substrate reduction therapy with genistein in clinical trials; substrate reduction therapy with miglustat in clinical trials; anti-inflammatory therapy in pre-clinical studies; Gene therapy in clinical development;
III B	Not usually recommended	–	In pipeline	Substrate reduction therapy with genistein in clinical trials; substrate reduction therapy with miglustat in clinical trials; gene therapy moving to clinical development;
III C	Not usually recommended	–	–	Substrate reduction therapy with miglustat in clinical trials; chaperone therapy with glucosamine proposed
III D	Not usually recommended	–	–	Substrate reduction therapy with miglustat in clinical trials
IV A	Not usually recommended	In clinical development	–	–
IV B	Not usually recommended	–	–	–
VI	Not usually indicated as ERT is available	Approved	Case report (spinal cord compression)	Gene therapy in pre-clinical development
VII	Case reports	Preclinical tests performed	–	Gene therapy in pre-clinical development
IX	–	–	–	–

when ERT is introduced), the importance of urinary GAGs in the evaluation of the long-term evolution and/or treatment outcome is limited, as its correlation with clinical parameters is poor, suggesting that new biomarkers are needed for the assessment and follow-up of treated and untreated patients.

Treatment

Bone Marrow Transplantation (BMT), which was proposed for the treatment of MPS diseases in the 1980s, was the first specific therapy to modify the natural history of these diseases. The types which benefit more from BMT or Haematopoietic Stem Cell Transplantation (HSCT) – in most instances using cord blood as cell source – are

MPS I and MPS VI. Experience with BMT/HSCT in MPS VII is limited and more information is needed to assess the role of HSCT in the treatment of MPS II. It is usually not recommended for MPS III and MPS IV and there is no experience for MPS IX. Enzyme replacement therapy (ERT) has, over the last decade or so, become available for MPS I (laronidase), MPS VI (galsulfase) and MPS II (idursulfase), and is in clinical development for MPS IV A. The inability of the recombinant enzymes administered by intravenous infusion to cross the blood–brain barrier and address the neurological disease is leading to the development of intrathecal ERT (in clinical development for MPS II and MPS III A). The use of inhibitors of GAG synthesis, such as the isoflavone, genistein, is also being tested. As the secondary storage of gangliosides seems to contribute to the pathology of some MPS, the use of miglustat to reduce the synthesis of gangliosides is also under evaluation. Gene therapy, which remains as a hope for the ultimate cure of these diseases, is finally coming to clinical development, as clinical trials for MPS III A and MPS III B are starting. Table 12.2 summarizes the present status of specific therapies for MPS disorders. Adjuvant and palliative therapies also play an important role. Upper airway obstruction should be adequately managed, and respiratory infections need to be vigorously treated. Surgery is frequently needed to correct hernias, to treat carpal tunnel syndrome, to relieve intracranial pressure, to replace heart valves, to improve ENT symptomatology and for skeletal complications. A corneal transplantation could restore visual ability. The global approach to the MPS patient requires a dedicated and experienced multi-professional team.

Treatment guidelines

The available guidelines recommend that children with the severe form of MPS I (Hurler syndrome) should be considered for BMT/HSCT if younger than 2 years of age, due to the possibility of preventing the cognitive decline when BMT/HSCT is performed before this age limit. Although it can have a positive result in MPS VI, BMT/HSCT is not routinely used for MPS VI because of the high mortality/morbidity and lack of cognitive impairment in this type, and also because ERT is available. In severe MPS I patients not suitable for BMT/HSCT, in attenuated cases of MPS I, in MPS II and in MPS VI, the treatment of choice is intravenous ERT. Treatment of markedly attenuated cases should be discussed, taking into consideration risks and benefits. The same considerations should be undertaken when discussing the treatment of severe patients with established neurological disease, as no benefit would be expected for the CNS component. The use of ERT immediately before and after the BMT/HSCT procedure seems to reduce transplantation-associated morbidity. Although no formal guideline is available, there is a growing body of evidence that the early commencement of therapy leads to improved outcome. In due course, the possibility of expanding newborn screening programs to include the MPS diseases is being considered.

Acknowledgements

The author is recipient of a CNPq investigator fellowship (grant 304618/2009-8). The author expresses his gratitude to Dr. Carolina Souza for the review of the clinical section and to Dr. Anthony H. Fensom for the careful review of the text and valuable suggestions.

References

1 Beck M. Therapy for lysosomal storage disorders. *IUBMB Life*, 2010; **62**(1): 33–40.

2 Clarke LA. The mucopolysaccharidoses: a success of molecular medicine. *Expert Rev Mol Med* 2008; **18**: 10e1.

3 Giugliani R, Federhen A, Rojas MV, et al. Mucopolysaccharidosis I, II, and VI: brief review and guidelines for treatment. *Genet Mol Biol* 2010; **33**(4): 589–604.

4 Giugliani R, Harmatz P, Wraith JE. Management guidelines for mucopolysaccharidosis VI. *Pediatrics* 2007; **120**(2): 405–418.

5 Hendriksz C. Improved diagnostic procedures in attenuated mucopolysaccharidosis. *Br J Hosp Med (Lond)* 2011; **72**(2): 91–95.

6 Martin R, Beck M, Eng C, et al. Recognition and diagnosis of mucopolysaccharidosis II (Hunter syndrome). *Pediatrics* 2008; **121**(2): e377–386.

7 Mendelsohn NJ, Harmatz P, Bodamer O, et al. Importance of surgical history in diagnosing mucopolysaccharidosis type II (Hunter syndrome): data from the Hunter Outcome Survey. *Genet Med* 2010; **12**(12): 816–822.

8 Muenzer J. The mucopolysaccharidoses: a heterogeneous group of disorders with variable pediatric presentations. *J Pediatr* 2004; **5** (Suppl): S27–34.

9 Muenzer J, Beck M, Eng CM, et al. Multidisciplinary management of Hunter syndrome. *Pediatrics* 2009; **124**(6): e1228–1239.

10 Muenzer J, Wraith JE, Clarke LA. Mucopolysaccharidosis I: management and treatment guidelines. *Pediatrics* 2009; **123**(1): 19–29.

11 Ponder KP, Haskins ME. Gene therapy for mucopolysaccharidosis. *Expert Opin Biol Ther* 2011; **7**: 1333–1345.

12 Prasad VK, Kurtzberg J. Transplant outcomes in mucopolysaccharidoses. *Semin Hematol* 2010; **47**(1): 59–69.

13 Pinto LLC, Viera TAV, Giugliani R, Schwartz IVD. Expression of the disease on female carriers of X-linked Lysosomal disorders: a brief review. *Orphanet J Rare Dis* 2010; **5**: 14.

14 de Ru MH, Boelens JJ, Das AM, et al. Enzyme replacement therapy and/or hematopoietic stem cell transplantation at diagnosis in patients with mucopolysaccharidosis type I: results of a European consensus procedure. *Orphanet J Rare Dis* 2011; **6**: 55.

15 Tomatsu S, Montaño AM, Oikawa H, et al. Mucopolysaccharidosis type IVA (Morquio A disease): clinical review and current treatment. *Curr Pharm Biotechnol* 2011; **12**(6): 931–945.

16 Wegrzyn G, Jakóbkiewicz-Banecka J, Gabig-Cimińska M, et al. Genistein: a natural isoflavone with a potential for treatment of genetic diseases. *Biochem Soc Trans* 2010; **38**(2): 695–701.

17 Wraith JE. Enzyme replacement therapy for the management of the mucopolysaccharidoses. *Int J Clin Pharmacol Ther* 2009; **47** (Suppl 1): S63–65.

CHAPTER 13

Pompe Disease

Arnold J.J. Reuser and Ans T. van der Ploeg

Center for Lysosomal and Metabolic Diseases, Erasmus MC University Medical Center, Rotterdam, The Netherlands

Pompe disease (glycogen storage disease type II, Acid Maltase Deficiency; OMIM #232300) is an autosomal recessive disease whereby a partial or complete deficiency of acid α-glucosidase, due to mutations in the *GAA* gene, results in the progressive storage of glycogen in the lysosomes. The clinical spectrum ranges from floppy babies with prominent cardiomegaly and a life expectancy of less than 1 year to 60–70 years old patients whose first symptoms are difficulty rising from a chair or climbing stairs. Three short case reports illustrate the clinical diversity and the challenge of making the correct diagnosis.

Case histories

Case history 1

A full-term female was born after an uneventful pregnancy. She had an abnormally high respiratory rate of 100 per minute during the first day. Her liver was palpable 2 cm below the costal margin. No other physical abnormalities were noted. A chest X-ray performed on day 2 postpartum revealed cardiomegaly; echocardiography was performed and a non-obstructive hypertrophic cardiomyopathy of both ventricles was demonstrated. Initially, diabetes gravidarum of the mother was suspected to be the cause of the cardiomyopathy, and the child was discharged. After 9 weeks, however, the child started to develop feeding difficulties and was re-admitted to the hospital for further evaluation. At that time, generalized hypotonia was noted and the child showed very little spontaneous movement. Otherwise, the girl presented as a normal baby without dysmorphic features. She had neither facial muscle weakness nor a protruding tongue as sometimes seen in patients with classic-infantile Pompe disease.

Additional tests revealed slightly elevated levels of: AST (182 U/L; normal 0–88), ALT (97 U/L; normal 0–59), and CK (456 U/L; normal 0–230). LDH (955 U/L; normal 0—1,099) was normal. The Glc_4 content of the urine was elevated. A muscle biopsy of the quadriceps femoris showed pathological changes with characteristic staining of lysosomal glycogen by Periodic Acid Schiff (PAS) reagent and lysosomes by increased acid phosphatase activity (Figure 13.1). The acid α-glucosidase activity in leukocytes was far below the normal range and fully deficient in cultured fibroblasts. Two pathogenic *GAA* mutations were identified in the patient's DNA: one was also identified in DNA from the mother and the other in paternal DNA, confirming the diagnosis.

Case history 2

A 23-year-old Caucasian man complained of difficulty in cycling and climbing stairs. After an uneventful childhood he had experienced difficulties with lifting heavy objects from the age of 14 years. From the age of 20 years he could no longer run due to progressive limb-girdle weakness. Neurological examination showed weakness of the proximal upper and lower extremities (MRC scores of 4/4 and 3/4, respectively). Sensation and tendon reflexes were normal. The patient had atrophy of the pectoral muscles, pseudo-hypertrophy of the calves, a lumbar hyperlordosis and scapular winging

Lysosomal Storage Disorders: A Practical Guide, First Edition. Edited by Atul Mehta and Bryan Winchester.
© 2012 John Wiley & Sons, Ltd. Published 2012 by John Wiley & Sons, Ltd.

(Figure 13.2). Furthermore, he had a waddling gait, and positive Trendelenburg and Gower signs. Blood tests revealed an elevated CK of 1,304 (normal < 200 U/L). Pulmonary examination showed an FVC of 75% in the sitting position and 65% in the supine position. The acid α-glucosidase activity in leukocytes was 4% of average normal, as measured with 4-MU-glucopyranoside in the presence of acarbose, and 13% of average normal in fibroblasts as measured with the same substrate. The muscle biopsy showed PAS positive inclusions in 3–12% of the muscle fibres and a punctated staining pattern of acid phosphatase. DNA analysis demonstrated heterozygosity for two pathogenic *GAA* mutations, c.-32-13 T > G and c.309 C > A, each located on a different allele.

Case history 3

A 6-year-old boy with atrophy of the shoulder muscles was referred to our "Pompe Centre" for a second opinion. The finding of an elevated plasma CK of 561 U/L (*vs* 0–200 U/L normal) and a reduced acid α-glucosidase activity in leukocytes of 0 nmole/mg.h (*vs* 33–160 nmole/mg.h normal) were the main reasons for his referral. Facioscapulohumeral muscular dystrophy (FSHD) had been excluded. He had started to walk at the age of 18 months. Dislocation of the shoulders had been noted at the age of 2.5 years. He had been under the care of an orthopaedic surgeon and a paediatrician, but no specific diagnosis had been made. At the age of 6 years a paediatric neurologist saw him because of his hanging shoulders. Clinical examination in our Centre revealed no weakness of the lower limbs, the hips, the paraspinal muscles, the abdominal muscles, the facial muscles or the respiratory muscles. We concluded that the clinical picture was not typical for a child with Pompe disease. No vacuolated lymphocytes were found in a PAS-stained blood smear. The Glc_4 level in urine was normal, and repeat enzyme analysis in leukocytes also did not confirm the diagnosis. The activity for glycogen substrate was 39 nmole/mg.h (normal range: 40–250) and for MU substrate 6.3 nmole/mg.h (normal range 6.7–27); both activities were measured in the presence of acarbose. DNA analysis revealed heterozygosity for the novel missense mutation c.1190 C > T (p.P397L) in the *GAA* gene. Mutation analysis by site-directed mutagenesis and transient expression showed p.P397L to cause loss of acid α-glucosidase function. A second mutation was not detected. Based on the combination of all findings, the diagnosis of Pompe disease was rejected.

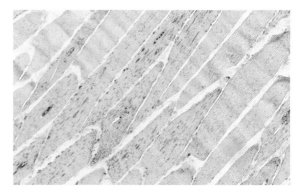

Figure 13.1 Muscle biopsy of a patient with Pompe disease. Routine staining with haematoxylin-eosin does not always reveal the pathologic abnormality but staining the lysosomes for acid phosphatase activity, as in this muscle biopsy specimen, usually reveals intensive staining (reddish colour).

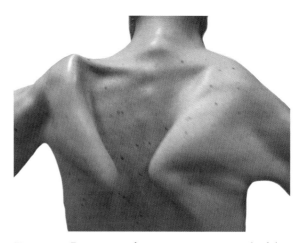

Figure 13.2 Extreme scapular winging in a patient with adult onset Pompe disease.

Confusing nomenclature

Unfortunately, the nomenclature used to cover the clinical spectrum of Pompe disease is confusing. Originally, Pompe disease or glycogenosis type II referred to infants with onset of symptoms shortly after birth, and the following characteristics: generalized hypotonia, cardiomegaly, and a life expectancy of less than one year. Later, "muscular variants" were described without cardiac involvement. In 1963, acid α-glucosidase deficiency was discovered as the very first lysosomal enzyme deficiency and as causative for Glycogen Storage Disease type II (Pompe disease). In 1968, the term Acid Maltase Deficiency became established among neurologists to describe adult, i.e. late-onset, variants of Pompe disease. Childhood and juvenile became widely accepted adjectives to bridge the gap between infantile-onset and late-onset disease.

The confusion started when, for the purpose of clinical trials of enzyme replacement therapy, patients with hypertrophic cardiomyopathy and onset of symptoms under the age of 1 year were said to have infantile-onset Pompe disease, and all with onset of symptoms above the age of 1 year to have late-onset disease. At present, veterans in the field adhere to the historic definition that late-onset Pompe disease, or Acid Maltase Deficiency, is typically a disease of adulthood. Others have adopted the new definition that late-onset Pompe disease is defined by onset of symptoms above the age of 1 year, and yet others argue that late-onset Pompe disease can manifest even before the age of 1 year.

Key message: information contained in publications on late-onset Pompe disease should be interpreted according to the definition of late-onset disease as set forth in that particular publication. Publications about patients with infantile onset Pompe disease may include patients who do not have the classic-infantile phenotype.

Epidemiology

Accurate numbers on the prevalence of rare diseases are difficult to obtain. Based on the birth prevalence of three common mutations in the Dutch population, an estimated frequency of 1:40,000 was obtained in the Netherlands, divided between 1:138,000 for the classic-infantile phenotype and 1:57,000 for the less progressive phenotypes. A study in the New York population based on a larger number of then known mutations came to a similar estimate. An Australian study counting the actual number of diagnosed and registered cases in that country indicated a much lower prevalence of 1:146,000. The birth prevalence of Pompe disease derived from two recently conducted newborn screening activities in Taiwan and Austria was 1:20,000 and 1:9,000, respectively.

Pompe disease is pan-ethnic. Certain pathogenic *GAA* sequence variations prevail in certain ethnic communities, and some are interestingly linked to migration patterns of people around the globe.

Genetic basis

The acid α-glucosidase gene (*GAA* ref seq Y00839/ M34424) is located on chromosome 17 q25.3 and encodes a protein of 952 amino acids that is glycosylated at seven different sites. As at June 2012, the Pompe Disease Mutation Data at www/pompecenter.nl lists 310 pathogenic sequence variations and 93 non-pathogenic variations. c.-32-13 T > G is by far the most common pathogenic sequence variation in the Caucasian population. The nonsense mutation c.2560 C > T (p.Arg854X) is the most common mutation in Afro-Americans, and c.1935 C > A (p.Asp645Glu) is widely encountered in Taiwanese, Chinese, and other Asian populations excluding the Japanese. In addition, a number of mutations are known to be more frequent in some countries than in others. Knowledge of the frequencies of mutations in ethnic populations has lost significance for diagnostic purposes, as it is presently more efficient and almost equally costly to perform whole gene sequencing than to selectively screen for specific mutations.

Pathophysiology

The acid α-glucosidase deficiency is genetically determined and almost always equally severe in all cell types. Consequently, the lysosomal glycogen storage manifests in all cell types. It is remarkable that symptoms related to central nervous system dysfunction do not dominate the clinical picture since massive glycogen storage has been demonstrated in motor neurons of severely affected infants. With regard to the preferential muscle pathology, some evidence has been presented that the muscle weakness followed by muscle wasting is brought about by the expanding lysosomal system within the muscle fibre. It hampers linear force transduction and ultimately damages the delicate organization of the contractile elements. Circumstantial evidence has been presented that genetic and non-genetic factors can modify the clinical course; patients with the same *GAA* genotype can have a widely different age of onset and rate of disease progression, provided that acid α-glucosidase is not fully deficient.

Clinical presentation

For practical reasons it is best to describe the disease by age category. Patients with classic-infantile Pompe disease present shortly after birth as floppy babies. They all have cardiac hypertrophy, feeding difficulties, and they do not achieve major developmental milestones including sitting, standing and walking. They typically succumb before the age of 1 year due to cardio-respiratory insufficiency. Severely affected infants with early-onset but without cardiac involvement survive longer. They usually develop a childhood phenotype characterized by

Box 13.1 **Typical signs and symptoms of Pompe disease according to age**

Newborns under 1 year of age
- Floppy babies.
- Failure to thrive.
- Cardiomegaly on X-ray.
- Poor cardiac function.
- Poor pulmonary function.
- Hepatomegaly and macro-glossia in some.
- Hearing impairment in all.

Children from 0 to 16 years old
- Developmental delay.
- Muscle weakness.
- Pulmonary deficit.
- Failure to keep up with their peers.
- Risk of scoliosis in puberty.

Adults
- Muscle weakness in most cases, and pulmonary deficit or fatigue in some cases as first complaints.
- Variable in age of onset from 20 to 70 years of age.

Box 13.2 **Diagnostic flow diagram**

First presenting case
Clinical investigation
Enzymes (blood): ALT AST, LDH, CK (often elevated).
Metabolites (urine): Glc_4 (often elevated in classic infantile Pompe disease).
Enzyme assay: Acid α-glucosidase (leukocytes, bloodspots, fibroblasts: deficient).

Confirmation of Diagnosis
Acid α-glucosidase deficient in leukocytes and/or fibroblasts *or*
A proven pathogenic mutation in both *GAA* alleles.

Follow-up
DNA analysis desirable for counseling and carrier detection in the family and for understanding genotype–phenotype correlation.

Familial case
Clinical investigation
Evident signs: Enzyme assay *or GAA* DNA sequence analysis (search for familial mutations).
No signs: *GAA* DNA sequence analysis (search for familial mutations; this enables clear distinction between affected homozygotes/compound heterozygotes, carriers and normals.

progressive skeletal muscle weakness affecting their pulmonary function and leading to ventilator dependency. There are also patients who are diagnosed in infancy, mostly based on poor motor development, but who progress very slowly and continue into adulthood without medical intervention. Using the historic nomenclature, adult-onset or late-onset cases of Pompe disease are typically diagnosed in early or late adulthood with an age range from 20 to 70 years at the time of diagnosis. They present with proximal muscle weakness, most prominently in the limb-girdle region, leading to a rather characteristic waddling gate and a Gower sign. Pulmonary function is usually compromised, especially when measured in the supine position. Some patients present with shortage of breath. Extreme fatigue or muscle cramps can also be the first sign of Pompe disease. Thus, Pompe disease patients may present to a range of clinical specialities in very different age categories (Box 13.1).

Natural history

The life expectancy for patients with classic-infantile Pompe disease is less than 1 year. The life expectancy for childhood cases is extremely variable. Those who become fully ventilator-dependent and immobile before the age of 5–10 years are at risk of developing fatal pulmonary infections. Young patients with minimal pulmonary involvement and a slowly progressive muscle weakness have a life expectancy that reaches beyond adulthood. Most patients with adult-onset Pompe disease have very slow disease progression. Their life expectancy is shortened compared to age-matched controls and their quality of life is substantially reduced. They are at risk of becoming wheelchair-bound and ventilator-dependent.

Enzymatic and molecular diagnosis

The deficiency of acid α-glucosidase in Pompe disease has been known since 1963 and up to now has been the best way to diagnose the disease in the proband (Box 13.2). Fibroblasts obtained by skin biopsy are the preferred material to use since the activity measured in this cell type has some prognostic value with regard to the expected clinical course. Furthermore, fibroblasts can serve as an unlimited source of material for follow-up studies and are most suitable for studies on the biosynthesis of acid α-glucosidase. In practice, however, leukocytes are easier to obtain and allow for a similar diagnostic accuracy if properly handled (see Case history 3). The enzyme assay in leukocytes has to be performed in the presence of acarbose to inhibit the interfering activity of glucoamylase. The assay in leukocytes does not discriminate amongst the various phenotypes of Pompe disease, whereas the assay in fibroblasts can. Bloodspot analysis has become an attractive alternative for the rapid screening for Pompe disease in suspected patients and for first tier new born screening, but the results need to be confirmed by an alternative methodology. *GAA* sequence analysis is the best method to establish the diagnosis of Pompe disease or carrier status in families known to be affected. However, it is not advised as the diagnostic tool in first presenting cases: pathogenic sequence variations can be missed and the effect of novel missense mutations is rarely predictable with 100% certainty. Muscle biopsies are conclusive if glycogen storage can be demonstrated with Periodic Acid Schiff (PAS) staining. Demonstration of enhanced acid phosphatase activity staining is very supportive. The finding of PAS-positive vacuoles in lymphocytes also supports the diagnosis.

Prenatal diagnosis in pregnancies at risk can be performed by measuring the acid α-glucosidase activity in either chorionic villi or in cultured amniocytes, or by foetal DNA analysis. In all instances it is strongly recommended to establish the acid α-glucosidase activity of the index patient and the parents, and to identify the pathogenic mutations of the index patient and the parents before the pregnancy is ongoing. DNA analysis is preferred if the familial mutations are known.

Treatment

Recombinant human acid α-glucosidase (Alglucosidase alfa; Myozyme/Lumizyme, Genzyme Corp.) has been available for enzyme replacement therapy (ERT) for Pompe disease since 2006. Myozyme was initially approved by the FDA in the USA for use in classic-infantile Pompe disease and by the EMA in Europe for use in all patients. Later, the FDA approved Lumizyme, which has a slightly different carbohydrate composition from Myozyme, for use in all patients across the clinical spectrum except those with classic-infantile Pompe disease.

The effect of ERT in classic-infantile Pompe disease is undisputed. Usually it resolves the hypertrophic cardiomyopathy rather quickly and thereby prolongs the life expectancy of the patients significantly. Most treated infants reach the key developmental milestones and/or acquire the ability to walk. However, response to treatment is negatively affected by the development of antibodies against the recombinant protein, which occurs mostly but not exclusively in acid α-glucosidase naïve patients (Cross Reactive Material-negative patients). Methods to prevent or counteract antibody formation are under investigation. Respiratory failure is the main threat to infantile patients. Once they become ventilator-dependent it is very difficult to wean them off the ventilator, and they tend to lose general strength after immobilization as a result of mechanical ventilation. So far about 50% of all the treated infants have survived without ventilation, but some form of residual disease has remained in virtually all cases.

In children, adolescents, and adults with less severe genotypes and less progressive phenotypes, ERT can stabilize the pulmonary function and improve the muscle strength. In all cases, the best results are obtained when the disease is diagnosed early and the treatment is started before an irreversible loss of muscle mass has occurred.

The recommended dose for ERT is 20 mg/kg body weight every second week but alternative dosing regimens of up to 40 mg/kg every week have been reported.

Patients seem to benefit from physiotherapy, muscle training and a high protein diet. Pulmonary infections are a great risk and need to be prevented, if possible. Prophylactic treatment with antibiotics may be of help in patients at risk for respiratory failure.

Treatment guidelines

There are no formal guidelines but case histories suggest that ERT is indicated in all Pompe-disease patients who manifest clear signs of muscle weakness or pulmonary dysfunction. With respect to the latter, the difference between FVC in upright and supine positions is very informative. In classic-infantile Pompe disease, a very early start of treatment, within 3 months after birth, seems mandatory for a long-term positive clinical outcome.

Acknowledgment

The authors would like to thank Carin van Gelder, Juna de Vries and Stephan Wens for providing the case reports, and Tom de Vries Lentsch for photographic artwork.

Selected literature

General

Hirschhorn R, Reuser AJJ. Glycogen Storage Disease Type II: acid alpha-glucosidase (Acid Maltase) deficiency. In: Scriver CR, *et al.* (eds.), *The Metabolic and Molecular Bases of Inherited Disease* (8th edn). New York: McGraw-Hill, 2001; pp. 3389–3420.

Engel AG, *et al*. 2004. Acid maltase deficiency. In: Engel AG, *et al*. (eds.), *Myology* (3rd edn.). McGraw-Hill; pp. 1559–1586.

Van der Ploeg AT, Reuser AJJ. Pompe's disease. *Lancet* 2008; **372**(9646): 1342–1353.

Baethmann M, Straub V, Reuser A (eds.). Pompe disease. *UNI-MED, Bremen* 2008.

Clinical spectrum

Engel AG, *et al*. The spectrum and diagnosis of acid maltase deficiency. *Neurology* 1973; **23**(1): 95–106.

Enzyme replacement therapy trials and antibody formation

Kishnani PS, *et al*. Chinese hamster ovary cell-derived recombinant human acid alpha-glucosidase in infantile-onset Pompe disease. *J Pediatr* 2006; **149**(1): 89–97.

Van der Ploeg AT, *et al*. A randomized study of alglucosidase alfa in late-onset Pompe disease. *N Engl J Med* 2010; **362**(15): 1396–1406.

Kishnani PS, *et al*. Cross-reactive immunologic material status affects treatment outcomes in Pompe disease infants. *Mol Genet Metab* 2010; **99**(1): 26–33.

De Vries JM, *et al*. High antibody titer in an adult with Pompe disease affects treatment with alglucosidase alfa. *Mol Genet Metab* 2010; **101**(4): 338–345.

Mendelson NJ, *et al*. Elimination of antibodies to recombinant enzyme in Pompe's disease. *N Engl J Med* 2009; **360**(2): 194–195.

Pathology

Hesselink RP, *et al*. Age-related morphological changes in skeletal muscle cells of acid alpha-glucosidase knock-out mice. *Muscle Nerve* 2006; **33**(4): 505–513.

Thurberg B. Insights into the pathophysiology of Pompe disease. *Clin Ther* 2008; **30**(Suppl 1): S3.

Raben N, Plotz PH. A new look at the pathogenesis of Pompe disease. *Clin Ther* 2008; **30** (Suppl C): S86–87.

Schoser BG, *et al*. Adult-onset glycogen storage disease type 2: clinico-pathological phenotype revisited. *Neuropathol Appl Neurobiol* 2007; **33**(5): 544–559.

Diagnosis and diagnostic guidelines

Reuser AJJ, *et al*. Enzymatic and molecular strategies to diagnose Pompe disease. *Expert Opin Med Diagn* 2010; **4**(1): 79–89.

Kroos MA, *et al*. Broad spectrum of Pompe disease in patients with the same c.-32-13 T > G haplotype. *Neurology* 2007; **68**(2): 110–115.

Kishnani PS, *et al*. Pompe disease diagnosis and management guideline. *Genet Med* 2006; **8**(5): 267–288.

Bembi B, *et al*. Management and treatment of glycogenosis type II. *Neurology* 2008; **71**(23 Suppl 2): S12–36. http://www.pompecenter.nl

CHAPTER 14

Glycoproteinoses

Dag Malm, Hilde Monica F. Riise Stensland and Øivind Nilssen

The Tromsø Centre of Internal Medicine (TIS as) and the Departments of Clinical Medicine and Medical Genetics, University and University Hospital of North-Norway, Tromsø, Norway.

The glycoproteinoses constitute a group of lysosomal disorders that result from deficiency of glycoprotein catabolism. It includes α-mannosidosis, β-mannosidosis, aspartyglucosaminuria (AGU), sialidosis, α-N-acetylgalactosaminidase deficiency (Schindler disease, Kanzaki disease) and fucosidosis, which are discussed in this chapter. Other disorders belonging to this group are mucolipidosis II and III, and galactosialidosis, caused by deficiencies of N-acetylglucosamine-1-phospotransferase and cathepsin A, respectively. These disorders, however, are described elsewhere (Chapters 15 and 16). All glycoproteinoses are genetic disorders, inherited in an autosomal recessive fashion.

Epidemiology

They are rare, but are expected to be found in populations worldwide. In the Czech Republic glycoproteinoses make up only 6.4% of the lysosomal storage disorders and their combined birth prevalence is less than 1 in 100,000, which is similar to the prevalence reported in the Netherlands and Australia [1]. Due to their low frequency, exact calculations on prevalence have been made only for a few of them. α-Mannosidosis shows a birth incidence of ~1:1,000,000 in The Netherlands, Portugal and Australia, a prevalence of 1:300,000 in the Czech Republic (reviewed in [1]) and ~1:600,000 in Norway [2]. No such prevalence estimates have been made for β-mannosidosis as less than 20 unrelated cases have been reported so far [3]. The incidence of aspartyglucosaminuria was reported to be 1:2,000,000 in Australia, ~1:800,000 in The Netherlands and ~1:600,000 in Portugal (reviewed in [1]). However, due to a strong founder effect, a prevalence as high as 1:18,000 was found in the Finnish population [4]. The sialidosis patients studied come from multiple origins, reflecting a wide geographic distribution of the disease. The majority of sialidosis type I patients reported have been Italian, whereas type II is relatively frequent in Japan [5]. The combined prevalence at birth for sialidosis (types I and II combined) has been estimated to be 1:2,500,000 [3]. α-N-acetyl galactosaminidase deficiency was found to have an incidence of 1:500,000 in The Netherlands [6], however, it is thought to be very rare elsewhere and no exact figures exist from other populations. The incidence of fucosidosis was reported to be 1:2,000,000 in The Netherlands [6]. World wide, about 100 cases have been reported [3] and patients have been identified in Europe, North and South America, Asia and Africa. Several of the reported patients originate from Italy, New Mexico and Colorado [7].

Pathophysiology

Common to the glycoproteinoses is the deficiency of one of the many lysosomal enzymes required for the ordered hydrolysis of glycoprotein carbohydrate moieties. Glycoproteins are degraded by proteases leaving only asparagine (Asn), serine (Ser) or threonine (Thr) linked to the glycan. Subsequently, the glycoprotein carbohydrate chain, as exemplified by an Asn-linked complex oligosaccharide in Figure 14.1, is degraded by sequential removal of monosaccharides. Each step in this catabolic pathway is governed by a specific glycosidase. α-Fucosidase cleaves off core and peripheral fucose residues, followed by glycosylasparginase, which removes the asparagine from the glycan moiety at the reducing

Lysosomal Storage Disorders: A Practical Guide, First Edition. Edited by Atul Mehta and Bryan Winchester.

© 2012 John Wiley & Sons, Ltd. Published 2012 by John Wiley & Sons, Ltd.

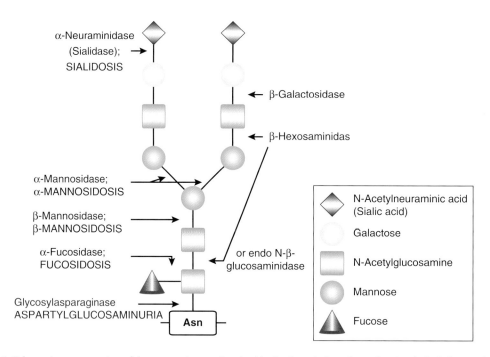

Figure 14.1 Schematic representation of the enzymatic steps involved in the degradation of complex Asn-linked oligosaccharides.

(a)   (b)

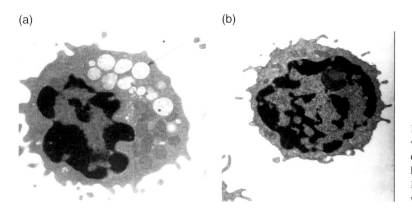

Figure 14.2 A lymphocyte with vacuolated lysosomes from a patient with α-mannosidosis (a), compared to a lymphocyte from a normal control (b). Reproduced from Malm and Nilssen [2] with permission from Biomed Central.

end. Subsequently, degradation takes place from the non-reducing end as the sialidase, β-galactosidase, N-acetyl β-hexosaminidase, α-mannosidase and β-mannosidase sequentially digest the remaining glycan. Since this process is highly ordered the deficiency of a single enzyme will compromise the pathway as a whole, resulting in the accumulation of undigested oligosaccharides or glycopeptides in the lysosomes. The spectrum of glycoconjugates accumulated and secreted into urine reflects the pathogenic step in the catabolic pathway; however, a variation in glycoconjugate content might be

seen among patients with the same enzyme deficiency. In patients with fucosidosis and aspartyglucosaminuria or α-N-acetyl galactosaminidase deficiency glycopeptides containing Asn and Ser/Thr, respectively, may be observed.

For many of these disorders the accumulation of undigested material results in vacuolization as seen in peripheral blood cells or fibroblasts cells under light or electron microscopy (Figure 14.2). Such accumulation of storage material may not only impair lysosomal function but, as seen in other lysosomal storage disorders, it may also cause pleiotropic effects on cellular functions such as vesicle maturation, synaptic release, endocytosis, exocytosis, Ca^{++} release and autophagy [8].

Genetic basis

The glycoproteinoses result from mutations in genes that encode the glycosidases involved in glycoprotein degradation (Figure 14.1). The different disorders and their corresponding loci, deficient genes and enzymes are displayed in Table 14.1. Most of the mutations reported in glycoproteinoses are private and occur in single or a few families only, however, exceptions exist. In α-mannosidosis the *MAN2B1* substitution p.Arg750Trp has been detected in 64 patients from 20 countries. It constitutes 27.9% of all unrelated disease alleles reported and shows a declining east–west gradient across Europe, indicating eastern European origin [9]. In β-mannosidosis 17 different *MANBA* mutations have been detected in patients from various ethnic origins. In patients with aspartyglucosaminuria the *AGA* substitution p.Cys163Ser (AGU$_{Fin}$) accounts for 98% of all AGU alleles in Finland, showing a carrier frequency of 1/30–1/40 [4]. More than 40 *NEU1* mutations have been reported in sialidosis patients of varying disease severity of which the substitution p.Gly227Arg appear to be the most frequent as it has been reported in four families from different countries. Seven *NAGA* mutations have been reported in patients with α-N-acetylgalactosaminidase deficiency, of which the substitution p.Glu325Lys has been detected in several families. In patients with fucosidosis, 29 different *FUCA1* mutations have been reported. Most mutations are found in homozygous form indicating a high rate of consanguinity in fucosidosis [6].

Genotype–phenotype relationship

The different glyoproteinoses show variation in clinical severity; however, in general there is no evident correlation between the genotype and the clinical phenotype. This is based on observations of extensive clinical heterogeneity among patients with the same mutation(s), the difference in clinical severity seen in affected siblings and variable clinical presentation in patients homozygous or compound heterozygous for null mutations. A possible exception is sialidosis. Based on cellular and biochemical analysis, Bonten and coworkers [10] classified mutant neuraminidases into three groups: (1) catalytically inactive and not localized to the lysosomes, (2) localized to the lysosomes but catalytically inactive, (3) localized to the lysosomes and with residual activity.

Patients with the mild type I form had at least one group 3 mutation. In contrast, patients with the juvenile, severe, type II had mutations belonging to group 1 or 2 [10].

Clinical presentation

The different glycoproteinoses show a wide variation in clinical severity. Accordingly α-mannosidosis (types I, II and III), sialidosis (types I and II), α-N-acetylgalactosaminidase deficiency (types I (Schindler), II (Kanzaki) and III) and fucosidosis (types I and II) have been divided into clinical subtypes. However, rather than specific subtypes, the clinical variation within each disorder appears to represent a continuum from the mild to the severe end of a clinical spectrum. Onset might be congenital but generally ranges from 3 months to 20 years of age. Most glycoproteinoses show infantile onset with a progressing disease course. The glycoproteinoses share in common several Hurler-like clinical features such as mental impairment, speech impairment, growth impairment, delay of motor development, hypotonia, dysostosis multiplex, scoliosis, organomegaly and facial dysmorphism, including macroglossia. Recurrent infections, hearing impairment, ataxia are common to most of these disorders. Additional features such as spasticity, neuroaxonal dystrophy and cortical blindness occur in α-N-acetylgalactosaminidase deficiency type I. However, progressive loss of visual acuity has also been reported in adult patients with other glycoproteinoses.

Laboratory diagnosis

For all glycoproteinoses, initial biochemical screening can be performed by analysis of the urinary oligosaccharide and/or glycopeptide profile by thin-layer or liquid chromatography-tandem mass spectrometry (LC-MS/MS). The oligosaccharide and/or glycopeptide composition will indicate glycoproteinosis and may be suggestive of a specific diagnosis. The exact diagnosis, however, will rely on direct measurement of the specific enzyme activity in white blood cells or cultured fibroblast cells. Diagnosis should always be confirmed by targeted sequencing of the patient DNA to identify the disease causing mutation(s) in the gene in question. The carrier status of the parents should be verified. Prenatal diagnosis can be performed by enzyme activity measurements in foetal cells, obtained by chorionic villus sampling at 10–12 weeks of gestation or by mutation analysis using DNA from the same source. Mutation analysis is to be preferred if the parental genotypes are known.

Table 14.1 Disorders of glycaprotein degradation

Phenotype	OMIM#	Gene	OMIM #	Symbol	Chromosomal localisation	#mutations (HGMDp July11)	Recurrent variants	Genotype-phenotype correlation
Alpha-mannosidosis	248500	lysosomal alpha-mannosidase	609458	MAN2B1	19p13.2	41	p.Arg750Trp	no
Alpha-N-acetylgalactosaminidase deficiency	609241 (Schindler); 609242 (Kanzaki)	N-acetyl-alpha-D-galactosaminidase	104170	NAGA	22q13.2	7 (only missense)	p.Arg325Lys	no
Beta-mannosidosis	248510	lysosomal beta mannosidase	609489	MANBA	4q22–q25	15		no
Aspartylgluconsaminuria (AGU)	208400	aspartylgulconsaminidase	613228	AGA	4q34.3	32	p.Cys163Ser (AGU$_{Fin}$)	no
Fucosidosis	230000	alpha-L-fucosidase	612280	FUCA1	1p34	29		no
Sialidosis	256550	neuraminidase 1	608272	NEU1	6p21.33	43	p.Glu227Arg	possible

(a)

(b)

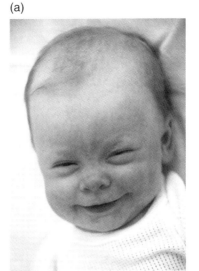 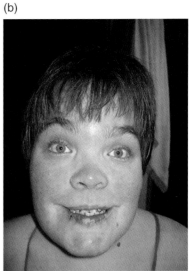

Figure 14.3 (a) Patient 1 year of age: note large head, prominent forehead, rounded eyebrows, saddle nose and broad mouth. (b) Patient 28 years of age: note large head, prominent forehead, rounded eyebrows, saddle nose, retrognathism, broad mouth with poorly healing sores and widely spaced teeth. Further notice the full hair on head and eyebrows. Normally, she would wear glasses and hearing devices.

Treatment

There is no specific therapy for glycoproteinoses, and treatment options are mainly directed towards ameliorating symptoms. Bone marrow transplantation (BMT) has only been reported for a few cases of fucosidosis, sialidosis and aspartylglucosaminuria. Whereas some cases of improvement have been shown regarding biochemical markers and MRI white matter signals, post-transplant complications have also been reported. In general, assessment of therapeutic efficiency is lacking since long-term follow-up studies have been performed in only a few cases. BMT in α-mannosidosis is discussed below. For the majority of these disorders there are animal models where therapeutic approaches are being investigated on a research level.

An example of glycoproteinosis: α-mannosidosis

Case history

From birth the girl was noted with coarse features, skeletal anomalies of the chest and continuous colds (Figure 14.3). At 9 months, she presented with a hydrocephalus, operated on with a ventriculoperitoneal shunt, which at the age of 3 had to be replaced with a ventriculocaval shunt due to insufficient peritoneal absorption. At the age of 1, otitis serosa and bilateral-deficient hearing for high tones was noted and stents and hearing aids were

provided. At age 3, umbilical and femoral hernias were operated on and ataxia, muscular hypotonia and mental impairment became evident. At age 6, the diagnosis of α-mannosidosis was made, based on deficient enzyme activity in leukocytes. At age 12, synovitis and a cystic lesion of the tallus occurred, forcing her to crawl on the floor. This was successfully treated orthopaedically with a triple arthrodesis. At the same time a bilateral genu valgus was operated with lateral epiphysisectomy with little success. During the first two decades of life, immunodeficiency was evident with several episodes of pneumonia. From the age of 14 there were yearly episodes of psychosis with various presentations like hallucinations, anxiety or depressions. At the same age, she started soiling herself, being unable to detect defecation signals, and a partial paralysis of the bladder was diagnosed. At the age of 25, the gait worsened, forcing the use of a wheelchair when walking more than 500 metres. She also presented with increasing dysphagia, making her aspirate certain food items. At this age, she lived in a flat on her own, but was dependent on help during daytime. She has a mild mental retardation, but is able to read and write. She has bilateral high tone deafness. Cardiac examination, ECG and echocardiogram are normal, except for some irregularities on the aortic valve.

Genetic basis

α-Mannosidosis is caused by mutations in the *MAN2B1* gene encoding lysosomal α-mannosidase. *MAN2B1* is located on chromosome 19 (19p13.2-p13.11) and is

(a)

(b)

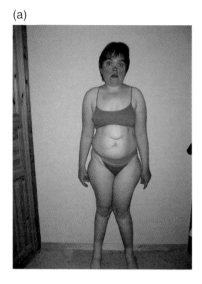

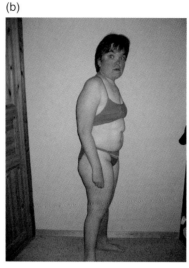

Figure 14.4 Patient 28 years of age. Whole body, front (a) and side (b); note short stature, large head, short neck, dysmorphic thorax, poorly healing scars after operations of umbilical hernia, kyphosis, muscular atrophy and genu valgus.

composed of 24 exons spanning 21.5 kb The *MAN2B1* mRNA has an open reading frame of 3,036 nucleotides (Genbank NM_000528.2) encoding a 1,011 amino acid protein. As judged by Northern blot analyses, the level of *MAN2B1* expression appears to be highest in lung, kidney, pancreas and peripheral blood leukocyte. In CNS the highest level of expression appears to be in the corpus callosum and spinal cord, whereas considerably lower levels are observed in the larger structures, which include cerebellum, cerebral cortex, frontal and temporal lobes. The significance (if any) of this variation is not clear [11].

Pathophysiology

Deficiency of the α-mannosidase enzyme, which normally is a component of the lysosomal glycoprotein degradation pathway, causes oligosaccharides to build up in all tissues. Whether this impairs cell function directly is not known. Complete absence of functional enzyme *per se* does not lead to death during early childhood. Measurement of low residual activity in tissues is most likely a result of Golgi or cytosolic α-mannosidase, which both show some activity at acidic pH.

Clinical presentation

α-Mannosidosis is characterized by immune deficiency, facial and skeletal abnormalities, hearing impairment, and intellectual disability. The children are often born apparently normal, and their condition worsens progressively. Some children are born with ankle equinus or

develop hydrocephalus in the first year of life. Main features are immune deficiency (manifested by recurrent infections, especially in the first decade of life), skeletal abnormalities (mild-to-moderate dysostosis multiplex, scoliosis and deformation of the sternum), hearing impairment (moderate-to-severe sensorineural hearing loss), gradual impairment of mental functions and speech, and often, periods of psychosis. Associated motor function disturbances include muscular weakness, joint abnormalities and ataxia. The facial traits include large head with prominent forehead, rounded eyebrows, flattened nasal bridge, macroglossia, widely spaced teeth, and prognathism (Figures 14.3 and 14.4). Slight strabismus is common. The clinical variability is significant, representing a continuum in severity [2]. The course of the disease is progressive.

Natural history

The life expectancy for patients with α-mannosidosis seems to be reduced by about 20–30 years, but data is scarce. The most common cause of death of the young is infectious diseases. Older patients seem to have an increased frequency of systemic lupus erythematosus (SLE), and further pneumonia due to aspiration.

Laboratory diagnosis

An efficient and reliable method of establishing the diagnosis of α-mannosidosis is the assay of acidic α-mannosidase activity in leukocytes or other nucleated cells using a fluorometric assay which is performed at low pH (usually at pH 4) with the substrate 4-methylumbelliferyl α-D-mannopyranoside. Enzyme activity measurements, however,are unreliable for carrier detection. Identification of disease causing mutations is carried out by *MAN2B1* DNA sequencing and prenatal genetic diagnosis can be established given that parental *MAN2B1* mutations are known in advance of pregnancy.

Treatment

There is some preliminary evidence that bone marrow transplantation (BMT) may stop/delay the disease progression. The rationale for BMT in α-mannosidosis is that enzyme-producing donor cells repopulate the host tissues and transfer enzyme to enzyme-deficient host cells. Because of the blood-brain barrier, the main question remained whether BMT could improve the pathology of the central nervous system. Early BMT was demonstrated to prevent neurological deterioration in a cat model [12]. A possible explanation for the neuronal benefits of BMT could be migration of donor-derived cells to the CNS of the recipient. Subsequently, BMT was performed in human patients. Of 17 patients who had undergone BMT 2.1–12.6 years earlier, 15 made developmental progress, although normal development was not achieved. Especially hearing improved to normal or near normal, but for speech frequencies only. However, BMT involves serious procedure-related complications and 2 patients died within 5 months [13]. The possible benefits of BMT must be weighed against the overall risk of procedure-related morbidity and mortality. The benefits are greater in younger patients before complications have developed, and also transplant-related complications are more frequent and severe in older patients. Therefore, BMT is a therapeutic option in the first decade of life, which makes early identification of affected patients critical.

Prognosis

The long-term prognosis is poor. There is an insidiously slow progression of neuromuscular and skeletal deterioration over several decades, making most patients wheelchair dependent. No patients manage to be completely socially independent. Many patients are over 50 years of age.

Unresolved questions

Enzyme replacement therapy (ERT) is a therapeutic modality in other lysosomal storage diseases, like Gaucher, Fabry or Pompe disease. In α-mannosidosis, experiments with ERT have been performed in an artificial knock-out mouse model [14] and in a naturally occurring guinea pig model [15]. The reduction in storage material was evident in almost all tissues in both models. However, whereas the first study found a reduction of mannose-containing oligosaccharides in the brain to less than 30% of that in control mice with α-mannosidosis [14], a similar cerebral improvement was not found in guinea-pigs [15]. The development of ERT in human is the long-term objective of the European ALPHA-MAN project [16].

Treatment guidelines

There are no formal treatment guidelines.

References

1 Poupetová H, Ledvinová J, Berná L, *et al.* The birth prevalence of lysosomal storage disorders in the Czech Republic: comparison with data in different populations. *J Inherit Metab Dis* 2010; **4**: 387–396.

2 Malm D, Nilssen Ø. *Orphanet J Rare Dis* 2008; **3**: 21. http://www.ojrd.com/content/3/1/21

3 Orphanet Report Series. Rare Disease collection. May 2011, #1. http://www.orpha.net/orphacom/cahiers/docs/GB/Prevalence_of_rare_diseases_by_alphabetical_list.pdf

4 Arvio M, Autio S, Louhiala P. Early clinical symptoms and incidence of aspartylglucosaminuria in Finland. *Acta Paediatr* 1993; **82**: 587–589.

5 Lowden JA, O'Brien JS. Sialidosis: a review of human neuraminidase deficiency. *Am J Hum Genet* 1979; **31**: 1–18.

6 Poorthuis BJHM, Wevers RA, Kleijer WJ, *et al.* The frequency of lysosomal storage diseases in The Netherlands. *Hum Genet* 1999; **105**: 151–156.

7 Willems PJ, Seo HC, Coucke P, *et al.* Spectrum of mutations in fucosidosis. *Eur J Hum Genet* 1999; **7**: 60–67.

8 Schultz ML, Tecedor L, Chang M, *et al.* Clarifying lysosomal storage diseases. *Trends Neurosci* 2011; **34**: 401–410.

9 Riise Stensland HMF, Klenow, HB, Nguyen LV, *et al.* Identification of 83 novel alpha-mannosidosis-associated sequence variants: Functional analysis of MAN2B1 missense mutations. *Hum Mutat*, 2012; **33**: 511–520.

10 Bonten EJ, Arts WF, Beck M, *et al.* Novel mutations in lysosomal neuraminidase identify functional domains and determine clinical severity in sialidosis. *Hum Mol Genet* 2000; **18**: 2715–2725.

11 Nilssen O, Berg T, Riise HM, *et al.* alpha-Mannosidosis: functional cloning of the lysosomal alpha-mannosidase cDNA and identification of a mutation in two affected siblings. *Hum Mol Genet* 1997; **6**: 717–726.

12 Walkley SU, Thrall MA, Dobrenis K, *et al.* Bone marrow transplantation corrects the enzyme defect in neurons of the central nervous system in a lysosomal storage disease. *Proc Natl Acad Sci USA* 1994; **12**: 2970–2974.

13 Mynarek M, Tolar J, Albert MH, *et al.* Allogeneic hematopoietic SCT for alpha-mannosidosis: an analysis of 17 patients. *Bone Mar Transpl* 2011 May; doi:10.1038/bmt.2011.99.

14 Roces DP, Lüllmann-Rauch R, Peng J, *et al.* Efficacy of enzyme replacement therapy in alpha-mannosidosis mice: a preclinical animal study. *Hum Mol Genet* 2004; **13**: 1979–1988.

15 Crawley AC, King B, Berg T, *et al.* Enzyme replacement therapy in alpha-mannosidosis guinea-pigs. *Mol Genet Metab* 2006; **89**: 48–57.

16 http://www.alpha-man.eu/index.htm

CHAPTER 15

Defect in Protective Protein/ Cathepsin A: Galactosialidosis

Alessandra d'Azzo and Erik J. Bonten

Department of Genetics, St. Jude Children's Research Hospital, Memphis, TN, USA

Galactosialidosis (Online Mendelian Inheritance in Man #256540) is a rare neurodegenerative lysosomal storage disorder caused by the combined deficiency of neuraminidase-1 (NEU1) and β-galactosidase (β-GAL), secondary to mutations in the protective protein/ cathepsin A gene (*CTSA*).

A case report

The following is one of the few clinical cases of early infantile galactosialidosis reported in the literature. A girl was the third child of healthy unrelated parents. Family history was unremarkable. Routine chromosome analysis of a chorion villus biopsy showed a normal karyotype. Pregnancy was complicated by a short period of maternal cholestasis in the sixth month. Ultrasound examination was normal. Thereafter the mother noticed a fast growth of the abdomen; however, further investigations were not performed. The patient was born at 35 weeks. Polyhydramnion with meconium containing amniotic fluid was found. The placenta weighed 1,320 g and was severely hydropic. The girl was asphyxic with bradycardia. After suction of the mouth and with oxygen supply she recovered rapidly. Apgarscores were 6, 4, and 10 after 1, 5, and 10 min. No facial dysmorphia was noticed at the time of birth. The liver was palpable 4 cm below the costal ridge. A great amount of ascites was present which led to mild tachypnea, respiratory distress, and feeding problems. Treatment with diuretics reduced the ascites; her lowest weight was 2,345 g. Hereafter her clinical condition improved, but she needed tube feeding.

Because of thrombopenia a platelet transfusion was given twice. Twice she needed intravenous antibiotics because of sepsis. Congenital viral infections, including parvo 19, cardiac anomalies, skeletal abnormalities, congenital nephrosis, arteriovenous malformations, and neuroblastoma were excluded as a cause for the polyhydramnion and the ascites. The patient was discharged from the hospital at 5 weeks. One week later she was brought moribund to the hospital and died due to a sepsis. Postmortem investigations were not performed. Mutation analysis of the patient's *CTSA* gene and biochemical assessment of the cathepsin A, β-GAL and NEU1 activities in cultured fibroblasts confirmed the diagnosis of early infantile galactosialidosis (patient #16 in Table 15.1).

Epidemiology and clinical presentation

Given the rarity of this disease, there is no comprehensive survey of the demographics and disease spectrum for galactosialidosis. All patients have clinical manifestations typical of a lysosomal disorder such as coarse facies, cherry-red spots, vertebral changes, foam cells in the bone marrow and vacuolated lymphocytes. Three phenotypic subtypes are recognized. The early infantile form is associated with foetal hydrops, edema, ascites, visceromegaly, skeletal dysplasia and early death. Hepatosplenomegaly, growth retardation, cardiac involvement and rare occurrence of important neurological signs characterize the late-infantile type. The majority of reported patients

Lysosomal Storage Disorders: A Practical Guide, First Edition. Edited by Atul Mehta and Bryan Winchester.
© 2012 John Wiley & Sons, Ltd. Published 2012 by John Wiley & Sons, Ltd.

Table 15.1 Galactosialidosis patients reported in the literature.

Patient/Gender	Origin	Age of onset	Reported age	Clinical type	Mutation 1	Protein	Mutation 2	Protein
1/F	Japanese	0 month	6 months	EI	1184 A > C	Y395C	268-269 TC > CT	S90L
2/M	Japanese	0 month	13 months	EI	1184 A > C	Y395C	?	?
3/F	French-German	3 months	18 years	LI	751 T > A	Y249N	?	?
4/F	Japanese	4 years	17 years	J/A	1184 A > C	Y395C	IVS7 A > G + 3	truncated
5/M	Japanese	6 years	27 years	J/A	146 A > G	Q49R	IVS7 A > G + 3	truncated
6/M	Japanese	7 years	15 years	J/A	1184 A > G	Y395C	IVS7 A > G + 3	truncated
7/F	Japanese	14 years	20 years	J/A	193 T > C	W65R	IVS7 A > G + 3	truncated
8/M	Italian	0 month	2.5 months†	EI	394 G > A	V132M	707 T > C	L236P
9/F	German	1 month	2 months†	EI	1315 G > A	G439S	?	?
10/F	American	0 month	3.5 years	LI/EI	1318 T > G	F440S	1217 T > C	M406T
11/M	Italian	14 months	22 years	LI	1318 T > G	F440S	1318 G > A	F440S
12/F	Canadian	2 months	20 years	LI	1318 T > G	F440S	745 T > A	Y249N
13/M	Canadian	1 year	19 years	LI	745 T > A	Y249N	?	?
14/F	American	8 months	24 years	LI	745 T > A	Y249N	112 del. C	truncated
15/M	Japanese/Dutch	8 years	48 years†	J/A	152 C > A	S51Y	IVS7 A > G + 3	truncated
16/F	Dutch	0 month	6 weeks	EI	253 G > A	G85S	889 ins. C	truncated
17/F	Dutch	0 month	8 months	EI	889 ins. C	truncated	889 ins. C	truncated
18/F	Arabic	?	7 years	LI	1357 A > G	K453E	?	?
19/F	Italian	0 month	52 days†	EI	IVS7 A > G +3	truncated	180 del. G	truncated
20/F	Polish/Italian/Canadian	7 months	18 years	LI	517 del. TT	truncated	IVS8 C > G + 9	truncated

F, female; M, male; ?, not reported, unknown, or not identified; EI, early infantile; LI, late infantile; J/A, juvenile/adult.

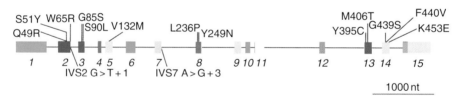

Figure 15.1 Genomic organization of the *CTSA* gene. Boxes represent exons 1 through 15; exons 1 and 15 contain UTRs. Two intronic splice mutations and 13 amino acid substitutions caused by missense exonic mutations are indicated below and above the gene, respectively.

belong to the juvenile/adult group and are mainly of Japanese origin. Myoclonus, ataxia, angiokeratoma, mental retardation, neurological deterioration, absence of visceromegaly and long survival are quite characteristic of this subtype.

Genetic basis

The gene encoding PPCA (*CTSA*, Genomic coordinates (GRCh37): 20:44 519 590–44 527 458) is located on chromosome *20q13*. The *CTSA* gene overlaps at its 5′and 3′

ends with two other genes both transcribed from the antisense strand relative to *CTSA*. The gene at the 3′ end (*PLTP*) encodes a phospholipid transfer protein whereas that at the 5′ end (*NEURL2*) encodes OZZ, a striated muscle-specific E3-ubiquitin ligase. Nineteen disease-causing mutations have been identified in the *CTSA* gene, the majority of which are missense mutations resulting in single amino acid substitutions (Table 15.1 and Figure 15.1). Other reported mutations include nonsense mutations, frameshift mutations or absence of the *CTSA* mRNA leading to either premature termination of the translated protein and a truncated protein product or the complete lack of the PPCA protein. The patients are either homozygous or compound heterozygous for the *CTSA* mutations (Table 15.1). Their parents are non-symptomatic heterozygous carriers. Generally, there is a good correlation between the type of *CTSA* mutation, the level of residual cathepsin A enzyme activity and the severity of the clinical phenotype. Mutations that result in up to 7% residual enzyme activity are typically associated with the juvenile or juvenile/adult phenotype (Table 15.1). Several of the identified amino acid substitutions were modelled into the tertiary structure of the PPCA precursor: none affected the catalytic machinery, but rather disrupted the integrity and stability of the enzyme. Notably two engineered active site mutations were shown not to affect the protective properties of the enzyme towards the two glycosidases (see below). This finding suggested that if such genetic mutations were to occur naturally, they would not result in a galactosialidosis phenotype.

Biochemistry

PPCA is a serine carboxypeptidase, which is synthesized as a 54-kDa zymogen and processed in lysosomes into a two-chain mature form of 32 and 20 kDa after endoproteolytic removal of a 2-kDa internal peptide. The enzyme carries two N-linked glycans, one on each chain, and is routed to the lysosome via the mannose-6-phosphate receptor pathway. PPCA has the unique capacity to specifically bind to β-GAL and NEU1 shortly after synthesis. Association of the three proteins in an early biosynthetic compartment assures the regulated trafficking of the two glycosidases to the lysosome as well as their intralysosomal activation and stable conformation in a multi-enzyme complex. Besides its chaperone-like function and protective properties, PPCA is catalytically active at both acidic and neutral pH and functions as cathepsin A/deaminase/esterase on a subset of neuropeptides, including substance P, oxytocin and endothelin-I. In a recent study multiple binding sites on the surfaces of both PPCA and NEU1 were identified that appear to be essential for the interaction of the two enzymes. One of these PPCA-binding sites on NEU1 can also bind to other NEU1 molecules, albeit with lower affinity. Therefore, in absence of PPCA, NEU1 tends to self-associate into chain-like oligomers and form insoluble aggregates. Thus, PPCA prevents aberrant self-association of NEU1 by promoting the formation of a PPCA–NEU1 heterodimeric complex. The proposed mechanism of interaction between NEU1 and PPCA provides a rationale for the secondary deficiency of NEU1 in galactosialidosis. In addition to a complete loss of NEU1 and a partial loss of β-GAL and N-acetylgalactosamine-6-sulfate-sulfatase activities, cathepsin A activity was found to be completely or partially deficient in cultured fibroblasts or lymphocytes of all tested patients with galactosialidosis.

Pathophysiology

Galactosialidosis belongs to the glycoproteinosis subgroup of lysosomal storage diseases (see Chapter 14) and affects primarily the reticuloendothelial system. In patients with this disease the secondary NEU1-deficiency, which preferentially targets the cleavage of α2-3- and α2-6-linked sialic acid residues on glycoproteins, leads to the accumulation of N-acetyllactosamine-type sialyloligosaccharides and glycopeptides in multiple tissues and body fluids. Fibroblasts and urine of galactosialidosis patients contain fully sialylated di- and triantennary N-linked oligosaccharides, and completely lack terminal galactose residues. Ultrastructural and histochemical analysis of patient-derived hepatocytes and Kupffer cells in the liver, glomerular and tubular epithelial cells in the kidney, as well as cultured fibroblasts has revealed the presence of numerous membrane-bound vacuoles filled with storage material. The severe secondary deficiency of NEU1, rather than the partial deficiency of β-GAL, is thought to be the primary contributing factor to the pathophysiology of galactosialidosis. This is supported by the fact that patients with galactosialidosis share several of the key clinical and biochemical features of patients with the lysosomal storage disease sialidosis (OMIM 256550), caused by structural lesions in the *NEU1* gene. In contrast, patients with GM1-gangliosidosis and Morquio B syndrome (OMIM 230500, 230650, 230600, 253010), with a primary defect in β-GAL, develop a glycosphingolipid storage disease that affects primarily the central nervous system, and a systemic disease without central nervous system involvement, respectively.

Diagnosis

The diagnosis of galactosialidosis can be suspected in patients with clinical features of a lysosomal storage disease who show Hurler-like facial features, growth retardation, sialyloligosacchariduria and vacuolated lymphocytes in their peripheral blood. The demonstration of a combined

Wild type   *Ctsa* knockout

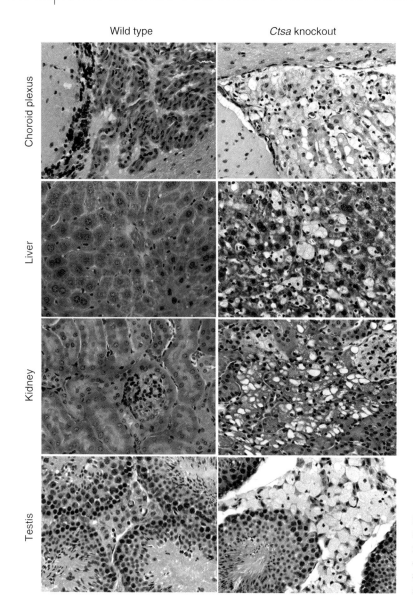

Choroid plexus

Liver

Kidney

Testis

Figure 15.2 H&E staining of tissue sections from galactosialidosis (*Ctsa*-knockout) mice showing extensive vacuolization of different cell types in multiple organs compared to the corresponding wild-type sections. Magnification 40×.

deficiency of β-GAL and NEU1 in lymphocytes and/or cultured skin fibroblasts is the preferred method of biochemical diagnosis. Mutation analysis based on DNA sequencing of the exons and the intron–exon junctions unequivocally establishes the diagnosis when a mutation is detected. In non-immune hydrops foetalis pregnancies, or when both parents are known heterozygous carriers, prenatal diagnosis may be performed by measuring cathepsin A and neuraminidase activities, or by DNA mutation analysis on either chorionic villi, amniotic fluid, and cultured amniotic cells.

Mouse model

Disruption of the *Ctsa* gene in mice results in systemic and CNS symptoms that resemble closely the early-infantile phenotype in galactosialidosis patients. Null mice have a shorter lifespan (~7–8 months) and present with signs of the disease soon after birth. Progressive and diffuse edema is accompanied by ataxic movements and tremor. Most tissues show characteristic vacuolization of specific cells attributable to lysosomal storage (Figure 15.2). The brain shows a regional distribution of

Kidney   Spleen

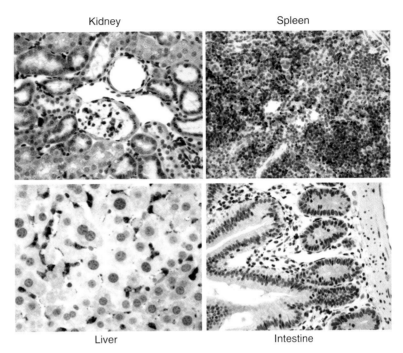

Liver   Intestine

Figure 15.3 Immunohistochemistry with PPCA antibody of tissue sections from galactosialidosis mice treated with insect cell-produced recombinant PPCA showing sustained expression of the PPCA protein in Kupffer cells of the liver and resident macrophages of the spleen, kidney, and intestine. Magnification 40×.

affected neurons and glial cells, and progressive loss of Purkinje cells in the cerebellum. Nephropathy, which is a major complication and cause of death in early-infantile patients, is also the most apparent cause of physical deterioration in affected mice. Excessive excretion of sialylated oligosaccharides in the urine is consistent with the severe reduction of NEU1 activity in all tissues tested.

Treatment

Currently, there is no treatment available for patients with galactosialidosis. Initial therapeutic studies in the galactosialidosis mouse model demonstrated complete reversal of systemic organ pathology when mutant mice were transplanted with bone marrow from transgenic mice over expressing human PPCA in the erythroid or myeloid lineages. Subsequent studies have shown that both the systemic and, to some extent, the CNS phenotypes could be corrected by transplanting mice with *Ctsa*-null bone marrow cells genetically-modified *ex-vivo* with a retroviral vector encoding PPCA. Complete reversal of the systemic organ pathology was also achieved by injecting 1-month-old galactosialidosis mice with recombinant insect cell-expressed PPCA. The enzyme was taken up by Kupffer

cells in the liver and by resident macrophages in other systemic organs (Figure 15.3), restoring cathepsin A activity and rescuing the secondary Neu1-deficiency. More recently, successful clearance of lysosomal storage in all systemic organs was obtained by intravenous injection of recombinant AAV (adeno-associated virus) vector encoding PPCA.

References

1 d'Azzo A, Andria G, Strisciuglio P, Galjaard H. Galactosialidosis. In: Scriver C, et al. (eds.), *The Metabolic and Molecular Bases of Inherited Disease* (8th edn.). New York: McGraw-Hill Publishing Co., 2001: pp. 3811–3826.

2 Zhou XY, Morreau H, Rottier R, *et al*. Mouse model for the lysosomal disorder galactosialidosis and correction of the phenotype with overexpressing erythroid precursor cells. *Genes Dev* 1995 Nov 1; **9**(21): 2623–2634.

3 Groener J, Maaswinkel-Mooy P, Smit V, *et al*. New mutations in two Dutch patients with early infantile galactosialidosis. *Mol Genet Metab* 2003 Mar; **78**(3): 222–228.

4 Galjart NJ, Gillemans N, Harris A, *et al*. Expression of cDNA encoding the human "protective protein" associated with lysosomal beta-galactosidase and neuraminidase: homology to yeast proteases. *Cell* 1988 Sep 9; **54**(6): 755–764.

5 Leimig T, Mann L, Martin Mdel P, *et al.* Functional amelioration of murine galactosialidosis by genetically modified bone marrow hematopoietic progenitor cells. *Blood* 2002 May 1; **99**(9): 3169–3178.

6 Bonten EJ, Campos Y, Zaitsev V, *et al.* Heterodimerization of the sialidase NEU1 with the chaperone protective protein/cathepsin A prevents its premature oligomerization. *J Biol Chem* 2009 Oct 9; **284**(41): 28430–28441.

7 Rudenko G, Bonten E, Hol W, d'Azzo A. The atomic model of the human protective protein/cathepsin A suggests a structural basis for galactosialidosis. *Proc Natl Acad Sci USA* 1998; **95**: 621–625.

CHAPTER 16

Multiple Enzyme Deficiencies

16.1 Defects in Transport: Mucolipidosis II alpha/beta, Mucolipidosis III alpha/beta and Mucolipidosis III gamma

Annick Raas-Rothschild,[1] Sandra Pohl[2] and Thomas Braulke[2]

[1] Department of Human Genetics and Metabolic Diseases, Hadassah Hebrew University Medical Center, Jerusalem, Israel
[2] Department of Biochemistry, Children's Hospital, University Medical Center Hamburg-Eppendorf, Hamburg, Germany

16.2 Multiple Sulfatase Deficiency

Graciana Diez-Roux and Andrea Ballabio

Telethon Institute of Genetics and Medicine, Naples, Italy

16.1 Defects in Transport: Mucolipidosis II alpha/beta, Mucolipidosis III alpha/beta and Mucolipidosis III gamma

Mucolipidosis type II (ML II) and mucolipidosis type III (ML III) are autosomal recessive disorders caused by defects in the N-acetylglucosamine-1-phosphotransferase (GlcNAc-1-phosphotransferase) complex, which is composed of three subunits, α, β and γ. Mutations in the gene encoding the alpha/beta subunits (*GNPTAB*) lead to ML II alpha/beta, which was also called I-cell disease (OMIM #252500), or to the clinically milder condition, ML III alpha/beta (OMIM #252600), which was formerly called pseudo-Hurler polydystrophy (ML IIIA – Table 16.1). ML III gamma (OMIM #252605), which was formerly called variant ML IIIC, arises from mutations in the gene encoding the γ subunit of GlcNAc-1-phosphotransferase (*GNPTG*) [1]. The GlcNAc-1-phosphotransferase complex catalyses the first step in the generation of the mannose 6-phosphate (Man6P) recognition marker required for efficient targeting of soluble lysosomal proteins (acid hydrolases and activator proteins) to lysosomes [2].

Case histories

Case history for ML II alpha/beta

Ultrasound examination of a foetus at week 24 of pregnancy showed a short femur with increased echogenicity and polyhydramnion. The child was born at week 37 and presented soon after birth with bowed legs, gingival hypertrophy, coarse face and respiratory difficulties (achydyspnea). X-ray examination of the bones showed osteopenia, wide ribs and other additional findings consistent with dysostosis multiplex. At 5 months she had growth deficiency with short stature (55 cm [–3SD]) and failure to gain weight (4.5 kg [–3SD]) (Figure 16.1). Echocardiogram revealed a thickened aortic and mitral valve. No hepatosplenomegaly was observed.

The activities of the serum lysosomal enzymes, arylsulfatase A, β-galactosidase and β-glucuronidase were elevated 10-fold. Mutation analysis of the *GNPTAB* gene showed a homozygous deletion (c.3503_4delTC) leading to a frameshift and a premature termination (p.L1168QfsX5). The constellation of the clinical,

Lysosomal Storage Disorders: A Practical Guide, First Edition. Edited by Atul Mehta and Bryan Winchester.
© 2012 John Wiley & Sons, Ltd. Published 2012 by John Wiley & Sons, Ltd.

biochemical and molecular findings permitted confirmation of the diagnosis of ML II.

Case history for ML III alpha/beta

A 3-year-old girl presented with severe claw hands, genu valgum, a severe kyphosis, and contractures of the hips and knees but without facial dysmorphism. The contractures of the fingers and large joints had been noticed as first symptoms by her parents at the time of consultation. Her psychomotor development was normal for her age. Her height was 80 cm (–3SD). She had no hepatosplenomegaly or gingival hypertrophy. Echocardiography revealed mitral valve thickening. X-rays of the spine showed kyphosis, platyspondyly, anterior–inferior beaking of L2; and the iliac wings were small. The girl presented with mild coxa valga of the femoral heads. The activities of the serum lysosomal enzymes arylsulfatase A, β-galactosidase and β-glucuronidase were elevated 20-fold. The combination of clinical findings and the elevated lysosomal serum enzyme activities led to the suspicion that the patient was affected with ML III because of the less severe phenotype than ML II. The patient was compound heterozygous for the mutations c.1120 T > C (p.F374L) and c.6565 C > T (p.R1189X) in the *GNPTAB* gene, which confirmed the diagnosis of ML III alpha/beta.

Case history for ML III gamma

A 12-year-old boy presented with claw hands, genu valgum, progressive stiffness of the fingers and reduced joint mobility of the knees and hips and shoulders. The claw hands had been observed as first symptoms at the age of 6 years. He had normal psychomotor development and went to a regular school. He had no facial dysmorphism. In addition he presented with a mild kyphosis and genu valgum (Figure 16.2). His height was 130 cm (–2SD). He had neither hepatosplenomegaly nor gingival hypertrophy. Echocardiography revealed mild mitral valve thickening. He had been followed up in the rheumatologic clinic for suspected rheumatoid arthritis since the age of 10 years. X-ray examination of the spine showed mild kyphosis, and mild platyspondyly. He had mild coxa valga of the hips and dystrophic changes of the femoral heads.

The activities of the lysosomal enzymes arylsulfatase A, β-galactosidase, and β-glucuronidase were elevated

15-fold in serum. The combination of relatively mild symptoms compared to patients with ML III alpha/beta and the elevated lysosomal enzyme activities led to the suspicion that the patient was affected with ML III gamma. This was confirmed by mutation analysis of the *GNPTG* gene which showed that the patient was homozygous for the mutation c.196 C > T, leading to a premature stop codon (p.Arg66X).

Epidemiology

ML II and ML III are rare lysosomal storage disorders with a variable prevalence of 0.16 (The Netherlands), 0.22 (Czech Republic), 0.31 (Australia), 0.4 (Japan) or 0.8 (north Portugal) per 100,000 live births for ML II. The highest ML II frequency, estimated at 16.2/100,000, has been found in Sanguenay-Lac-Saint-Jean (Quebec, Canada). The prevalence of ML III was reported to be 0.08 and 1.89 per 100,000 in The Netherlands and north Portugal, respectively.

Genetic basis

The GlcNAc-1-phosphotransferase complex is composed of three different subunits α, β, and γ in a molar ratio of 2:2:2 and is encoded by two genes. The *GNPTAB* gene, which is located at chromosome 12q23.3, encodes a 145 kDa α/β subunit precursor [3] that is catalytically activated by proteolytic cleavage by the site-1 protease involved in the cholesterol homeostasis [4] (Figure 16.3 [5]). The *GNPTG* gene, which is located at chromosome 16p13.3, encodes the soluble 36 kDa γ subunit of unknown function [6]. ML II alpha/beta and ML III alpha/beta patients carry mutations in *GNPTAB* whereas ML III gamma patients have mutations in the *GNPTG* gene.

Table 16.1 Classification of mucolipidosis types II and III.

	Former nomenclature	New nomenclature
I-cell disease	ML II	ML II alpha/beta
pseudo-Hurler Polydystrophy	ML IIIA	ML III alpha/beta
ML III variant	ML IIIC	ML III gamma

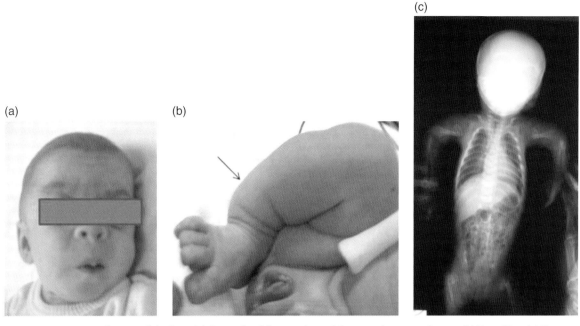

Figure 16.1 Patient with ML II alpha/beta. (a) Coarse facial features, long philtrum and antevarted nares. (b) Bowed leg. (c) X-ray of the spine showing severe hip dysplasia, and dysostosis multiplex of the lower limbs bones.

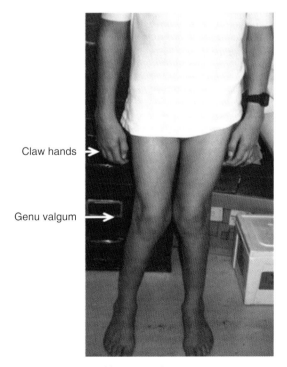

Figure 16.2 12-year-old patient with ML III gamma.

Pathophysiology

Defects in GlcNAc-1-phosphotransferase lead to missorting of multiple lysosomal hydrolases in mesenchymal cells especially fibroblasts and the lysosomal accumulation of different non-degraded macromolecules, lipids, amino acids or sugars (e.g. glycosaminoglycans, GM2-gangliosides, cholesterol, cystine or sialic acid). Many other cultured cells such as hepatocytes, Kupffer cells, and leukocytes exhibit normal levels of lysosomal enzyme activities. Therefore, peripheral leukocytes are not suitable for ML II and ML III diagnostics. In addition, in liver, kidney, spleen, and brain tissue of ML II patients nearly normal activities of lysosomal enzymes are detectable. The cellular consequences of the accumulating material are still unclear and appear to depend on the composition and extent of storage and the type of storing cells.

Clinical presentation

Neonates with ML II alpha/beta might show craniofacial abnormalities with striking gingival hypertrophy. Importantly, patients with clinical phenotypes intermediate between the ML II alpha/beta and ML III alpha/beta phenotypes have been reported with slower progression

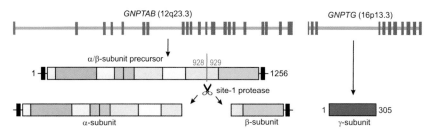

Figure 16.3 Organisation of the *GNPTAB* and *GNPTG* genes and their encoded α/β subunit precursor membrane protein (1,256 amino acids) and the soluble γ subunit (305 amino acids), respectively. The α/β subunit precursor is cleaved by the Golgi-resident site-1 protease into mature and enzymatically active α and β subunits (modified from Kollmann *et al.* 2010 [5]).

Table 16.2 Clinical findings and symptoms of mucolipidosis types II and III.

Typical time of onset	Disorder	Signs and symptoms
Prenatal	ML II alpha/beta	Short and bowed lower limbs; hips and knees contractures; bone fracture; transient alveolomaxillary defect (TAD); osteopenia; periosteal new bone formation ("cloaking").
Postnatal	ML II alpha/beta	**Dysmorphism**: coarse facies; gingival hypertrophy, short neck **Neurology**: Developmental delay; intellectual disabilities; hypotonia **Eyes**: corneal clouding **Skeletal**: short bowed limbs; joint contractures; pectus carinatum; thoracal asymmetry; congenital hip dislocation; osteopenia **Abdomen**: hepatosplenomegaly; umbilical hernia; inguinal hernia **Heart**: mitral valve thickening; dilated cardiomyopathy transient neonatal hyperparathyroidism
Early infancy and adulthood	ML III alpha/beta & ML III gamma*	**Skeletal**: progressive joint stifness; stiffness of the small joints; claw hand; carpal tunnel syndrome; tarsal tunnel syndrome; scoliosis; kyphosis; hyperlordosis; genu valgum; shoulder, decreased mobility and/or contractures of knees and hip joints; upper limb paraesthesia; progressive growth retardation; C1-C2 instability; progressive bone dystrophy **X-rays**: progressive development of "J" shaped sella turcica; oar-shaped ribs; anterior inferior beaking of lower thoracic to upper lumbar vertebral bodies; flared iliac wings; progressive dysplasia of the femoral heads and necks; coxa valga; "bullet-shaped" proximal phalanges and central pointing of proximal metacarpals **Eyes**: hyperopic astigmatism and corneal clouding; retinal and optic nerve abnormalities **Heart**: aortic and /or mitral valve thickening; dilated cardiomyopathy **Abdomen**: umbilical hernia; inguinal hernia

*The ML III gamma patients seems to have a milder clinical picture than the ML III alpha/beta patients.

than ML II alpha/beta and more severe progression than ML III alpha/beta phenotypes (Table 16.2).

ML III alpha/beta and ML III gamma are slowly progressive disorders mainly affecting skeletal, joint and connective tissues. Clinical onset is in early childhood with restricted joint mobility, and skeletal changes that mainly affect the pelvis and spine. ML III gamma seems to be less severe than ML III alpha/beta.

Natural history

ML II alpha/beta is a severe disease with onset of signs and symptoms at birth and a fatal outcome most often in early childhood. ML III alpha/beta patients show first clinical symptoms at approximately 3 years of age whereas data on life expectancy are missing. The onset of first symptoms in ML III gamma patients is in

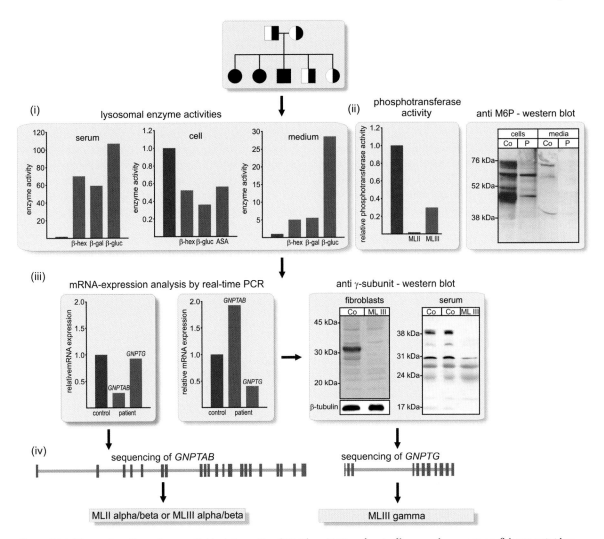

Figure 16.4 Diagnostic pathway for mucolipidosis types II and III. The activities of a set of lysosomal enzymes, e.g. β-hexosaminidase (β-hex), β-glucuronidase (β-gluc), β-galactosidase (β-gal), and arylsulfatase A (ASA) should be measured in the serum, in extracts of cultured fibroblasts and conditioned media. In comparison to controls (black column) the activities of the lysosomal enzymes are decreased in patient cells but increased in serum and conditioned cell media, demonstrating the missorting of lysosomal enzymes. (ii) Defects in the generation of the Man6P recognition marker can be analyzed by radioactive measurement of GlcNAc-1-phosphotransferase activity in extracts of cultured cells, or by Man6P-western blotting of cell extracts and aliquots of conditioned media. Both experimental approaches support the diagnosis of ML II or ML III. (iii) Since many of the known mutation in *GNPTAB* or *GNPTG* lead to frameshift and unstable transcripts due to "nonsense-mediated mRNA decay", the mRNA expression of *GNPTAB/GNPTG* is performed in fibroblasts. Reduced *GNPTG* mRNA levels have been reported to be accompanied by compensatory up-regulation of *GNPTAB* mRNA. The decreased expression of *GNPTG* mRNA can be confirmed by western blotting for the human γ subunit. (iv) The direct sequencing and DNA analysis of the *GNPTAB* or *GNPTG* genes allow the diagnosis of ML II alpha/beta or ML III alpha/beta or gamma.

infancy as well and they are known to survive to the fourth or fifth decades; the oldest reported patient was 86 years old [7]. ML III might be misdiagnosed as rheumatoid arthritis.

Laboratory diagnosis

Increases (5- to 25-fold) in lysosomal enzyme activities in patient serum or dried blood compared to controls are typical and reflect the biochemical missorting and subsequent hypersecretion of lysosomal enzymes (such as β-hexosaminidase, β-galactosidase, α-L-fucosidase, β-glucuronidase). In cultured fibroblasts, the levels of lysosomal enzyme activities are elevated 5- to 20-fold in the medium but decreased intracellularly. ML II is distinguished from ML III on the basis of the clinical severity and time of first symptoms and not on the basis of the hydrolase activities.

The GlcNAc-1-phosphotransferase activity can be directly determined in white blood cells and fibroblasts using the metabolically labelled [^{32}P]UDP-GlcNAc substrate. Recently, a specific and non-radioactive tool, a single-chain antibody fragment recognizing Man6P-residues, has been introduced in laboratory diagnosis of ML II and ML III allowing the fast and sensitive immunodetection of Man6P-containing proteins. However, both radioactive GlcNAc-1-phosphotransferase activity measurements and Man6P western blotting are available in only a few research laboratories. Furthermore, decreases in *GNPTAB* or *GNPTG* mRNA levels may be indicators of mutation-induced mRNA instability, which requires the sequencing of the respective genes. It is useful to examine both the *GNPTAB* and *GNPTG* genes at the genomic and cDNA levels to identify intronic splice mutations and deletions as well. Patients with a severe phenotype should be directly examined for mutations in the *GNPTAB* gene (Figure 16.4).

Prenatal diagnosis in families at risk is done by analysis of DNA extracted from foetal cells obtained by chorionic villus sampling (CVS) at approximately 11 weeks of gestation or amniocentesis usually performed at approximately 17 weeks of gestation. The disease-causing mutations in the family must have been identified before prenatal testing is performed. Preimplantation genetic diagnosis (PGD) may be available for families in which the disease-causing mutations have been identified.

Treatment

1. Therapy depends on the severity of the disease and treatment is essentially symptomatic. Physiotherapy might be helpful if gentle, especially aquatherapy.

2. Surgery might be indicated in the following situations:
   (a) inguinal and umbilical hernia
   (b) carpal and tarsal tunnel syndromes
   (c) recurrent otitis media with myringotomy
   (d) joint replacement when needed

3. There is a need for special care regarding anesthesia in patients with mucolipidosis II/III.

4. Symptomatic treatment with cyclic intravenous pamidronate, with the aim of preventing or treating osteopenia/osteoporosis, is a possible adjunctive therapy that has been evaluated for a few patients with ML III alpha/beta [8].

5. It is recommended that families are referred to genetic clinics to receive genetic counselling for family planning.

References

1 Cathey SS, Kudo M, Tiede S, *et al.* Molecular order in mucolipidosis II and III nomenclature. *Am J Med Genet A* 2008; **146A**: 512–513.

2 Kornfeld S, Sly WS. I-cell disease and pseudo-Hurler polydystrophy: disorder of lysosomal enzyme phosphorylation and localization. In: Scriver CR, *et al.* (eds.), *The Metabolic and Molecular Bases of Inherited Disease*. New York: McGraw-Hill Inc., USA; pp. 3421–3452.

3 Tiede S, Storch S, Lübke T, *et al.* Mucolipidosis II is caused by mutations in GNPTA encoding the α/β GlcNAc-1-phosphotransferase. *Nat Med* 2005; **11**: 1109–1112.

4 Marschner K, Kollmann K, Schweizer M, *et al.* A key enzyme in the biogenesis of lysosomes is a protease that regulates cholesterol metabolism. *Science* 2011; **333**: 87–90.

5 Kollmann K, Pohl S, Marschner K, *et al.* Mannose phosphorylation in health and disease. *Eur J Cell Biol* 2010; **89**: 117–123.

6 Raas-Rothschild A, Cormier-Daire V, Bao M, *et al.* Molecular basis of variant pseudo-Hurler polydystrophy (mucolipidosis IIIC). *J Clin Invest* 2000; **105**: 673–681.

7 Leroy JG. Oligosaccharidoses, disorders allied to the oligosaccharides. In: Rimoin DL (eds.), *Emery and Rimoin's Principles and Practice of Medical Genetics* (5th edn.). Philadelphia, PA: Churchill Livingstone, 2007: pp. 2413–2448.

8 Robinson C, Baker N, Noble J, *et al.* The osteodystrophy of mucolipidosis type III and the effects of intravenous pamidronate treatment. *J Inherit Metab Dis* 2002; **25**: 681–693.

16.2 Multiple Sulfatase Deficiency

MSD (Online Mendelian Inheritance in Man #272200) is a rare autosomal recessive disorder (prevalence 1 in 1.4 million births) in which affected individuals present a complex phenotype due to the impaired activity of all sulfatases. The lack of sulfatase activities in MSD patients leads to the accumulation of sulfated lipids and glycosaminoglycans resulting in a clinical phenotype that combines the features of at least six diseases due to individual sulfatase deficiencies: metachromatic leukodystrophy (ML D), X-linked ichthyosis, and mucopolysacccharidoses type II, IIIA, IIID, IVA and VI ([1]).

Clinical presentation

The first case of MSD was described in 1963 by Austin. MSD patients are characterized by a complex phenotype that includes features observed in single sulfatase deficiencies such as multisystemic features, rapid neurological deterioration and developmental delay [1]. Increased amounts of glycosaminoglycans are found in several tissues and there is excessive excretion of glycosaminoglycans and sulfatide in the urine. Cerebrospinal fluid protein is increased. Peripheral nerves show metachromatic degeneration of myelin on biopsy.

Genetic basis

MSD is due to mutations in the sulfatase modifying factor 1 (SUMF1) gene (3p26.1). This gene was discovered by two completely independent and complementary approaches, one biochemical and the other genetic [2, 3]. A mutational analysis of SUMF1 in 20 MSD patients of different ethnic origin identified a total of 22 *SUMF1* mutations, including missense, nonsense, microdeletion, and splicing mutations [4]. The results showed lack of a direct correlation between the type of molecular defect and the severity of phenotype. However, other studies demonstrated that the phenotypic outcome in MSD depends on both the residual activity and stability of the SUMF1 protein [5]. In all MSD patients, residual sulfatase activities are detectable, at variable levels. To correlate the nature of the residual sulfatase activities detected in MSD patients with residual SUMF1 activity, four SUMF1mutants (i.e. p.S155P, p. 224W, p.R345C, p.R349W) found in homozygosity in MSD patients were analyzed. Using viral-mediated gene delivery, these mutants were over-expressed in mouse embryonic fibroblasts (MEFs) from a *Sumf1* KO mouse line that is completely devoid of all sulfatase activities ([6]. The results obtained indicated that mutant *SUMF1* cDNAs encode stable *SUMF1* proteins that are of the appropriate molecular weight and are properly localized in the endoplasmic reticulum. Expression of these cDNAs in *Sumf1-/-* MEFs resulted in partial rescue of sulfatase activities. These data indicate that MSD is due to hypomorphic *SUMF1* mutations [7] and suggest that a complete lack of SUMF1 function in humans could be lethal.

Biochemistry

Interestingly, the study of MSD led to the discovery of a novel biological mechanism. The landmark of this disorder, impaired activity of all known sulfatases, suggested that these enzymes not only shared a common biochemical role but also a common regulation of their activity. The first experimental evidence suggesting that the defect underlying MSD did not directly affect sulfatase genes was a series of complementation studies performed by fusing MSD cells with cells from patients with a single sulfatase deficiency, in these experiments the activity for each deficiency was restored demonstrating that the genes for sulfatases are not affected [8–10].

Further experiments demonstrated that the expression of sulfatase cDNAs in MSD fibroblasts yielded sulfatases with severely diminished enzymatic activity. These results strongly suggested that the defect in MSD did not affect the transcription or translation of sulfatase genes and supported the hypothesis that the molecular defect is a co- or post-translational mechanism that is common to all sulfatases and is required for their catalytic activity [11]. The search for the protein modification present in active sulfatases but absent in the inactive MSD sulfatases revealed that sulfatases undergo a unique post-translational modification of an active site cysteine residue to 2-amino-3-oxopropanoic acid (α-formylglycine) [12]. The modification involves the conversion of a thiol into an aldehyde group. This finding strongly suggested that MSD was caused by a mutation of a gene, or genes, implicated in the cysteine-to-formylglycine conversion machinery. The modified cysteine residue is highly conserved across evolution and present in all sulfatases, with the exception of a few bacterial sulfatases, which have a serine, instead of the cysteine, at the same location. Interestingly, this serine also gets modified into α-formylglycine using a different mechanism [13].

Further studies *in vitro* demonstrated that the post-translational modification occurs on unfolded sulfatase polypeptides within the endoplasmic reticulum

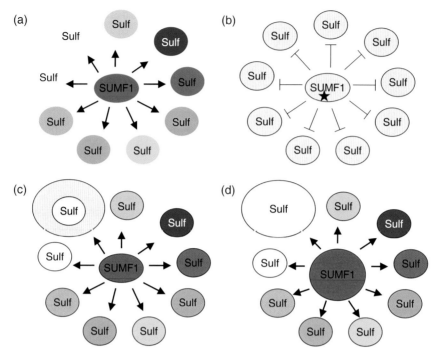

Figure 16.5 SUMF 1 is both an essential and a limiting factor for the activity of sulfatases: (a) SUMF1 activates sulfatases in physiological conditions; (b) if SUMF1 is mutated, as in MSD, the activity of all sulfatases is impaired; (c) if a sulfatase is overexpressed, the activity is partial (coloured circle) due to the limiting amount of SUMF1 protein; (d) a complete activation of a sulfatase only occurs when both the sulfatase and SUMF1 are overexpressed. (Reproduced from Cosma *et al.* [10] with permission from Elsevier.)

immediately after translation [14]. A thorough analysis consisting of multiple or single amino acid substitutions on the minimal sequence necessary for the modification to occur revealed that a sequence determinant directs the conversion of cysteine to formylglycine in eukaryotic sulfatases [15]. Only 11 amino acid residues beginning at the cysteine to be modified to FGly are necessary to direct the conversion. Mutation and truncation of this targeting sequence revealed that a core motif, C(X/T)P(X/S)R, is the minimum sequence required to obtain modest amounts of modification [16, 17]. Only the cysteine that is modified to FGly is required for the modification to occur, if this cysteine is modified there is no activity, if any other amino acid in the core sequence is modified some activity is retained. The cysteine to FGly post-translational modification of sulfatases is carried out by the formylglycine generating enzyme, which is encoded by the SUMF1 gene. The crystal structure of the formylglycine-generating enzyme revealed that it is a single-domain monomer, which adopts a unique fold but otherwise has a surprising

paucity of secondary structure. In addition, this crystal structure revealed two crucial cysteine residues in the active site, one of which is thought to be implicated in substrate binding. The other cysteine residue partakes in a novel oxygenase mechanism whereby FGE utilizes molecular oxygen to generate FGly via a cysteine sulfenic acid intermediate [18].

The functional analysis of SUMF1 revealed that co-expression of SUMF1 with sulfatases resulted in a strikingly synergistic increase in enzymatic activity, indicating that SUMF1 is both essential and a limiting factor for sulfatases [2] (Figure 16.5). The sulfatase activity of all three sulfatases tested (ARSC, ARSA and ARSE arylsulfatases A C and E) showed a dramatic increase (20 to 50 fold) when co-expressed with SUMF1 [2]. Further studies demonstrated that SUMF1 enhances sulfatase activities *in vivo* in five sulfatase deficiencies [19]. These results indicate that a sulfatase overexpressed alone is only partially activated; the threshold for the full activation of all the overexpressed sulfatases is the limiting amount of

SUMF1. These data have significant implications for the *in vitro* production of sulfatases for enzyme replacement therapy, which currently relies on the use of SUMF1.

Pathophysiology

A mouse line carrying a null mutation in the *Sumf1* gene (*Sumf1*(-/-)) recapitulates the human syndrome phenotype and displays early mortality, congenital growth retardation, skeletal abnormalities, and neurological defects [6]. The thorough analysis of tissues from these mice showed progressive cell vacuolization and significant lysosomal storage of glycosaminoglycans. A generalized inflammatory process characterized by a massive presence of highly vacuolated macrophages also characterized the knockout mice. Astroglyosis and neuronal cell loss were detected in the cerebellum and brain cortex associated to activated microglia. At later stages, there was a strong increase in the expression levels of inflammatory cytokines and of apoptotic markers in both the CNS and liver. Further studies showed that there is an accumulation of autophagosomes in MSD brain and in cultured MSD cells. This accumulation is due to an impaired autophagosome-lysosome fusion and a block of the autophagic pathway leads to the accumulation of dysfunctional mitochondria and of polyubiquitinated proteins [20, 21].

Diagnosis

A complex clinical phenotype is observed in MSD patients. The clinical phenotype may include features of single sulfatase deficiencies including rapid neurodegeneration and developmental delay gargoyle-like features, visceromegaly, skeletal involvement (dysostosis multiplex), ichthyosis, and chondrodysplasia punctate [1]. Biochemical confirmation of a diagnosis of MSD is made measuring the pattern of sulfatase activities in leukocytes, plasma and cultured fibroblasts from individual patients [1]. Molecular diagnosis can be made by searching for mutations in the SUMF1 gene [4].

Treatment

There is to date no effective treatment for MSD. Recent studies, performed in the MSD mouse model, showed that the combined, administration of an rAAV9 vector encoding the *SUMF1* gene into intracerebral ventricles and systemically resulted in the global activation of sulfatases, near-complete clearance of glycosaminoglycans

(GAGs) and decrease of inflammation in both the central nervous system (CNS) and visceral organs. Furthermore, behavioural abilities were improved by this combined treatment [22]. In addition, a novel approach based on the transcriptional activation of lysosomal exocytosis rescued pathologic storage and restored normal cellular morphology both *in vitro* and *in vivo* in multiple sulfatase deficiency [23].

References

1 Hopwood JJ, Ballabio A. Multiple sulfatase deficiency and the nature of the sulfatase family. In: Scriver CR, *et al.* (eds.), *The Metabolic and Molecular Basis of Inherited Disease*. New York: McGraw-Hill, 2001; pp. 3725–3732.

2 Cosma MP, Pepe S, Annunziata I, *et al.* The multiple sulfatase deficiency gene encodes an essential and limiting factor for the activity of sulfatases. *Cell* 2003 May 16; **113**(4): 445–456.

3 Dierks T, Schmidt B, Borissenko LV, *et al.* Multiple sulfatase deficiency is caused by mutations in the gene encoding the human C(alpha)-formylglycine generating enzyme. *Cell* 2003 May 16; **113**(4): 435–444.

4 Cosma MP, Pepe S, Parenti G, *et al.* Molecular and functional analysis of SUMF1 mutations in multiple sulfatase deficiency. *Hum Mutat* 2004 Jun; **23**(6): 576–581.

5 Schlotawa L, Ennemann EC, Radhakrishnan K, *et al.* SUMF1 mutations affecting stability and activity of formylglycine generating enzyme predict clinical outcome in multiple sulfatase deficiency. *Eur J Hum Genet* [Research Support, Non-U.S. Gov't]. 2011 Mar; **19**(3): 253–261.

6 Settembre C, Annunziata I, Spampanato C, *et al.* Systemic inflammation and neuro-degeneration in a mouse model of multiple sulfatase deficiency. *Proc Natl Acad Sci USA* 2007 Mar 13; **104**(11): 4506–4511.

7 Annunziata I, Bouche V, Lombardi A, *et al.* Multiple sulfatase deficiency is due to hypomorphic mutations of the SUMF1 gene. *Hum Mutat* 2007 Sep; **28**(9): 928.

8 Horwitz AL. Genetic complementation studies of multiple sulfatase deficiency. *Proc Nat Acad Sci USA* 1979; **76** (No. 12): 6496–6499.

9 Chang PL, Davidson RG. Complementation of arylsulfatase A in somatic hybrids of metachromatic leukodystrophy and multiple sulfatase deficiency disorder fibroblasts. *Proc Natl Acad Sci USA* 1980; **77**(10): 6166–61670.

10 Ballabio A, Parenti G, Napolitano E, *et al.* Genetic complementation of steroid sulphatase after somatic cell hybridization of X-linked ichthyosis and multiple sulphatase deficiency. *Hum Genet* 1985; **70**: 315–317.

11 Rommerskirch W, von Figura K. Multiple sulfatase deficiency: catalytically inactive sulfatases are expressed from retrovirally introduced sulfatase cDNAs. *Proc Nat Acad Sci USA* 1992; **89**: 2561–2565.

12 Schmidt B, Selmer T, Ingendoh A, von Figura K. A novel amino acid modification in sulfatases that is defective in multiple sulfatase deficiency. *Cell* 1995 Jul 28; **82**(2): 271–278.

13 Miech C, Dierks T, Selmer T, *et al.* Arylsulfatase from Klebsiella pneumoniae carries a formylglycine generated from a serine. *J Biol Chem* 1998; **273**(9): 4835–4837.

14 Dierks T, Schmidt B, von Figura K. Conversion of cysteine to formylglycine: a protein modification in the endoplasmic reticulum. *Proc Natl Acad Sci USA* 1997; **94**(22): 11963–11968.

15 Dierks T, Lecca MR, Schlotterhose P, *et al.* Sequence determinants directing conversion of cysteine to formylglycine in eukaryotic sulfatases. *Embo J* 1999; **18**(8): 2084–2091.

16 Waldow A, Schmidt B, Dierks T, *et al.* Amino acid residues forming the active site of arylsulfatase A. Role in catalytic activity and substrate binding. *J Biol Chem* 1999; **274**(18): 12284–12288.

17 Recksiek M, Selmer T, Dierks T. Sulfatases, trapping of the sulfated enzyme intermediate by substituting the active site formylglycine. *J Biol Chem* 1998; **273**(11): 6096–6103.

18 Dierks T, Dickmanns A, Preusser-Kunze A, *et al.* Molecular basis for multiple sulfatase deficiency and mechanism for formylglycine generation of the human formylglycine-generating enzyme. *Cell* [Research Support, Non-U.S. Gov't] 2005 May 20; **121**(4): 541–552.

19 Fraldi A, Biffi A, Lombardi A, *et al.* SUMF1 enhances sulfatase activities in vivo in five sulfatase deficiencies. *Biochem J* 2007 Apr 15; **403**(2): 305–312.

20 Settembre C, Fraldi A, Jahreiss L, *et al.* A block of autophagy in lysosomal storage disorders. *Hum Mol Genet* 2008 Jan 1; **17**(1): 119–129.

21 Settembre C, Fraldi A, Rubinsztein DC, Ballabio A. Lysosomal storage diseases as disorders of autophagy. *Autophagy.* 2008 Jan 1; **4**(1): 113–114.

22 Spampanato C, De Leonibus E, Dama P, *et al.* Efficacy of a combined intracerebral and systemic gene delivery approach for the treatment of a severe lysosomal storage disorder. *Mol Ther* [Research Support, Non-U.S. Gov't]. 2011 May; **19**(5): 860–869.

23 Medina DL, Fraldi A, Bouche V, *et al.* Transcriptional activation of lysosomal exocytosis promotes cellular clearance. *Dev Cell* 2011; 21: 421–430.

CHAPTER 17

Lysosomal Membrane Defects

Michael Schwake and Paul Saftig

Biochemical Institute, Christian-Albrechts-University Kiel, Kiel, Germany

Introduction

There is increasing evidence that apart from the known disease-causing role of mutated lysosomal hydrolases, mutations in genes encoding for protein components of the lysosomal membrane are also of importance for the development of lysosomal disorders. Lysosomal membrane proteins are required for lysosomal biogenesis, autophagy, phagocytosis, acidification of the lysosomal lumen, cholesterol homeostasis, metabolite export and fusion events with other organelles. We briefly summarize the major clinical features of typical diseases caused by mutations in this class of proteins (Figure 17.1). On account of their non-enzymatic nature, defects in lysosomal membrane proteins cannot yet be corrected by conventional therapeutic approaches used for the treatment of classical lysosomal storage disorders. The in-depth analysis of these proteins by biochemical and functional studies may also provide new ideas of how to treat this novel class of lysosomal disorders.

Whereas the biogenesis and function of many lysosomal hydrolases are well characterized and the diseases caused by lack of their lysosomal delivery or enzymatic functions are extensively studied, little is known about the physiological role of proteins residing in the lysosomal membrane. The severe diseases caused by the impaired function of lysosomal membrane proteins dramatically underline the central role of these proteins for lysosomal and cellular physiology. More than 30 lysosomal membrane proteins are required to mediate a multitude of lysosomal functions including transport of metabolites and proteins across the membrane, membrane fusion and cellular trafficking of certain hydolases [1–3]

(Figure 17.2). We are only beginning to understand their role and function and how diseases develop in the case of mutated lysosomal membrane proteins. Genetic disorders of these proteins [4] cause a wide array of neurological and visceral symptoms and some of the important and most recently described diseases are summarized below.

Cystinosis

Genetic basis

CTNS, which is located at 17q13, encodes for cystinosin, which mediates the H^+-driven transport of cystine. Cystinosis (Online Mendelian Inheritance in Man #219800, #219900, #219750) is caused by intralysosomal storage of crystals of the amino acid cystine [5]. It is estimated that there are around 2000 patients worldwide and that the disease affects approximately 1 in 100,000 to 200,000 newborns with somewhat higher incidence in the North of France. A large number of different mutations, both homozygous and compound heterozygous, have been described. The most common mutation is a large deletion, which is responsible for about 50% of cystinosis cases in people of European descent.

Pathophysiology

Proximal tubule function in the kidney is impaired due to the intracellular accumulation of cystine crystals. The cellular pathology leads to a disturbed reabsorption of small molecules (Fanconi renal tubulopathy) very early in life.

Clinical presentation

Three clinical forms of cystinosis are known: infantile, adolescent and adult cystinosis. The majority of patients

Lysosomal Storage Disorders: A Practical Guide, First Edition. Edited by Atul Mehta and Bryan Winchester.
© 2012 John Wiley & Sons, Ltd. Published 2012 by John Wiley & Sons, Ltd.

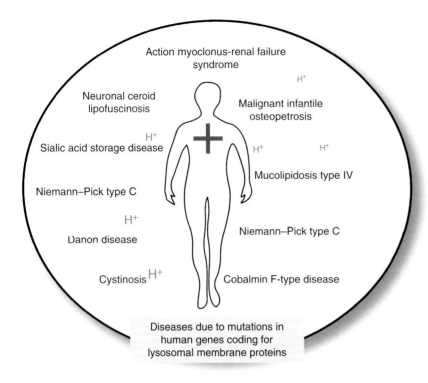

Figure 17.1 Brief overview of diseases caused by mutations in lysosomal membrane proteins. Most disorders are described in detail in this chapter. In addition, Mucolipidosis type IV (ML IV) is characterized by symptoms such as delayed psychomotor development and ocular aberrations. The disorder is caused by mutations in the MCOLN1 gene, which encodes a non-selective cation channel, mucolipin1. Mutations in the lysosomal membrane proteins ClC-7, a major chloride ion transporter or/and its subunit Ostm1 lead to malignant infantile osteopetrosis.

(around 95%) suffer from classical infantile or nephropathic cystinosis.

Laboratory diagnosis
Measurement of cystine levels in polymorphonuclear leukocytes and cultured fibroblasts is typically used for diagnosis. The prenatal diagnosis of cystinosis is based genetic analyses or on the determination of increased amount of free-cystine present in amniotic fluid cells.

Sialic acid storage disease
Genetic basis
Mutations in the SLC17A5 (solute carrier family 17 (anion/sugar transporter), member 5) gene, which is localized on chromosome 6q14–15, cause the different forms of sialic acid storage disease (SASD, Online Mendelian Inheritance in Man #604369, #269920). The gene product, sialin, transports free sialic acid out of the lysosomes. Sialin can also transport glucuronic and iduronic acids across the lysosomal membrane. Approximately 20 mutations have been identified in the *SLC17A5* gene. The majority of patients are from Finland, Sweden or the Netherlands. These mutations result in

loss of synthesis of the protein or defective transport of the protein to the lysosomal membrane.

Pathophysiology.
Mutations in the *SLC17A5* gene that reduce or eliminate sialin transport activity result in an accumulation of the acidic monosaccharide, sialic acid, in lysosomes, which increase in number and become swollen. It is still unexplained how this defect in the transport of sialic acid leads to a brain developmental defect and to neurodegeneration.

Clinical presentation.
Sialic acid storage disease [6] primarily affects the nervous system. Patients with sialic acid storage disease have signs and symptoms that may vary widely in severity. Infantile free sialic acid storage disease (ISSD) is the most severe form of this disorder. Severe developmental delay, coarse face, hypotonia, failure to thrive, the development of ascites, nephrosis, seizures, multiple dysostosis, hepatosplenomegaly, and cardiomegaly are hallmarks of ISSD. Affected infants may have foetal hydrops and hydrocephalus. Children with this severe form of the condition

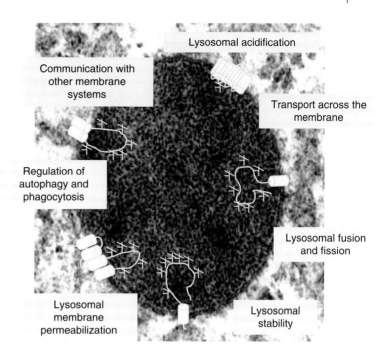

Figure 17.2 Multiple functions of lysosomal membrane proteins.

usually live only into early childhood. Salla disease is a less severe form of sialic acid storage disease, which leads to hypotonia during the first year of life and progressive neurological symptoms, intellectual disability, developmental delay, seizures, ataxia, spasticity and athetosis. Individuals with Salla disease usually survive into adulthood. People with a phenotype intermediate between that of classic Salla disease and ISSD have been described.

Laboratory diagnosis

The increased excretion of free sialic acid in the urine forms the basis of a screening test for SASD. Diagnosis is confirmed by quantitative measurement of of free sialic acid in the patient´s urine or fibroblasts and by mutation analysis of the sialin gene. Prenatal diagnosis is available for pregnancies known to be at risk by measurement of free sialic acid in amniotic fluid supernatant (AFS) or mutation analysis. The measurement of free sialic acid in AFS is also used to screen for SASD in cases of foetal hydrops. Prenatal diagnosis of a new case of Salla disease can be made by measuring the amount of sialic acid in fetal cells followed preferably by genetic testing.

Danon disease
Genetic basis
LAMP2, which is located at Xq24, encodes for one of the most abundant lysosomal membrane proteins

LAMP-2, which can be expressed in three isoforms (LAMP-2A, LAMP-2B and LAMP2-C). Danon Disease (Online Mendelian Inheritance in Man #300257) is caused by premature truncation of the LAMP-2 protein [7]. About 35 different mutations (frameshifts, stopcodons, and splicing site mutations) over the whole gene have been described to date. Most mutations are private, being reported in just a single family with the notable exceptions of recurrent mutations in exons 3 and 7.

Pathophysiology
The disease manifests as a serious skeletal and cardiac myopathy associated with morbidity and early mortality. A hallmark is the accumulation of autophagic vacuoles with sarcolemnal features in myofibres. LAMP-2 has been postulated to control the autophagic flux, lysosomal motility and lysosomal degradation of certain cytoplasmic proteins. All three known LAMP-2 isoforms (LAMP-2-A, B and C) have the same large luminal domain whereas the transmembrane and short cytosolic domains differ. Whereas the LAMP-2A isoform has been implicated in the direct transport of cytosolic proteins into the lysosome (chaperone-mediated autophagy) the LAMP-2B isoform seems to be more important for regulating macroautophagy.

Clinical presentation

Due to the X-linked nature of inheritance men are more severely affected, displaying cognitive disabilities, hypertrophic cardiomyopathy and muscle weakness. Without cardiac transplantation these patients rarely reach the age of 25. Women are less severely affected with cognitive disabilities, muscle problems leading to dilated and hypertrophic cardiomyopathy. Retina and liver defects are also less regularly observed.

Laboratory diagnosis

Diagnosis is based on sequence analysis or analysis of leukocyte or tissue samples by immunoblotting, which detects the absence of LAMP-2 protein expression in patient samples. Prenatal diagnosis is possible once the disease-causing mutation has been established.

Action myoclonus renal failure syndrome
Genetic basis

SCARB2 (Scavenger Receptor Class B) is located on 4q21.1 and encodes for a ubiquitiously expressed lysosomal membrane protein, which translocates the lysosomal membrane twice (also called LIMP-2). Null mutations in SCARB2 cause action myoclonus renal failure syndrome (Online Mendelian Inheritance in Man #254900). To date only few families have been indentified carrying mutations in the *SCARB2* gene [8]. Mutations were first identified in a French-Canadian isolate. However, the disorder has also been recognized in other countries.

Pathophysiology

The renal pathology is of focal glomerulosclerosis, sometimes with features of glomerular collapse. Brain pathology shows unusual and uncharacterized storage material.

Clinical presentation

AMRF is a lethal inherited form of progressive myoclonus epilepsy associated with renal failure. It typically presents at 15–25 years with proteinuria evolving into renal failure or with neurological symptoms (tremor, action myoclonus, seizures, and later ataxia).

Laboratory diagnosis

SCARB2 has a recognized role as a lysosomal transport receptor for the lysosomal enzyme β-glucocerebrosidase. Therefore, a low or almost absent activity of β-glucocerebrosidase in fibroblasts but not leukocytes can be used to diagnose AMRF. Available antibodies are useful to monitor the presence or absence of SCARB2 in leukocytes or tissue biopsies. Genetic testing can be used for pre- and postnatal diagnosis, when the mutations in the index case are known.

Juvenile Ceroid Lipofuscinosis (see Chapter 18)
Genetic basis

Mutations in the *CLN3* gene are responsible for the autosomal recessive inheritance of Juvenile Ceroid Lipofuscinosis (Online Mendelian Inheritance in Man #204200) [9]. A 1.02-kb deletion in the *CLN3* gene is found in about three quarters of all patients. However, a number of additional mutations have been described. The frequency of the disease ranges from 1:25,000 (Finland) to 1:100,000 live births.

Pathophysiology

Juvenile Ceroid Lipofuscinosis (Batten disease) is the most common progressive neurodegenerative disorder of childhood. The pathological lysosomal storage of autofluorescent material and a 'fingerprint' profile can be found in all type of tissues especially in the central nervous system. In the latter tissue a severe neuronal degeneration, retinal atrophy, massive loss of brain substance and accumulation of lipofuscin in neuronal cells are observed.

Clinical presentation

The first presenting symptom of the disease is a loss of vision followed by subtle behavioural changes, slow learning or regression, repetitive speech, clumsiness, or stumbling. Later seizures, mental retardation, and loss of motor skills are regularly observed.

Laboratory diagnosis

Apart from a genetic analysis a test to detect vacuolation in lymphocytes in blood smears is recommended.

Cobalmin-F transporter disease
Genetic basis

The causative gene of cobalamin F type disease (Online Mendelian Inheritance in Man #277380) has been identified as *LMBRD1* [10], which is located on chromosome 6q12-q13. It encodes a lysosomal membrane protein of 540 amino acids and 61.4 kDa, which probably has 9 transmembrane domains. To date only few homozogous and compound heterozygote mutations have been identified.

Pathophysiology

The disease is characterized by the inability to transport free cobalamin from the lysosome into the cytoplasm.

Cobalamin is trapped in the lysosomes and is lacking for synthesis of coenzymes. This leads to hyperhomocysteinemia and methylmalonic aciduria.

Clinical presentation

Patients are often small for gestational age on presentation, develop feeding difficulties in infancy, and show failure to thrive, persistent stomatitis and developmental delay of varying degree from mild to more severe. Facial abnormalities and heart defects have also been noted.

Laboratory diagnosis

The detection of elevated propionyl carnitine in newborn screening and elevated homocysteine and methylmalonic acid concentrations in blood or urine samples may be a first sign of a defect in cobalamin metabolism. Sequence analysis to demonstrate mutations in the *LMBRD1* provides a definitive diagnosis.

Niemann–Pick disease (NPC1) (see Chapter 11)

Genetic basis

Niemann–Pick disease type C is a recessive neurodegenerative disorder [11]. It is genetically heterogenous and numerous mutations, including nonsense and missense mutations, insertions, deletions and dublications in two genes, *NPC1* on chromosome 18q11 (Online Mendelian Inheritance in Man #257220) and *NPC2* on chromosome 14q24.3 have been described. *NPC1* encodes for a proton-driven transporter, with 13 transmembrane domains. The mutated transporter leads to intralysosomal accumulation of cholesterol and glycolipids.

Pathophysiology

An accumulation of cholesterol and sphingomyelin within lysosomes is observed in the macrophage-monocyte phagocyte lineage. Affected cells become enlarged, secondary to the distention of lysosomes with sphingomyelin and cholesterol. Histology demonstrates lipid laden macrophages in the marrow. Small vacuoles of uniform size are created displaying a foamy cytoplasmic appearance.

Clinical presentation

Clinical symptoms of Niemann–Pick disease type C include cholestatic jaundice, hepatic dysfunction, supranuclear vertical gaze palsy, ataxia, extrapyramidal deficits, spasticity and dementia.

Laboratory diagnosis

The demonstration of vesicle-bound intracellular cholesterol accumulation by filipin staining of cultured fibroblasts allows an early diagnosis with confirmation by genetic testing. Prenatal diagnosis is possible by genetic analysis and the inspection of fetal skin fibroblast cultures.

Conclusions

The number of protein components of the lysosomal membrane may vary from cell type to cell type and the type of sub-proteomic analysis. However, it is estimated that between 30 and 120 lysosomal membrane proteins are needed to mediate the numerous functions of the lysosomal membrane. Accordingly, the number of diseases caused by mutations in genes encoding lysosomal membrane proteins is increasing and it is likely that hitherto unrecognized diseases may be linked to mutated integral proteins of the lysosomal compartment. Despite the fact that for the majority of known disorders the pathogenic events are still poorly understood at a molecular and cellular level, it is expected that new molecular tools and animal models will help to resolve the function of these proteins. This will hopefully also pave the way for the development of urgently required new ideas of how to treat these currently incurable diseases.

Acknowledgements

This work was supported by the Deutsche Forschungsgemeinschaft GRK1459 to P.S. and M.S.

References

1 Eskelinen EL, Tanaka Y, Saftig P. At the acidic edge: emerging functions for lysosomal membrane proteins. *Trends Cell Biol* 2003; **13**: 137–145.

2 Saftig P, Klumperman J. Lysosome biogenesis and lysosomal membrane proteins: trafficking meets function. *Nat Rev Mol Cell Biol* 2009; **10**: 623–635.

3 Schroder BA, Wrocklage C, Hasilik A, Saftig P. The proteome of lysosomes. *Proteomics* 2010; **10**: 4053–4076.

4 Ruivo R, Anne C, Sagne C, Gasnier B. Molecular and cellular basis of lysosomal transmembrane protein dysfunction. *Biochim Biophys Acta* 2009; **1793**: 636–649.

5 Wilmer MJ, Emma F, Levtchenko EN. The pathogenesis of cystinosis: mechanisms beyond cystine accumulation. *Am J Physiol Renal Physiol* 2010; **299**: F905–916.

6 Mancini GM, Havelaar AC, Verheijen FW. Lysosomal transport disorders. *J Inherit Metab Dis* 2000; **23**: 278–292.

7 Boucek D, Jirikowic J, Taylor M. Natural history of Danon disease. *Genet Med* 2011; **13**: 563–568.

8 Berkovic SF, Dibbens LM, Oshlack A, *et al.* Array-based gene discovery with three unrelated subjects shows SCARB2/LIMP-2 deficiency causes myoclonus epilepsy and glomerulosclerosis. *Am J Hum Genet* 2008; **82**: 673–684.

9 Cooper JD. Moving towards therapies for juvenile Batten disease? *Exp Neurol* 2008; **211**, 329–331.

10 Rutsch F, Gailus S, Suormala T, Fowler B. LMBRD1: the gene for the cblF defect of vitamin B metabolism. *J Inherit Metab Dis* 2011; **34**: 121–126.

11 Rosenbaum AI, Maxfield FR. Niemann–Pick type C disease: molecular mechanisms and potential therapeutic approaches. *J Neurochem* 2011; **116**: 789–795.

CHAPTER 18

Neuronal Ceroid Lipofuscinoses

Jonathan D. Cooper[1] and Ruth E. Williams[2]

[1] Centre for the Cellular Basis of Behaviour, King's Health Partners Centre for Neurodegeneration Research, Institute of Psychiatry, King's College London, London, UK
[2] Department of Paediatric Neurology, Evelina Children's Hospital, Guy's and St Thomas' NHS Foundation Trust, London, UK

Batten disease or Neuronal Ceroid Lipofuscinosis (NCLs) is the collective name for a group of at least 11 fatal inherited storage disorders that share similar pathological and clinical features. The characteristic pathology common to all these disorders is the accumulation of autofluorescent storage material within the lysosome and the widespread death of neurons. Clinically these disorders typically involve visual failure, medically refractory epilepsy and relentless declines in motor and cognitive skills, invariably ending in premature death. Each NCL is caused by mutations in a different gene. Confusingly, these genes are called "CLN" genes, but more commonly the forms of NCL are referred to by the age of onset, e.g. infantile, late-infantile or juvenile NCL. A new classification scheme has been proposed (*http://www.ucl.ac.uk/ncl/ newnomenclature.shtml*), which includes the name of the mutated gene (e.g. CLN1 disease, etc) and the age of onset seen in that individual. It is likely that all forms of nomenclature will remain in use, and this may vary between clinicians, affected families and the scientists investigating these disorders.

The most common NCLs in the UK are CLN1 disease, infantile (also known as infantile NCL, INCL); CLN2 disease, late-infantile (late-infantile NCL, LINCL) and CLN3 disease, juvenile (juvenile NCL, JNCL). In addition there are less common late-infantile variants (CLN5 disease, CLN6 disease, CLN7 disease and CLN8 disease), and the very rare congenital (CLN10 disease, CNCL) and adult-onset forms (ANCL).

Typical case scenarios

CLN2 disease, late infantile

A child is healthy and achieves developmental milestones as expected in the first year of life and there are no concerns. At 2 years she is walking independently but is not gaining fine motor skills as quickly as peers, and is not yet putting words together or able to point to body parts on demand. Just after her third birthday, the child has an unexplained sudden fall to the ground with rapid recovery. A few weeks later the child has a generalized convulsion lasting 3 minutes during an intercurrent febrile illness. The child goes on to have recurrent febrile and afebrile generalized motor seizures and is started on medication. However, the seizures are not easily controlled and within 12 months, she is on combination therapy for seizures, which include motor seizures, drop attacks and absences. Meanwhile developmental gains have slowed and the child has not learned any new words. At 5 years the child is becoming increasingly jerky and clumsy, is just able to sit without support, has lost all vocabulary and fine motor skills, and chewing and swallowing is becoming difficult. At this stage there are concerns that visual behaviour is deteriorating. The child is still visually responsive to large coloured objects and bright lights, and parents are clear that hearing and personality are retained. The seizures continue, but can be managed. Over the next few years, limb myoclonus

Lysosomal Storage Disorders: A Practical Guide, First Edition. Edited by Atul Mehta and Bryan Winchester.
© 2012 John Wiley & Sons, Ltd. Published 2012 by John Wiley & Sons, Ltd.

with or without an EEG correlate, becomes more and more obvious. The jerks settle completely in sleep and are aggravated with moving and handling. By 6 years old, most children with CLN2 disease, late infantile, are completely dependent for all their everyday care needs, and vision is limited to light/dark differentiation. Feeding by nasogastric or gastrostomy tube is necessary. There is increasing pyramidal tract involvement with evolving limb spasticity and joint contractures. Head control is lost. Gut and chest problems increase and death occurs prematurely before or around adolescence.

The diagnosis is usually made when seizures become intractable and developmental standstill or regression is recognized, often a year or more after the onset of symptoms. CLN2 disease should be suspected if there is an occipital spike/wave response to slow photic stimulation on the EEG. It is confirmed by the finding of TPP1 deficiency in blood or fibroblasts and mutations on both alleles of the *CLN2* gene.

CLN3 disease, juvenile

A child is healthy and achieves normal developmental milestones in the pre-school years. Between 4 and 7 years of age, vision deteriorates dramatically over a period of around 6–12 months. This is noticed as children struggle in the classroom, sit closer to the TV at home, start to not notice objects of interest or to look for things using hands in preference to vision. Low vision aids are useful for a while, but vision gradually declines further, reaching the level of light/dark awareness by the early teens. Children remain in good health for a number of years following the initial visual symptoms, but short-term memory and rate of learning may decline towards the end of primary school. The average age at the first seizure is around 10 years, but there may be long time intervals of many months or even years before subsequent seizures occur. During the early teenage years there is further slowing of thought and learning, and a slowly evolving Parkinsonian movement disorder, which affects speech as well as ambulation. There is a characteristic emotional/psychiatric phenotype but this is not seen universally. Many teenagers and young adults have episodes of acute anxiety, which may be associated with visual or sensory hallucinations. Restricted interests and topics of conversation are very common. Seizures gradually become more troublesome, requiring medical treatment, alongside deteriorating gait, speech and feeding skills. Understanding is preserved far longer than the ability to communicate easily with others and skilled care is

needed. Personality and hearing are preserved until the end. Myoclonus, tremor and asymmetrical motor signs are seen occasionally. There is evidence to suggest that other systems are involved in the disease process, and some specialist centres advocate cardiac surveillance for rhythm abnormalities. Young adults become increasingly dependent for all their care needs, and death occurs at any time from early teenage to the fifth decade.

The diagnosis is now made most often soon after presentation with rapid sight impairment in the early school years. Sometimes children are given an initial diagnosis of a retinal dystrophy and CLN3 disease is not diagnosed until after the first seizure several years later. With a history of vision deteriorating over 6–12 months and an abnormal electroretinogram in a school-aged child there are few differential diagnoses. Blood can be sent for microscopic examination of a thick film to look for the presence of vacuolated lymphocytes. If these are present the diagnosis may be confirmed genetically. Over 80% of affected individuals are homozygous for a common 1-kb deletion of the *CLN3* gene.

Epidemiology

Collectively the NCLs are considered the most common inherited neurodegenerative disorder of childhood, but accurate incidence and prevalence rates are hard to obtain. Recent data from the British Paediatric Surveillance Unit reveals the NCLs to be the largest single cause of progressive childhood motor and intellectual decline in the UK, with between 10 and 12 cases diagnosed each year. Of these, approximately one-half have CLN2 disease, about one-quarter CLN3 disease and the remainder one of the rarer forms. With the exception of the recently identified autosomal dominant adult-onset NCL, all forms of NCL display a classic recessive Mendelian inheritance with asymptomatic heterozygous carrier parents. Although certain genetic types of NCL were once thought to be most prevalent in particular geographic populations, it is now evident that all NCLs occur more widely.

Genetic basis

The genetic basis of 13 of the different forms of NCL has now been identified. Broadly these disease-causing genes fall into two categories, either encoding a soluble lysosomal protein (CLN1, CLN2, CLN5, CLN10 diseases) or a transmembrane protein that may be expressed in the lysosome (CLN3, CLN7 diseases) or elsewhere in the endosomal–lysosomal system (CLN6, CLN8 diseases). The nature of the defective protein has significant therapeutic implications for what types of curative therapies may be feasible in the future (see below), but it remains unclear how mutations in any of these genes lead to the devastating effects upon affected individuals. Many different disease-causing mutations have been identified in each "CLN" gene and this high degree of genetic variability and the lack of clear phenotype–genotype correlations can make it difficult to obtain a genetic diagnosis and predict the prognosis in an individual. A comprehensive database of the mutations documented in the different forms of NCL is available (*http://www.ucl.ac.uk/ncl/*) and is regularly updated. Recently, the genetic basis of adult-onset NCL has finally been clarified, with mutations in *CLN6* being revealed as causing some cases of autosomal recessive ANCL, and mutations in *DNAJC5* causing some dominant forms of ANCL, now also referred to as CLN4 disease. New disease-causing genes are still being identified, with up to 14 different genes suggested so far.

Pathophysiology

Despite now knowing the genetic basis of nearly all forms of NCL, our understanding of the mechanisms that underlie these disorders remains incomplete. Indeed, with very little known about the normal function of the disease-causing gene products, it has been difficult to draw conclusions about how these are compromised by disease-causing mutations. In this respect, a series of genetically modified and spontaneously occurring experimental models of NCL have proved particularly valuable. These have been generated in many different species, ranging from yeast and zebrafish, or found naturally in large animal models like sheep and cows. However, the mainstay of these efforts has been mouse models of each form of NCL. These are typically "knock-out" mice that bear a null mutation in the relevant gene. "Knock-in" mice that recreate a specific human disease-causing mutation have also been used. Large animal models are especially valuable, since their complex brains more closely resemble the human nervous system, and overcome the limitations of the relatively simple nervous system of mice.

Studying these animal models has revealed a number of important new features of these diseases, and provided detailed behavioural and pathological landmarks that are invaluable for testing the efficacy of a range of experimental therapies (see below). We have also learnt that some of the basic assumptions about these diseases were incorrect. For example, neuron loss is far more selective than previously thought, especially in the earliest stages of disease progression. It has become apparent that there may be no direct relationship between the build-up of storage material and neuronal death. A better predictor of subsequent neuron loss is the activation of either astrocytes or microglia, which occurs very early in pathogenesis. The specific relationship between these events is being investigated in cell culture models, but is likely to vary between the different NCLs. Indeed, despite their broadly superficial pathological appearance, it now seems more likely that different disease mechanisms will be identified in each disorder. It remains a mystery how these converge to result in similar pathological endpoints.

Natural history

Although the different forms of NCL share the major clinical features, the age at which symptoms are first detected, the order of symptoms and the rapidity of disease progression vary greatly between these different forms. In addition to genetic and allelic heterogeneity, there is clinical variability between and within families. The age at which first symptoms appear gives an important clue to which gene may be mutated, but obtaining accurate complete biochemical and molecular diagnosis as well as a clinical diagnosis is now imperative.

The first presentation of disease varies between the different forms of NCL, and is reviewed in detail elsewhere. Briefly, this tends to be a slowing in development and then developmental regression in CLN1 disease, seizures in CLN2 disease and loss of vision in CLN3 disease. With no curative or disease-modifying treatment available, the disease follows a degenerative course in all NCLs. Typically for individuals presenting early in life, disease progression is more rapid than in those presenting later. There may however be periods of plateau before subsequent deterioration. As supportive care has improved many young adults with CLN3 disease, they now survive into their twenties or thirties. As described below, the practical management of children and young people is of great importance for maintaining quality of life for as long as possible.

Laboratory diagnosis

Since protocols for enzymatic and genetic testing are now widely available, the rapid genetic and biochemical diagnosis of most forms of NCL is theoretically straightforward (*http://www.ucl.ac.uk/ncl/algorithms.shtml*). There is now less dependence on the electron microscopic analysis of skin or rectal biopsy samples. The presence of vacuolated lymphocytes in thick films of peripheral blood that is specific to CLN3 disease is still valuable and widely used, followed by genetic confirmation of mutations in *CLN3*. Testing for deficiencies of CTSD, PPT1 and TPP1 is relatively simple and can be performed on saliva or blood samples. Tests for most of the more common mutations are now readily available (e.g. the major 1-kb mutation in *CLN3* that is present in 85% of mutated alleles). These routine tests will not identify the less common or unique mutations, and more detailed testing including gene sequencing may be required in individual cases.

Treatment

At present there is no curative or disease-modifying treatment available for any form of NCL, and clinical care is limited to symptom control and supportive approaches. Nevertheless, a number of different experimental therapies have been tested in animal models, some of which have reached phase I clinical trials. The type of therapeutic approach that might be attempted is directly linked to the type of protein that is defective. For enzyme-deficient forms of NCL this depends upon the principle of cross-correction that underlies the successful treatments of lysosomal enzyme defects in other storage disorders. A proportion of synthesized lysosomal enzymes is secreted extracellularly, but this enzyme can be scavenged and returned to the lysosome via mannose-6-phosphate receptors that are present on the surface of every cell type. This phenomenon means that therapeutically supplied enzyme can be taken up by deficient cells to correct their disease. Theoretically the enzyme may be supplied in a number of ways, by direct administration of the recombinant protein (ERT), from grafts of transplanted of neural stem cell, or by gene therapy vectors. Each of these approaches has been tested in mouse models of CLN1 and CLN2 diseases, displaying various effects on behaviour, pathology, neurological disease and lifespan.

Enzyme replacement may be able to correct systemic disease, but access to the central nervous system is compromised due to the presence of the blood–brain barrier. Direct grafts of human neural stem cells (HuCNS-SC) into a mouse model of CLN1 disease delivered the missing PPT1 enzyme into the brain, reduced storage material, protected vulnerable neuron populations and led to a modest improvement in the motor performance of the mice. On the basis of these promising pre-clinical data, a phase I trial of these HuCNS-SC cells in patients with identified mutations in either *CLN1* or *CLN2* was undertaken in the USA. Gene therapy has proved much more effective in mice with CLN2 disease, especially if this therapy is initiated early in disease progression using the newer generations of adeno-associated vectors (AAVs). A phase I trial of AAV2-mediated CNS gene therapy was recently conducted at Cornell University and, despite limited efficacy, has paved the way for a subsequent trial using the AAV.rh10 vector that was so effective in mice with CLN2 disease. In contrast, gene therapy for CLN1 disease has been much less successful in mouse models, with limited improvements in pathological and behavioural measures and only modest effects upon lifespan. It appears that combined therapeutic strategies may be required to target both CNS and visceral manifestations of disease. This idea is supported by the recent report that combining CNS-directed gene therapy and a bone marrow transplant doubles the lifespan of mice with CLN1 disease. The challenge will now be to find a way to translate this successfully into clinical practice.

Compared to these experimental advances, treatment options for forms of NCL that are caused by defects in transmembrane proteins are even more challenging. Being present in the membrane of various different intracellular organelles, these proteins cannot be released to cross-correct deficient cells and it has also been suggested that over-expression may be toxic. Despite the normal function of the CLN3 protein remaining elusive, much useful information has come from studying the pathological cascade in the *Cln3*-deficient mouse model of human disease. Two key events appear to be the elevated levels of glutamate present in the brains of mice with CLN3 disease, which may cause excitotoxicity, and the presence of an autoimmune response in these mice and in human CLN3 disease. Different classes of glutamate receptor antagonists have shown some moderate improvements in pathological and behavioural phenotypes of *Cln3*-deficient mice, but are yet to reach clinical testing. Genetic blockade of the autoimmune response showed similar improvements, and treatment with the immunosuppressant mycophenylate mofetil (CellCept) had similar beneficial effects, leading to a phase I trial of this drug in patients with mutations identified in *CLN3* and a classical juvenile-onset phenotype, which is currently underway in the USA. Indeed, it is important to note that although significant advances have been made in testing experimental therapies for several forms of NCL, none is yet suitable for routine clinical use.

Treatment guidelines

With no curative or disease-modifying treatment approach available for any form of NCL, medical care is palliative and aimed at minimizing the distressing and disabling symptoms of these disorders, and maintaining skills for as long as possible. Seizure management can be challenging and requires that children and young people are reviewed regularly by experts. The effects of medications should be monitored closely and drug regimes modified appropriately. Because of the progressive nature of the disease, goals of medical and educational interventions should be discussed and agreed with the family, school, therapy teams and community services. Informed and expert multidisciplinary and interagency working is essential.

Helpful further reading and websites

Mole SE, Williams RE, Goebel HH (eds.), *The Neuronal Ceroid Lipofuscinoses (Batten Disease)*, Oxford University Press 2011, provides a much more comprehensive and up-to-date reference for all aspects of these disorders than can be provided in this brief guide.

Mole SE, Williams RE. Neuronal ceroid lipofuscinoses. *GeneReviews*, NCBI Bookshelf (http://www.ncbi.nlm.nih.gov/books/NBK1428/)

- www.bdfa-uk.org.uk
- www.bdsra.org
- www.ucl.ac.uk/ncl
- www.bartimeus.nl
- www.seeability.org
- http://tinyurl.com/newpsdl

CHAPTER 19

Other Lysosomal Disorders

Bryan Winchester[1] and Timothy M. Cox[2]

[1] Emeritus Professor of Biochemistry, UCL Institute of Child Health at Great Ormond Street Hospital, University College London, London, UK

[2] Professor of Medicine, University of Cambridge, Addenbrooke's Hospital, Cambridge, UK

Introduction

This chapter includes sections on two typical storage disorders that have not been covered in other chapters – Farber disease and acid lipase deficiency – and a possible new lysosomal nucleoside transporter defect. There is also a discussion of the function and pathology of lysosomal proteases, the cathepsins, deficiencies of which lead to a wide range of phenotypes. Sections on disorders of biogenesis of lysosome-related organelles and the possible contribution of defects in the formation of the lysosomal recognition marker, mannose-6-phosphate, to non-syndromic stuttering, provide further evidence for the wide role of lysosomes.

Farber disease: acid ceramidase deficiency (OMIM: 228000)

Farber disease is a rare (less than 100 cases reported), autosomal recessive, lysosomal sphingolipid storage disorder caused by a deficiency of acid ceramidase (*N*-acylsphingosine amidohydrolase, ASAH1: EC 3.5.1.23). The genetically distinct alkaline ceramidase activity present in most cells is not affected in this disorder. The deficiency of acid ceramidase (OMIM: 228000) leads to the intralysosomal accumulation of ceramide in most tissues, including heart, liver, lung and spleen. Farber disease is also called Farber lipogranulomatosis because of the formation of the subcutaneous nodules near joints and other pressure points. Despite the small number of patients, Farber disease has been classified into seven subtypes according to age of onset, severity and which

tissues are affected by the accumulation of ceramide. Types 1–5 are called classic, intermediate, mild, neonatal and neurologic progression, respectively. Type 6 arises from a serendipitous combination of Farber and Sandhoff diseases. In Type 7 a defect in prosaposin leads to a functional deficiency of acid ceramidase together with deficiencies of β-galactocerebrosidase and β-glucocerebrosidase activities. These patients present neonatally with a rapidly progressing neurovisceral lipid storage disease. Acid ceramidase is activated by saposin D *in vitro* but no patients with an isolated deficiency of saposin D have been reported. A mouse with a mutation in the saposin D domain of the prosaposin gene accumulated ceramide in the kidney and brain suggesting a role for saposin D in sphingolipid metabolism *in vivo*.

The characteristic features of Farber disease include progressive hoarseness due to laryngeal involvement, painful swollen joints, subcutaneous nodules and pulmonary infiltrations. Initial signs appear between 2 and 4 months of age except in the mild type 3. Death usually occurs within the first years of life but prolonged survival is known in patients without severe CNS involvement. Psychomotor development is mostly normal, although deterioration has been observed in the later phases of this disorder. Very severe forms, with corneal clouding, hepatosplenomegaly, marked histiocytosis, with death before 6 months of age (type 4) or death *in utero* have been reported.

Pathophysiology

Ceramide is formed during the catabolism of all sphingolipids within the lysosomes and the deficiency of acid ceramidase

Lysosomal Storage Disorders: A Practical Guide, First Edition. Edited by Atul Mehta and Bryan Winchester.
© 2012 John Wiley & Sons, Ltd. Published 2012 by John Wiley & Sons, Ltd.

leads to the accumulation of ceramide exclusively in lysosomes in most tissues. Extremely high levels of ceramide have been observed in the urine, but it is not increased in the plasma of patients. The accumulated intralysosomal ceramide does not appear to interfere directly with the regulatory roles of ceramide and its derivatives in other subcellular compartments, e.g. in apoptosis. The accumulation of ceramide may alter membrane fluidity and raft formation and, consequently, receptor-mediated signalling.

Genetics

The acid ceramidase gene (*ASAH1*) has been cloned and about 20 mutations have been identified in patients. It is not possible to make any deductions about a genotype–phenotype correlation because of the small number of patients analysed. The clinical severity does not correlate with the residual activity measured under non-physiological conditions, but there is a good correlation with the level of lysosomal storage of ceramide.

Diagnosis

Historically Farber disease was diagnosed by the measurement of the accumulation of ceramide in cultured fibroblasts either by including [^{14}C]stearic acid-labelled sulfatide or sphingomyelin in the medium for 1–3 days or by the enzymic determination of extracted, unlabelled ceramide. Acid ceramidase activity can also be measured in leukocytes and cultured fibroblasts using synthetic substrates in the presence of added detergent. Recently a simple fluorigenic assay using a synthetic substrate incorporating umbelliferone has been developed for the measurement of acid ceramidase activity in cells. It should make the diagnosis of Farber disease more accessible and supersede the radioactive methods. A novel mass spectrometric method for quantifying sphingolipids in extracts of cultured fibroblasts may also be applicable to the diagnosis of Farber disease. Carrier detection is based on mutation analysis. Prenatal diagnosis has been carried out by measuring the ceramidase activity in CV and CAC or by lipid-loading tests in CAC. Genetic testing is the method of choice when the family mutations are known.

Treatment

There is improvement in the peripheral manifestations of infantile Farber disease after bone marrow transplantation but neurological deterioration continues even in mildly symptomatic patients. However, in patients without neurological involvement, allogeneic stem cell transplantation results in almost complete resolution of granulomas and joint contractures and considerable improvement in mobility and joint motility. Gene therapy is in the preclinical stage in large animals using Farber patient haematopoietic cells transduced with a lentivirus vector that overexpresses human acid ceramidase.

Acknowledgement

The authors would like to thank Prof. Thierry Levade for reviewing this section.

Lysosomal acid lipase deficiency: Wolman Disease and Cholesteryl Ester Storage Disease (OMIM: 278000)

A deficiency of the lysosomal enzyme acid lipase (LAL) (EC 3.1.1.13) leads to two main phenotypes, Wolman Disease and Cholesteryl Ester Storage Disease (OMIM: 278000). There is a complete absence of acid lipase activity in Wolman disease, or primary familial xanthomatosis with involvement and calcification of the adrenals. It is a rapidly progressing disease marked by severe failure to thrive, diarrhoea, vomiting and hepatosplenomegaly evident in the first few weeks of life with death usually occurring within 6–8 months from cachexia, complicated by peripheral oedema. Most patients have calcification of the adrenals, which can be detected readily by radiology. Foam cells are found in the bone marrow and later in peripheral blood. The organs contain cells loaded with neutral lipids, especially cholesterol esters and triglycerides, but the levels of cholesterol and triglycerides are normal in plasma.

The presence of some residual acid lipase activity results in the more attenuated disease, cholesteryl ester storage disease (CESD), with a wide spectrum of clinical presentation. It is characterized by liver enlargement, which may be the sole symptom early on and for many years, short stature, chronic gastrointestinal bleeding, chronic anaemia, headaches and abdominal pain. The hepatic fibrosis often leads to atherosclerois. There is not usually any calcification of the adrenals but patients may have sea-blue histiocytosis. Some patients live to adulthood with unpredictable presentation, making diagnosis relatively difficult, whereas others die in their juvenile years. Levels of cholesterol esters are markedly elevated in the liver, whereas the levels of triglycerides are only moderately elevated. There is hyperlipidaemia with a marked decrease in plasma high-densitylipoprotein (HDL) and a slight elevation of liver enzymes.

Pathophysiology

The failure to release cholesterol from cholesteryl esters due to a deficiency of LAL results in upregulation of endogenous cholesterol synthesis and expression of the LDL-receptor gene. There is also increased synthesis of apo-B lipoproteins, which increases delivery of lipoproteins into the lysosomes, particularly in the liver. The clinical features of Wolman disease and CESD result from the deposition of cholesteryl esters and triglycerides in tissues and secondary effects such as the toxicity of lipoprotein oxidation.

Genetics and epidemiology

Lysosomal acid lipase is encoded by the *LIPA* gene, which is localized on chromosome 10(10q23.2-q23.3) and has been cloned, permitting identification of mutations in Wolman and CESD patients (see Lugowska and Tylki Szymanska, 2012, for list). In general those mutations that abolish acid lipase activity are found in Wolman disease and those that result in some residual activity are found in CESD. There are no recurrent mutations in Wolman disease, which is very rare in the general population with a frequency as low as 1 in 350,000 births. However, in the Iranian – Jewish community (in which the disease was first described) an incidence as high as 1 in 4,200 newborns has been predicted by screening for carriers of a specific mutation, pG87V. The common splice site mutation del254–277 found in CESD patients produces residual LAL activity, which is sufficient even in heterozygosity to prevent the severe Wolman phenotype. The frequency of CESD among newborns in Germany has been predicted to be 25 cases per million from measurement of the frequency of the common mutation, del254–257 in the population and an estimate of the frequency of this mutation in all cases of CESD. This suggests that CESD is under-diagnosed because this frequency is higher than reported in the literature.

Diagnosis

There is a marked deficiency of acid lipase activity (EC 3.1.1.13) in all tissues of patients with both Wolman disease and CESD. Diagnosis is made by demonstrating a deficiency of acid lipase in leukocytes or cultured skin fibroblasts using a variety of substrates, including radiolabelled triglycerides and cholesterol esters as well as synthetic fatty acid esters of 4-methylumbelliferone and *p*-nitrophenol. The diagnosis should be confirmed by mutation analysis if possible. Prenatal diagnosis is possible by direct enzyme assay of foetal samples using the synthetic substrates or radiolabelled cholesterol oleate, but molecular testing is the preferred method if the disease-causing mutations have been identified in the family.

Treatment

There are several reports of successful haematopoietic stem cell transplantation in cases of Wolman disease by BMT or unrelated umbilical cord blood transplantation. Based on encouraging pre-clinical data from ERT in acid lipase-deficient rats and mice, trials of enzyme replacement therapy in both Wolman disease and CESD patients are in progress using human recombinant enzyme produced in eggs.

Defects in equilibrative nucleoside transporter 3 – a new lysosomal transporter defect?

Mutations in the human equilibrative nucleoside transporter 3 (ENT3/*SLC29A3 gene*) have been found in patients with familial Rosai–Dorfman disease, Faisalabad histiocytosis, H syndrome and pigmented hypertrichosis with insulin-dependent diabetes (PHID), all of which are characterized by histiocytosis. Macrophages, which cannot synthesize nucleosides *de novo*, are highly phagocytic and need to redistribute the nucleosides derived from the lysosomal breakdown of phagocytosed DNA/RNA. It is postulated that a defect in lysosomal ENT3 and the accumulation of nucleosides in the lysosomes could initiate a cascade of secondary events leading to the altered macrophage function observed in these disorders. However, ENT3 has been localized to the mitochondrial as well as the lysosomal membrane and its role in the intracellular transport of nucleosides is not fully understood.

Defects in the lysosomal proteases, cathepsins

At least 15 genetically distinct lysosomal proteases or cathepsins have been described. Most have a catalytic cysteine residue in the active site and are called cysteine proteases, but cathepsins C and E and cathepsins A and G have catalytic aspartic acid and serine residues, respectively. They are predominantly endopeptidases, i.e. cleave the polypeptide chain at internal sites, but cathepsins C (dipeptidyl peptidase I) and X are true exopeptidases and cathepsins B and H have both exo- and endopeptidase activities. Cathepsins are found in all vesicles of the endocytic pathway with some also showing tissue- or cell- or vesicle-specific expression, e.g. cathepsin E in endosomes, cathepsin G in azurophilic granules in neutrophils, whereas cathepsins B, C, H and L are expressed ubiquitously. Cathepsins may be secreted from certain cells for specific functions such as turnover of the extracellular matrix. In addition to the lysosomal catabolism of proteins, specific cathepsins play a role in antigen processing, processing of proteins at various points in the endosomal/lysosomal pathway, and in apoptosis. Other non-cathepsin lysosomal proteases have also been described.

Collectively the lysosomal proteases have the capacity to degrade all polypeptides to their constituent amino acids and possibly to a few dipeptides. A general failure in the lysosomal breakdown of proteins has not been reported, presumably because a deficiency of one cathepsin can be compensated for by another cathepsin due to redundancy in substrate specificity. Very little is known about the specific substrates for cathepsins, and synthetic or purified peptides have usually been used for substrate specificity studies. However, deficiencies of single cathepsins are associated with diseases, reflecting the failure to hydrolyse specific, unknown, polypeptide substrates: cathepsin C in Papillon–Lefèvre syndrome, cathepsin D in NCL10, cathepsin K in immune disorders, and cathepsin K in pycnodysostosis.

Undoubtedly defects of cathepsins and other lysosomal proteases will be shown to contribute to a wide range of diseases because of their involvement in so many key cellular processes unrelated to bulk protein turnover in the lysosome. The potential multifunctional role of cathepsins is illustrated by the deficiency of cathepsin A in galactosialidosis, where cathepsin A has a stabilizing role in the formation of a multiple enzyme complex unrelated to its proteolytic activity (see Chapters 15). As the predominant biochemical feature of galactosialidosis is a defect in the catabolism of glycoproteins, it has been classified as a glycoproteinosis.

Disorders of biogenesis of lysosome-related organelles

(Contributed by Timothy M Cox)

Numerous genetic defects affect protein complexes implicated in the biogenesis and function of lysosomes and their related secretory organelles such as melanosomes; partial albinism is thus a common feature. Several distinct organelles with specialized functions closely resemble lysosomes and are known as lysosome-related organelles. These include δ-granules in platelets; Weibel–Palade bodies of endothelial cells; lytic granules and vesicles implicated in the immune "synapse" in lymphocytes; basophil and azurophil granules in polymorphonuclear leucocytes; lamellar bodies in type 2 pneumocytes; neuromelanin granules in the catecholaminergic neurones of the nigro-striatal pathway, and the melanosomes of the iris, choroid and skin. Most of these organelles are also maintained at an acidic pH and have a membrane composition with many similarities to those of lysosomes.

Disturbances of the endosome–lysosome vesicular trafficking network occur at several distinct steps. Disrupted vesicular traffic observed in these albinism syndromes resembles some of the consequences of other lysosomal disorders but there is additionally defective biogenesis of lysosomes and abnormal trafficking of allied organelles and their related proteins – sometimes with impaired extrusion of specialized granules or their contents. These disorders most characteristically affect melanosomes and platelet dense granules but may or may not affect the other related organelles. Pigmentary abnormalities, including the distribution of pigment in hair shafts (as in Chédiak–Higashi syndrome), and impaired platelet function and/or structure are often the first indication of the diagnosis.

Genetic defects in the processes required for the organization of membranes and trafficking of vesicles that lead to the formation of functional lysosomes and lysosome-related organelles, also illustrate their common biogenesis – and reveal much about their complex molecular physiology in differentiated cells.

Hermansky–Pudlak disease(s)

The Hermansky–Pudlak syndrome (HPS) is a group of autosomal recessive disorders affecting specialized secretory organelles. HPS is characterized by a bleeding tendency due to abnormal platelets; reduced pigmentation of the skin, iris and hair – and diverse inflammatory complications including granulomatous colitis, cardiomyopathy and severe fibrosis of the lung. The basic cause of this group of disorders is mis-sorting of molecules typically destined for lysosomes or related organelles; albinism reflects mis-targeting of the tyrosinase-related proteins either to early endosomes or if they are delivered to the melanosome, defective exocytosis leads to their pathological retention. There is accumulation of ceroid lipofuscin pigment in lymphocytes, monocytes, and macrophages in bone marrow. In the lung, defective release of surfactant phospholipid by type 2 pneumocytes leads to inflammatory injury, emphysema and pulmonary fibrosis. Deficient secretion of ADP, which promotes platelet clumping, occurs because the platelet δ-granules are absent: this causes easy bruising, bleeding in the mucous membranes and severe bleeding after injuries and surgery. In women there may be excessive menstruation and bleeding complications in pregnancy and childbirth. Oculocutaneous albinism results from defective formation of melanosomes.

Clinical diagnosis is suggested by the occurrence of colitis or granulomatous colitis often masquerading as Crohn's disease in patients with fair skin, blue irides and white or blonde hair; increased pigmentation of the hair may occur after puberty. These patients frequently have a tendency to bruise or bleed with prolonged bleeding time and abnormal platelet-function tests. Bone marrow examination shows pigmentary granules in macrophages and autofluoresence due to ceroid material in urinary sediment, and autofluorescent material in oral mucosa biopsy specimens may be detected. Chronic exposure to light is strongly associated with skin injury and cancer; they may also have moderate visual impairment with jerky eye movements due to nystagmus and ocular photophobia. Fortunately, blindness is rare and loss of vision does not usually progress beyond childhood. In later life, the occurrence of fatal lung fibrosis with respiratory failure may alert physicians to the diagnosis of this autosomal recessive disease, sometimes confirmed by a careful family history.

Nine genetically distinct types of Hermansky–Pudlak syndrome have been identified. The affected proteins in type 1 and types 3–9 belong to the biogenesis of lysosome-related organelles complexes 1–3 (BLOC1–3). Definitive diagnosis of these forms of HPS relies upon molecular analysis of genes of the members of the BLOC1–3 families. Hermansky–Pudlak type 2 (HP2), has been shown to be due to mutations in the *ADTB3A* gene, which encodes the β3A subunit of the adaptor protein complex AP3 involved in the formation of vesicles between the trans-Golgi network and late endosomes. Patients with HPS2 have an immunodeficiency due to congenital neutropenia, as well as platelet defects and partial albinism.

HPS is very rare in most populations, affecting 1 in 500,000 to 1 in 1,000,000 individuals worldwide. Type 1 is more common in northwest Puerto Rico, where the prevalence is about 1 in 1,800 persons; Hermansky–Pudlak syndrome type 3 is also frequent in central Puerto Rico, in Japan, and in an isolated community in Switzerland.

Chédiak–Higashi syndrome

This disorder is also characterized by oculocutaneous albinism, easy bruising and bleeding caused by defective platelet dense bodies but recurrent infections, with neutropenia, impaired chemotaxis and bactericidal activity and abnormal natural killer-cell function, also occur. Most patients experience a phase with lymphohistiocytic infiltration of multiple organs, which resembles lymphoma and appears to be induced by Epstein–Barr viral infection. Death often occurs in childhood from infection,

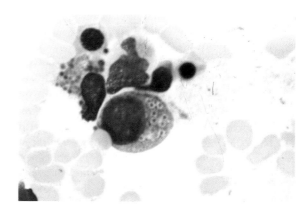

Figure 19.1 Photomicrograph of vacuolated lymphocytes from a patient with Chédiak–Higashi syndrome.

bleeding, or development of this accelerated phase of illness. Chédiak–Higashi syndrome is suggested by partial oculocutaneous albinism, photophobia, nystagmus, large eosinophilic, peroxidase-positive inclusion bodies in the myeloblasts and promyelocytes of the bone marrow, neutropenia, abnormal susceptibility to infection, and development of malignant lymphoma. Death often occurs before the end of the first decade.

Large cytoplasmic granules or giant lysosomes are present in circulating granulocytes and other cells (Figure 19.1): in the case of melanocytes, giant melanosomes are formed. Chédiak–Higashi disease impairs the ability of neutrophils and macrophages to kill microbes in phagolysosomes as a result of disordered intracellular trafficking; degranulation of lysosomes on fusion with phagosomes is defective so that bacteria are not digested. Secretion of lytic secretory granules by cytotoxic T cells is also affected. Patients with Chédiak–Higashi disease have impairments in both innate and adaptive immunity with immunodeficiency. Inhibition of T-cell activation is impaired as a result of mistargeting of regulatory molecules and, once initiated by a stimulus such as EBV infection, may lead to uncontrolled macrophage–lymphocytic proliferation and inflammatory cytokine release – haemophagocytic lymphohistiocytosis – characterized by expanding hepatosplenomegaly, pancytopenia and the presence of macrophages demonstrating haemophagocytosis within the marrow (Figure 19.2).

Homozygous or compound heterozygous mutations in the lysosomal trafficking regulator gene (*CHS1/LYST*) have been reported to underlie the disease. The gene encodes a cytosolic protein involved in membrane fusion, and mutations disrupt interactions with the microtubule cytoskeleton, thus interfering with intracellular transport of proteins

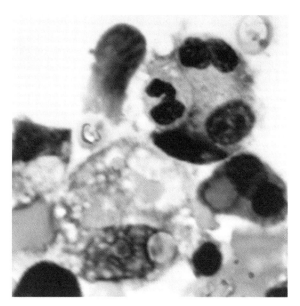

Figure 19.2 Photomicrograph of macrophages laden with cellular debris from a bone marrow aspirate in a patient with haemophagocytic lymphohistiocytosis (HLH). (Reproduced from Mehta A, Hoffbrand, V, *Haematology at a Glance* (2nd edn.). Oxford: Blackwell Publishing Ltd, 2005: p. 88, with permission.)

to specialized endosomes and lysosomes. Uncontrolled fusion or fission induces formation of giant secretory lysosomes and other organelles, which interfere with the delivery of other cellular cargo. Antigen presentation requires appropriate vesicular trafficking and the Major Histocompatibility Complex (MHC) class II-loading compartment of antigen-presenting cells in Chédiak–Higashi disease is expanded with commensurate delays in antigen processing and presentation. Impaired delivery of major histocompatibility complex class II molecules to the plasma membrane thus appears to alter antigen presentation.

Griscelli syndrome(s)

There are three variants of this syndrome: one is a simple form of albinism (type III), while the other two also have defective immunity (type II) or neurological deficits (type I). Griscelli syndrome type II with immunological defects is caused by mutations in Rab27a, a soluble GTPase, which regulates the movement of melanosomes to the periphery of melanocytes and regulates exocytosis of lytic granules in cytotoxic T lymphocytes. The lack of Rab27a thus causes pigment anomalies and dysfunctional T lymphocytes. The Griscelli syndrome type I, which also has neurological symptoms, is caused by mutations in the motor protein, myosin Va, which may cooperate with

Rab27a to transport melanosomes along actin filaments but apparently does not participate in the exocytosis of lytic T-cell granules. Patients with the Griscelli type III syndrome only have pigment abnormalities without additional features. They have mutations in melanophilin, which interacts with the Rab and myosin Va solely in pigment cells to form a complex involved in vesicle transport and membrane trafficking, including transport of melanosomes in melanocytes. Elejalde syndrome is a rare variant in which peripheral neuropathy is prominent but without the lymphocytic defect or immune deficiency.

Treatment of disorders of lysosomal biogenesis

These diseases are often severe and affect many systems; after some years of apparent stability, patients may become rapidly unwell and present with an acute illness that is a challenge to diagnosis. In outline below are some of the principles of care that merit consideration in these complex patients.

• *Oculo-cutaneous albinism* is variable in these syndromes but where appropriate, aids for poor vision due to retinal photoinjury, especially in the school environment and cutaneous protection against high-intensity ultraviolet and visible light-induced damage, and skin carcinoma, should be offered.

• The *bleeding manifestations* may require platelet transfusions and parenteral administration of desmopressin (DDAVP – 1-desamino-8-D-arginine vasopressin) may also be used to improve platelet function in the short term – especially to prevent serious bleeding associated with minor surgical procedures such as dental extraction and during obstetric delivery. Given the association with defective platelet function, aspirin and other non-steroidal drugs should be avoided.

• Children and adults with Chédiak–Higashi syndrome are susceptible to serious *microbial infections* with *Staphylococcus aureus* and *Streptococci as well as* Gram-negative bacteria; fungal infections due to *Candida* or *Aspergillus* also occur. Immunization for common viral and bacterial infections, including influenza, *Haemophilus influenzae* and pneumococci, should be instituted. Prompt use of appropriate antimicrobial agents (including parenteral antifungal agents and antivirals where indicated) is recommended to limit the consequences of infections.

• In the Hermansky–Pudlak syndromes, *granulomatous colitis* may cause perforation or severe bleeding; it appears to respond well to anti-inflammatory agents, including corticosteroids. *Pulmonary fibrosis* (which may in part be related to impaired surfactant release from type 2 pneumocytes) progresses rapidly and may require treatment with supplemental oxygen in the home; there are a few reports of successful lung transplantation. A smoke-free environment and prompt treatment of respiratory infections with anti-pneumococcal immunization may preserve lung function and prolong symptom-free survival. The role of prophylactic antimicrobial therapy is, as yet, not established.

• Patients with Chédiak–Higashi disease and Griscelli syndrome type 2, can develop a fulminating illness – **haemophagocytic lymphohistiocytosis** – which may not be immediately recognized but is related to impaired natural killer and cytotoxic T-cell function. This leads to life-threatening and uncontrolled proliferation of activated lymphocytes and histiocytes accompanied by release of inflammatory cytokines causing fever, hepatosplenomegaly and pancytopenia. The illness is triggered by viral infections, particularly Epstein–Barr virus. The immediate goal of therapy is suppression of the accelerated inflammation with immunosuppressive and immunomodulatory agents and cytostatic drugs. Successful use of rituximab and cyclosporin has been reported in a patient with Chédiak–Higashi disease who failed to respond to corticosteroids, cyclosporine and etoposide. When the accelerated phase has been controlled, haematopoietic stem-cell transplantation to replace cellular components of the defective immune system with normally functioning effector cells, if safely accomplished, reduces the risk of recurrence.

Conclusion

As an emerging field of investigation, disorders of lysosomal biogenesis and lysosome-related organelles represent a highly specialized area of medical practice. Strong communication links with centres able to advise and provide wide-ranging clinical care – including appropriate high-dependency units, genetic counselling, with access to diagnostic, haematological and transplantation services – are of crucial value. In the event of difficulties, expert advice should be sought from the best international centres of expertise for example, Dr William Gahl and colleagues based in the Section on Human Biochemical Genetics, Medical Genetics Branch at the National Institutes of Health, Maryland, USA.

Stuttering

A very interesting new aspect to lysosomal dysfunction is the report that mutations in the three genes encoding enzymes that catalyse the formation of the lysosomal recognition marker, mannose-6-phosphate, have been found in patients with non-syndromic stuttering [24]. A missense mutation, Glu1200Lys, in the N-acetylglucosamine-1-phosphate transferase gene (*GNPTAB*), was associated with stuttering in a large consanguineous Pakistani family. Most affected members of the family were either homozygous or heterozygous for the mutation, but some individuals carrying one or two copies of the mutation were currently unaffected, suggesting non-penetrance and that the mutation does not show absolute segregation with trait. Three affected members of the family did not have mutations in the *GNPTAB* gene. Three other mutations in the *GNPTAB* gene were found in unrelated individuals with stuttering. None of these mutations was found in control subjects. Three mutations in the *GNPTG* gene, which encodes the gamma subunit of GlcNAc-1-phosphotransferase GNPT, were found in affected individuals of Asian and European descent but not in control subjects. Three mutations were also identified in the uncovering enzyme, N-acetylglucosamine-1-phosphodiester alpha-N-acetylglucosaminidase (NAGPA), in six unrelated individuals with stuttering, one homozygote and five heterozygotes. Each of the mutations in the *NAGPA* gene has been shown to lower the cellular activity of NAGPA [25]. Thus it seems that defects in the pathway for the formation of the lysosomal recognition marker, may predispose towards non-syndromic stuttering as well as leading to ML II/III phenotype.

Further reading

Farber disease: acid ceramidase deficiency

1 Bär J, Linke T, Ferlinz K, *et al*. Molecular analysis of acid ceramidase deficiency in patients with Farber disease. *Hum Mutat* 2001; **17**: 199–209.

2 Bedia C, Camacho L, Abad JL, *et al*. A simple fluorogenic method for determination of acid ceramidase activity and diagnosis of Farber disease. *J Lipid Res* 2010; **51**: 3542–3547.

3 Burek C, Roth J, Koch HG, *et al*. The role of ceramide in receptor- and stress-induced apoptosis studied in acidic ceramidase-deficient Farber disease cells. *Oncogene* 2001; **20**(45): 6493–6502.

4 Ehlert K, Frosch M, Fehse N, *et al*. Farber disease: clinical presentation, pathogenesis and a new approach to treatment. *Pediatr Rheumatol* 2007; **5**: 15.

5 Levade T, Enders H, Schliephacke M, Harzer K. A family with combined Farber and Sandhoff, isolated Sandhoff and isolated fetal Farber disease: postnatal exclusion and prenatal diagnosis of Farber disease using lipid loading tests on intact cultured cells. *Eur J Pediatr* 1995; **154**(8): 643–648.

6 Levade T, Sandhoff K, Schulze H, Medin JA. Acid ceramidase deficiency: Farber lipogranulomatosis The online metabolic and molecular bases of inherited disease; 0. http://www.ommbid.com

7 Matsuda J, Kido M, Tadano-Aritomi K, *et al.* Mutation in saposin D domain of sphingolipid activator protein gene causes urinary system defects and cerebellar Purkinje cell degeneration with accumulation of hydroxy fatty acid-containing ceramide in mouse. *Hum Mol Genet* 2004; **13**(21): 2709–2723.

8 Neschadim A, Lopez-Perez O, Alayoubi A, *et al.* Autologous transplantation of lentivector/acid ceramidase-transduced hematopoietic cells in nonhuman primates. *Hum Gene Ther* 2011; **22**(6): 679–687.

Lysosomal acid lipase deficiency

9 Lugowska A, Tylki-Szymanska A. Lysosomal acid lipase deficiency: Wolman disease and cholesteryl ester storage disease. *CML – Lysosomal Storage Diseases* 2012; **10**: 1–8.

10 Muntoni S, Wiebusch H, Jansen-Rust M, *et al.* Prevalence of cholesteryl ester storage disease. *Arterioscler Thromb Vasc Biol* 2007; **27**: 1866–1868.

11 Valles-Ayoub Y, Esfandiarifard S, No D, *et al.* Wolman disease (LIPA p.G87V) genotype frequency in people of Iranian-Jewish ancestry. *Genet Test Mol Biomarkers* 2011; **15**(6): 395–398.

Defects in equilibrative nucleoside transporter 3

12 Hsu C-L, Lin W, Seshasayee D, *et al.* Equilibrative nucleoside transporter 3 deficiency perturbs lysosome function and macrophage homeostasis. *Science* 2012; **335**(6064): 89–92.

13 Kang N, *et al.* Human equilibrative nucleoside transporter-3 (hENT3) spectrum disorder mutations impair nucleoside transport, protein localization, and stability. *J Biol Chem* 2010; **285**: 28343–28352.

14 Morgan NV, *et al.* Mutations in SLC29A3, encoding an equilibrative nucleoside transporter ENT3, cause a familial histiocytosis syndrome (Faisalabad histiocytosis) and familial Rosai-Dorfman disease. *PLoS Genet* 2010; **6**: e1000833.

Defects in the lysosomal proteases, cathepsins

15 Brix K. Lysosomal proteases: revival of the sleeping beauty. In: Saftig P (ed.), *Lysosomes*. Landes Bioscience/Springer Science + Business Media, USA.

16 Repnik U, Stoka V, Turk V, Turk B. Lysosomes and lysosomal cathepsins in cell death. *Biochimica Biophysica Acta* 2012; **1824**: 22–33.

Disorders of biogenesis of lysosome-related organelles

17 Bonifacino JS. Insights into the biogenesis of lysosome-related organelles from the study of the Hermansky–Pudlak syndrome. *Ann NY Acad Sci* 2004; **1038**:103–14.

18 Cullinane AR, Curry JA, Carmona-Rivera C, *et al.* A BLOC-1 mutation screen reveals that PLDN is mutated in Hermansky–Pudlak syndrome type 9. *Am J Hum Genet* 2011; **88**: 778–787.

19 Dell'Angellico EC. AP-3-dependent trafficking and disease: the first decade. *Curr Opin Cell Biol* 2009; **21**: 552–559.

20 Huizing M, Helip-Wooley A, Westbroek W, et al. Disorders of lysosome-related organelle biogenesis: clinical and molecular genetics. *Annu Rev Genom Hum Genet* 2008; **9**: 359–386.

21 Kaplan J, De Domenico I, Ward DM. Chediak–Higashi syndrome. *Curr Opin Hematol* 2008; **15**: 22–29.

22 Stinchcombe J, *et al.* Linking albinism and immunity: the secrets of secretory lysosomes. *Science* 2004; **305**: 55–59.

23 Van Gele M, Dynoodt P, Lambert J. Griscelli syndrome: a model system to study vesicular trafficking. *Pigment Cell Melan Res* 2009; **22**: 268–282.

Stuttering

24 Kang C, Riazuddin S, Mundorff J, et al. Mutations in the lysosomal enzyme-targeting pathway and persistent stuttering. *N Engl J Med* 2010; **362**(8): 677–685.

25 Lee WS, Kang C, Drayna D, Kornfeld S. Analysis of mannose 6-phosphate uncovering enzyme mutations associated with persistent stuttering. *J Biol Chem* 2011; **286**(46): 39786–39793.

PART 3

Therapy and Patient Issues

CHAPTER 20

Current Treatments

Timothy M. Cox

Department of Medicine, University of Cambridge, and Addenbrooke's Hospital, Cambridge, UK

Introduction

The burden of disease

The lysosomal disorders critically affect well-being, life quality and survival at all ages. With a birth frequency of one in every 5,000–7,500 live births and with illness often lasting many years, the individual and societal burden of these conditions is very great. The lysosome interacts dynamically with other cellular components and is a central point of convergence in countless functions that are crucial for health: thus lysosomal diseases can affect all systems of the body, with potential consequences in the skeleton and major organs, as well as the blood-forming and immune systems; most of the diseases also affect the brain. So far, effective treatments have been developed for only a few lysosomal conditions; but for many patients and their families, these provide a tangible focus of hope – and at the same time emphasize the importance of comprehensive clinical care and management in circumstances where definitive therapy is, as yet, unavailable. Furthermore, few really striking treatment effects have been observed in lysosomal diseases other than Gaucher disease: even many aspects of this condition, including established skeletal manifestations and the neurological features, remain beyond reach. Familiar strictures about early diagnosis and prompt introduction of treatments are highly relevant to the lysosomal diseases and there is much to be done to improve diagnostic awareness and thus access to care for patients with these rare conditions.

General considerations

Supportive and palliative treatment

"To cure sometimes; to relieve often – but comfort always." Despite advanced knowledge about the molecular cell biology of the lysosome and much biopharmacological investment, for most patients, no specific or curative therapy is available. The diseases – especially those with neurological manifestations – are relentless and cruel; and despite optimism that the outlook may improve, the hackneyed expression, "unmet medical need", retains a chilling significance.

In this context, the social burden and psychological strain experienced by patients and their immediate families are hard to bear: beyond diagnosis, even where specific therapies cannot be introduced, it is incumbent on health professionals to address these aspects and as far as possible provide appropriate continuity of care.

Comprehensive clinical care

The lack of specific treatment for most lysosomal diseases is a harsh truth, but those experienced in arts of nursing and medicine, and in the professions allied to medicine, bring a wealth of resources with which to ameliorate symptoms and support disabled patients who are unable to care for themselves. Much can be gained by team-working among diverse professionals – and particularly to establish strong practical links with those delivering clinical care at the point of need whether it be in the home, a hospice, local hospital – or, in unfortunate cases, custodial institutions.

Lysosomal Storage Disorders: A Practical Guide, First Edition. Edited by Atul Mehta and Bryan Winchester.
© 2012 John Wiley & Sons, Ltd. Published 2012 by John Wiley & Sons, Ltd.

Genetic counselling

In the management of all these conditions, their hereditary basis should be considered for at-risk first-degree relatives. Siblings of affected patients should be evaluated either by appropriate assay of lysosomal enzyme activities in white blood cells or cultured fibroblasts or by molecular genetic testing (once disease-causing mutations in the family have been identified) in order to start therapy at the most reasonable time early in the course of the disease.

General measures

Attention should be given to simple measures to identify and relieve constipation, flexion deformities, cough, pressure sores, urinary infection and other indignities frequently encountered by those unable to care for themselves. Tonsillectomy and adenoidectomy for Eustachian tube malfunction and/or upper airway obstruction, even tracheostomy for sleep apnoea may be required. Pulmonary hypertension and right heart failure may result from ventilatory defects; and tracheostomy for sleep apnoea may prevent pulmonary hypertension and right heart failure.

Apart from ventilatory support, numerous ingenious motorized mobility aids are available for patients with severe disability: these contribute a great deal to the quality of life and improve the immediate burden on carers to transport and enliven the immediate environment for the patient.

Sleep disturbance, agitation, mood and seizure control

Melatonin and the judicious use of tranquillizers, mood-stabilizing agents and anticonvulsants such as carbamazepine may be helpful for the treatment of sleep disturbance. However, pharmacological intervention is often disappointing. A safe and comforting location, with minimal changes in the immediate environment, supported by experienced long-standing carers – including familiar objects as well as diverting visual and other stimuli, plus visits from relatives – and the ready accessibility of welcome sound and music, are frequent adjuncts to success.

Seizures of many types are frequently encountered. Careful attention to pharmacological principles of careful dose-titration with appropriate monitoring and the engagement of specialists with expertise in paediatric or adult neurology (as appropriate) is advised for the long-term control of epilepsy. With several new anticonvulsants available, the therapeutic armamentarium has expanded; combination therapies are often successful in seizure management.

Surgical interventions and other procedures for specific disorders

(For details see individual sections)

Particular symptoms and signs of disease (bone pain, ligamentous injury, sinus and middle-ear disorders, corneal opacities, optic nerve compression; abdominal hernias, hydrocephalus, spinal cord and other compression neuropathies – including carpal tunnel syndrome, respiratory failure, renal failure, hepatic disease with portal hypertension, stroke, gallstones and their complications, marrow failure, cardiomyopathy) will require management. Interventions, which may involve standard surgical procedures such as joint-replacement surgery or insertion of a ventricular shunt for raised intracranial pressure, can be highly successful. When operating on patients who are very disabled by their disease, attention must be given to the use of agreed ethical principles of care and the maintenance of the quality of life.

Patients with individual lysosomal diseases often have special requirements in relation to surgery and anaesthesia: to avoid catastrophes, these must be considered before any procedure is carried out. Space here is sufficient only to outline some areas of concern in considering surgery. Patients with Chédiak–Higashi and Hermansky–Pudlak syndromes, Gaucher disease and Niemann–Pick diseases A and B are examples of disorders where failure to consider the haemorrhagic tendency may be disastrous. Similarly, many patients with mucopolysaccharidoses have a significant risk from anaesthesia: cardiomyopathy; infiltration of the soft tissues in the larynx, tonsils, upper and lower airways; and fragility of the atlanto-occipital joint all may cause perioperative catastrophes. Before patients are advanced for elective surgery, the expertise of those who thoroughly understand the disease should be sought.

Neurological support

Patients with neurological disease require support for loss of given functions – bulbar palsy and the inability to swallow or initiate swallowing, will require consideration of either enteral (feeding gastrostomy) or parenteral nutrition and hydration (using indwelling intravenous access). Behavioural difficulties, including aggression, hyperactivity and insomnia, occur in those neurodegenerative disorders in which dementia advancing slowly in childhood rather than rapidly in infancy, is a feature; often these are major features of the Sanfilippo diseases (MPS III A–D) and may be accompanied by seizures. Patients with late-onset forms of metachromatic leukodystrophy, Krabbe and the GM2-gangliosidoses (Tay–Sachs and

Sandhoff diseases) often present with florid psychological disorders, including frontal-type dementia with loss of memory, insight and inhibitions. Behavioural manifestations can be particularly challenging and are distressing, especially for carers and others close at hand.

Specific strategies for treating lysosomal diseases

Cell complementation

Cellular complementation is the use of haematopoietic stem cells to supply deficient function present in the bone marrow and bone marrow-derived cells in the tissues of the recipient. In this category, other transplantation techniques are utilized, e.g. renal transplantation in Fabry disease, cardiac transplantation in Danon disease.

Treatment of many metabolic diseases has followed empirical developments in transplantation – specifically, bone marrow transplantation, which allows engraftment of haematopoietic stem cells (HSCs) into the immuno-suppressed recipient. Transplantation has the potential to supply complementing enzyme activity over the long-term, but often the lack of suitable donors and procedural complications with significant morbidity and mortality, encourage the search for improved alternatives. The European Group for Bone Marrow Transplantation has reported transplantation-related mortality risk from 10% (HLA-antigen identical) to 20% to 25% (HLA-antigen mismatched) in more than 60 patients with lysosomal diseases who have received haematopoietic stem cells, principally from bone marrow transplants [1].

After early success with bone marrow as a source of HSCs, the procedure today usually involves the harvesting of peripheral blood enriched with HSCs after treating the donor with colony-stimulating haematopoietic growth factors such as G-CSF to stimulate the release of stem cells from the marrow. Latterly, stored umbilical cord blood harvested from HLA-matched donor infants that are unrelated to the recipient has become a useful source of stem cells; occasionally stored umbilical cord blood from a matched younger sibling donor has been utilized. Staba et al. [2] have suggested that cord-blood stem cells obtained from unrelated donors can usefully be administered to patients with severe MPS1 under 2 years of age. An 85% event-free survival rate and reports of improved growth velocity and neurocognitive performance were noted; bone disease remained stable after the procedure. Several factors related to cord-blood transplantation may affect outcome, including the donor status, especially if the donor is a heterozygous carrier-sibling, the extent and persistence of donor chimerism,

and complications, such as graft-versus-host disease, which occur after the procedure has been carried out.

HSC transplantation supplies a complement of cells competent in lysosomal degradative and recycling functions but may also serve as a source of functional lysosomal proteins lacking in the recipient and which may be secreted by the donor cells and taken up at a distance to restore function in recipient tissues. While it cures the systemic defect in Gaucher disease and has benefit for some of the peripheral manifestations of the MPS syndromes, HSC transplantation has little effect on the neurological manifestations; the procedure is also valuable for the haematological and immune defects associated with the lysosomal biogenesis disorders, particularly Hermansky–Pudlak, Chédiak–Higashi and Griscelli syndromes. Several patients in northern Sweden, with the Norrbottnian variant of Gaucher disease, have received marrow transplants and while any effect on the neurological disease in type 3 Gaucher patients is unlikely (or at best controversial), clear benefit has been shown compared with those untreated. With the advent of successful enzyme treatment, haematopoietic stem-cell therapy has become largely obsolete for Gaucher disease in the context of most modern health care systems.

Haematopoietic stem cell transplantation in mucopolysaccharidoses

MPS I

HSCT is a long-established procedure in MPS I offering clear evidence of systemic benefit (but less correction of the osseous disease and growth failure) in patients with MPS1 [3]. The procedure may arrest progression of the neurological disease, and improves the outcome of infiltrative heart or liver disease; it prolongs the life of affected children. Even prompt use of stem-cell transplantation in early infancy fails to correct the principal skeletal deformities, although odontoid dysplasia may be improved and disturbed growth and dwarfism may be partially ameliorated. Many ocular abnormalities improve but complications in the lung commonly follow and are related to pre-existing risk factors. Enzyme therapy given in advance of transplantation may improve difficulties with engraftment and reduce the risk of these respiratory complications. Overall long-term survival in many centres exceeds 70%.

MPS II

Although haematopoietic stem cell transplantation (HSCT) using stem cells in pooled umbilical cord blood or bone marrow might provide sufficient enzyme activity to affect the progression of Hunter disease (MPS II), no results from systematic controlled trials are available to make an informed judgement. The position of HSCT in other mucopolysaccharidoses is hence controversial. In Hunter syndrome (MPS II) poor initial results [4] led, as a result of the influence of patient-based organizations, to a widespread moratorium on its use in UK children in the 1980s. Improved outcomes have been reported using haematopoietic stem-cell transplantation in a few very young MPS II patients but, as in other severe neurological diseases, this stratagem cannot generally be advocated because of poor cognitive outcomes, a high rate of graft failure and the other sequelae.

MPS VI

HSCT was used in MPS VI (Maroteaux–Lamy syndrome), but with the comparative success of enzyme augmentation it is no longer advocated. Herskhovitz *et al.* [5] reported long-term outcomes of HSCT in 4 patients with MPS VI; facial dysmorphism and some cardiac manifestations were improved but skeletal changes persisted or progressed. The procedure offers little benefit for the neurological disease with cognitive impairment in MPS VI and, given that enzyme therapy is safe, well-tolerated and effective for many of the systemic manifestations, there appears to be little clinical merit in its use [6].

Haematopoietic stem-cell transplantation in neurological disorders

Over about 30 years there have been efforts to utilize transplantation of haematopoietic cells as a means to correct the neurological component of lysosomal diseases. HSCT will lead to the replacement of microglia and other non-neuronal cells by healthy cells of donor origin; thereafter, cell or enzymatic complementation is postulated to improve the lysosomal defect in the nervous system. This approach has strong advocates – especially in the case of disorders such as globoid-cell leukodystrophy (Krabbe disease) and, to a lesser degree, metachromatic leukodystrophy [7]. In the former, there is overt evidence of diseased central macrophage-like cells and microglia – but in both conditions, peripheral nerve (and in the case of Krabbe, nerve root) disease may contribute significantly to the disability. There are reports of benefit and continued developmental progress as determined by neuropsychological testing, with improved hearing in several patients with alpha-mannosidosis treated by bone marrow transplantation. Currently this exceptionally rare disease is the object of clinical research into enzymatic complementation and reports of experience with HSCT are likely to involve only sporadic cases. Recently two siblings were transplanted at different ages and follow-up studies indicate that the therapeutic benefit was significantly greater in the sibling treated presymptomatically at 6 months of age rather than at 13 years [8].

After early reports suggesting benefit from marrow transplantation in children (and a few adults) with Krabbe disease, more recent attempts have been made to use HSCT (in most cases from umbilical cord-blood) in the neonatal period. The first results of these studies indicate a better outcome than would be expected in untreated Krabbe infants born to families with previously identified cases, but despite the heroic nature of the treatment, cognitive and motor deficits persist [9].

In metachromatic leukodystrophy the results have been even more disappointing and in late-infantile variants most centres avoid the procedure. Clearly the severity and extent of disease at the time of transplantation are critically important for determining outcomes.

Haematopoietic stem-cell therapy in disorders of lysosomal biogenesis (see Chapter 19)

The absence of the secondary aggregation response in platelets in Hermansky-Pudlak and Chédiak-Higashi syndromes, renders correction by haematopoietic stem-cell transplantation attractive. Successful transplantation completely obviates the risk of the EBV-associated accelerated phase characterized by haemophagocytic lymphohistiocytosis since it provides a source of healthy donor macrophages, lymphoid cells and megakaryocytes.

Enzyme enhancement

Enzyme replacement therapy

This stratagem seeks to enhance enzyme function in lysosomes – it includes enzymatic augmentation with appropriate targeting to diseased tissues commonly called enzyme replacement therapy (ERT), gene therapy and the use of pharmacological chaperones. These latter agents are designed to enhance the activity of unstable lysosomal enzymes by promoting their intracellular delivery to the site of action in the lysosome – thus preventing their premature destruction.

From the earliest days it was realized that lysosomes would be accessible to molecules presented at the cell surface, and thus specific defects, especially of soluble acid hydrolases, should be accessible to facile therapeutic complementation. The supposition proved correct: mutual and reciprocal secretion of factors that restore the biochemical abnormality in individual lysosomal diseases was shown in fibroblasts cultured from genetically distinct mucopolysaccharidoses (now known as MPS I and II). Proteins destined for the lysosome are sorted on the basis of a molecular signature – the mannose-6-phosphate moiety – which serves as a lysosomal recognition signal. Specific proteins bearing the correct targeting signal thus have the potential to complement inherited defects of lysosomal enzyme function. Later identification of the defect in patients with inclusion body disease due the presence of lysosomes engorged with diverse cellular debris – I-cell disease (mucolipidoses II and III) – led to the discovery of the mechanism by which lysosomal glycoproteins are decorated with mannose-6-phosphate.

Enzymatic augmentation has been introduced with preparations authorized for several lysosomal disorders, including Gaucher disease, Fabry disease, Pompe disease and Mucopolysaccharidoses types I, II and VI; promising late-stage clinical studies are underway for Niemann–Pick disease type B, α-mannosidosis and Mucopolyscaccharidosis type IV. Additional trials of enzyme replacement have been carried out in challenging diseases with neurological manifestations such as metachromatic leukodystrophy; are underway in Sanfilippo disease type B (MPS type IIIB); and planned in Krabbe disease. A notable exception to the process was harnessed in the first (and most successful) therapy for a lysosomal disease: uptake of therapeutic imiglucerase (Cerezyme™, partially deglycoslyated human β-glucocerebrosidase) by the diseased tissues in patients with Gaucher disease is mediated by mannose-binding lectins expressed on the macrophage surface. Accordingly, remodelling of human tissue-derived β-glucocerebrosidase glycoforms was undertaken to reveal terminal mannose residues; after years of fruitless research, this stratagem proved to be decisive for therapeutic targeting *in vivo* and for the approval of highly effective enzymatic augmentation in Gaucher disease [10]. Targeting of the modified enzyme molecule (derived from human placenta and as the genetically-engineered recombinant protein) to the affected viscera and marrow with preferential uptake by the pathological macrophages has been demonstrated in living patients with Gaucher disease [11].

Table 20.1 lists those enzyme preparations based on mannose and mannose-6-phosphate receptor targeting that are either licensed or are in the late phase of clinical development for lysosomal disease.

Enzyme therapy for individual disorders
Gaucher disease (see Chapter 6)
After remodelled human placental β-glucocerebrosidase (alglucerase, Ceredase™, Genzyme Corporation, Cambridge, MA, USA) was found to be safe and effective,

Table 20.1 Licensed Enzyme Preparations for Lysosomal Diseases.

Approved enzyme treatments for lysosomal diseases

- Gaucher disease types 1 and 3 (imiglucerase, velaglucerase alfa, taliglucerase alfa)*
- Anderson-Fabry disease (agalsidase alfa and agalsidase beta)
- Mucopolysaccharidosis type I (laronidase)
- Mucopolysaccharidosis type II (idursulfase)
- Mucopolysaccharidosis VI (galsulfase)
- Glycogenosis type ll A/Pompe (alglucosidase alfa)

Diseases for which enzyme therapy is in clinical development

○ Niemann-Pick disease B
○ Sanfilippo A and B (MPS 3A & 3B)
○ Morquio A and B (MPS 4A & 4B)
○ Metachromatic leukodystrophy
○ Alpha mannosidosis

*only imiglucerase licensed for use specifically in type 3 Gaucher disease

it gained marketing approval in 1991 but is now obsolete. Recombinant human β-glucocerebrosidase, expressed in Chinese hamster ovary cells – also modified to yield a mannose-terminated protein – was approved as imiglucerase (Cerezyme™, Genzyme Corporation) in 1995. Imiglucerase reverses or ameliorates many of the manifestations of type 1 Gaucher disease and sets the standard of care. A report from the International Gaucher Registry in 2002 included 1,028 patients with serial improvements in measurements of haemoglobin concentration, platelet count, liver and spleen volumes, and the occurrence of bone pain and bone crises.

Velaglucerase (VPRIV™, Shire Human Genetic Therapies) a recombinant human β-glucocerebrosidase expressed after activating the endogenous GBA1 gene in human fibrosarcoma cells cultured in the presence of an inhibitor of glycoprotein processing (kifunensine) to yield a highly mannosylated product was approved in 2010 for marketing in the USA and Europe. In May 2012, a mannose-terminated preparation of human β-glucocerebrosidase (taliglucerase-alfa; Elelyso) manufactured in genetically engineered carrot cells has been approved by the US Food and Drug Administration for the treatment of adult patients with type 1 Gaucher disease. Elelyso is manufactured and distributed by Pfizer Inc., under license from Protalix BioTherapeutics Inc

(Carmiel-Israel). The most common side effects reported during clinical studies were infusion reactions and allergic reactions.

Generally the infusion-related reactions are mild and, in treatment-naïve patients, occurred mostly during the first months of treatment; they tend to occur less frequently with time. Therapeutic goals in Gaucher disease, as well as guidelines for monitoring, were published by an expert panel in 2004; these guidelines are used to generate an individualized plan of treatment to optimize the management of the disease. While often useful in practice, these therapeutic goals may not be sensitive to all health changes during monitoring and should not be regarded as fixed points of care for a given patient.

Fabry disease

Fabry disease (see Chapter 7) has been treated with α-galactosidase A since 2001 and two competing enzyme preparations – agalsidase alfa (Replagal™) and agalsidase beta (Fabrazyme™) – are authorized for use in Europe whereas in the United States, at the time of writing, only agalsidase beta is authorized. Enzyme therapy showed efficacy in clinical trials, principally in male hemizygous patients at an early phase of disease; treatment has effects on myocardial hypertrophy, renal impairment, pain, and quality of life. However, no conclusion can be drawn from direct comparison of the therapeutic responses between the two available enzyme preparations – even though the licensed dose of agalsidase alfa (0.2 mg/kg/month) is materially less than agalsidase beta (1.0 mg/kg/month). Male patients with Fabry disease frequently develop antibodies associated with infusion reactions; while there may be a greater antigenic response to agalsidase beta, cross-reactivity between the two preparations is often found.

Mucopolysaccharidoses (see Chapter 12)

MPS I (Hurler–Scheie disease)

Enzyme therapy with laronidase (Aldurazyme™), licensed for treatment of the systemic manifestations of MPS I, improves liver size, linear growth, joint mobility, breathing, and sleep apnea in persons with the attenuated form of disease. The timing at which enzyme therapy is started is likely to influence the outcome.

MPS II (Hunter disease)

After early development by Transkaryotic Therapies Inc., to augment the impaired capacity of tissues in Hunter patients to digest sulfated glycosaminoglycans, including heparan sulfate, the enzyme preparation, idursulfase (Elaprase™), has been marketed for MPS II by Shire Human Genetic Therapies. Idursulfase contains eight asparagine-linked glycosylation sites occupied by complex oligosaccharide chains decorated by mannose-6-phosphate residues to allow specific binding of the enzyme to the cognate receptors on the cell surface and subsequent cellular internalization of the enzyme and delivery to lysosomes. As with other sulphatases, the enzyme activity of idursulfase is dependent on the post-translational modification of an active-site cysteine to formylglycine. Elaprase™ is approved in the United States and the European Union and marketed in many countries. Idursulfase has principally been studied in individuals with the attenuated form of Hunter disease and limited information is available on the outcome of enzyme therapy in young children (< 5 years) or individuals with respiratory difficulties or severe neurological disease. Since proteins do not materially traverse the blood–brain barrier, enzyme treatment would not be expected to improve the cognitive and related features of disease affecting the brain.

MPS IV A (Morquio disease)

Enzyme treatment of Morquio A syndrome (MPS IVA) using N-acetylgalactosamine-6 sulphatase (Biomarin Pharmaceuticals) is expected to clear keratan sulphate from the lysosomal compartment and arrest progression of the disease; it may ameliorate other manifestations. The enzyme preparation harbours mannose-6-phosphate residues on the glycan chains, thus allowing cellular uptake by the mannose-6-phosphate receptor and delivery to the lysosomes. A randomized, placebo-controlled double-blind phase 3 study is currently under way to evaluate the efficacy and safety of 2.0 mg/kg/week and 2.0 mg/kg/alternate weeks. The primary outcome will be based on the 6-minute Walk test and with secondary outcome measures change from baseline in endurance as measured by the 3-minute Stair-Climb test as well as changes from baseline in urine keratan sulfate excretion.

MPS VI (Maroteaux–Lamy disease)

Galsulfase (Naglazyme™), which has been developed by the Biomarin Pharmaceutical company, is a recombinant version of N-acetylgalactosamine 4-sulphatase(arylsulphatase B), and was licensed in 2005/6 in the United States and Europe (and latterly in many other countries); the agent has been shown to improve walking and stair-climbing capacity in patients with MPS VI [3].

Pompe disease (acid maltase deficiency; glycogen storage disease type 2 – see Chapter 13)

The doses of recombinant human acid α-glucosidase displaying mannose-6-phosphate residues used to treat Pompe disease exceed by an order of magnitude those used in other lysosomal disorders (20–40 mg/kg, compared with 0.1–2 mg/kg). This, combined with the absence of endogenous acid α-glucosidase cross-reacting antigen (CRIM^{-ve}) in many infants with the condition contributes to the development of important immune reactions which frequently complicate therapy. It is becoming clear that infants showing little or no clinical response to the treatment lack expression of endogenous acid α-glucosidase antigen (CRIM^{-ve}). They generate high-titre IgG antibodies which may inhibit the enzyme *in vitro*. Those who develop IgE antibodies to alglucosidase alfa are at a high risk of severe allergic reactions and even anaphylaxis; close monitoring of enzyme infusions is mandatory. These and others who are severely compromised may require radical immunomodulatory intervention – including the use of rituximab or omalizumab – in attempts to overcome the barrier to life-saving treatment [12]. As described in Chapter 13, however, Myozyme™ prolongs life when administered to very young infants with Pompe disease who do not develop high-titre antibodies, and in a controlled clinical trial shows clear benefit when given to adults, preventing respiratory failure and with improvement in skeletal muscle function [13]. The long-term health outcome in severely affected infants after life-saving treatment has yet to be reported.

Alpha-mannosidosis (see Chapter 14)

After the cloning and expression of human α-mannosidase and several years of promising preclinical animal studies into the use of enzyme therapy for human α-mannosidosis, phase 1/2 clinical trials have been announced and recruitment is now closed for a single centre, randomized open-label, multiple-dose study of the efficacy and long-term safety of recombinant human alpha-mannosidase (Lamazym™). The manufacturer of this enzyme preparation is the Zymenex company and the results of this clinical trial in such a severely disabling and rare disorder are awaited eagerly.

Niemann–Pick disease type B (see Chapter 10)

The Genzyme Corporation has two approved clinical research studies for individuals with Niemann–Pick disease caused by acid sphingomyelinase deficiency (types A and B). Clinical studies are long-awaited and significant delays in the testing of the recombinant human enzyme are in part the result of dose-related toxicity in preclinical studies using genetically modified mice. The author considers it possible that increased intracellular concentrations of ceramide, a recognized cell-death signal released directly from sphingomyelin by the action of acid sphingomyelinase, may have caused toxicity and thus contributed to entirely appropriate delays in the clinical development of enzyme therapy by Drs Schuchmann and Desnick at Mount Sinai hospital in New York.

Substrate restriction therapy ("substrate reduction therapy")

Mode of action

This stratagem seeks to compensate for the impaired ability of a lysosomal enzyme to break down its physiological target molecules. The use of an inhibitor to decrease the rate of formation of the specific material, the breakdown of which is defective in a given disorder, depends upon identifying very selective compounds which modulate substrate formation at early steps in their production, thus allowing the residual activity of the degradative enzyme system to cope with new incoming material for digestion. Inhibitors that influence sphingolipid biosynthesis have received considerable attention for pharmaceutical development; if suitable compounds can be found for other molecular pathways, the approach could be applied more generally.

Sphingolipidoses: general considerations

The inhibitory action is directed to UDP-glucose: N-acylsphingosine glucosyltransferase, the first committed step for the biosynthesis of β-glucosylceramide and its derivatives. β-Glucosylceramide is the precursor of several hundred glycolipid products of combinatorial reactions catalyzed by the addition of simple sugar moieties. According to the nature of the inherited biochemical defect in lysosomal breakdown and recycling, members of this complex sphingolipid family accumulate in Gaucher disease, Fabry disease, and the GM1 and GM2 gangliosidoses. Inhibition of UDP-glucose: N-acylsphingosine glucosyltransferase (UDP-glucosylceramide transferase) was predicted by Norman Radin to serve as the immediate target of therapy in Gaucher disease.

The sugar mimetic, miglustat (N-butyldeoxynojirimycin), is approved for the treatment of Gaucher disease and Niemann–Pick C disease (the latter in the EU). This iminosugar inhibits glycosidases, including α-glycosidases and at micromolar concentrations inhibits

N-acylsphingosine glucosyltransferase, and consequently the biosynthesis of β-glucosylceramide (glucocerebroside) in cultured cells. It is likely that the action of miglustat arises from its monosaccharide structure and that it serves as an inhibitory mimic of the sugar nucleotide substrate.

Eliglustat tartrate (Genz-112638) is in late clinical development by the Genzyme Corporation for the treatment of Gaucher disease – with possible application to cognate glycosphingolipidoses. It is also a potent, specific and orally active inhibitor (Ki ~25 nM) of its molecular target, N-acylsphingosine glucosyltransferase).

Application to specific diseases

Gaucher disease

Miglustat

After encouraging preclinical studies, a clinical trial of miglustat (Zavesca®) in patients with mild-to-moderate type I Gaucher disease, using 100 mg thrice daily, showed that the agent reduced visceral enlargement and improved haematological parameters, as well as the plasma biomarker of storage macrophages, chitotriosidase.

As a small iminosugar molecule that penetrates the blood–brain barrier, miglustat was explored in children with chronic neuronopathic (type 3) Gaucher disease. Unfortunately, this trial failed to meet its clinical end points and the drug is not recommended for neurological manifestations in Gaucher disease.

Eliglustat tartrate

In healthy volunteers, plasma glucocerebroside concentrations were diminished after oral dosing with eliglustat tartrate, and in open-label phase II clinical trials in patients with type 1 (non-neuronopathic) Gaucher disease, spleen and liver volumes were decreased together with impressive haematological responses.

Eliglustat tartrate appears to be effective and hitherto relatively safe. It also would have the convenience of an orally active agent for Gaucher disease. Clearly the mode of action suggests possible application in Fabry disease, but it is unlikely to benefit glycosphingolipidoses affecting the brain. The outcome of several ongoing phase 3 multicentre trials, including those involving a switch from enzyme therapy in adult Gaucher type 1 patients with stable disease, are awaited with great interest.

Niemann–Pick disease type C

Miglustat (Zavesca™) has recently received approval from EMA for treating Niemann–Pick disease type C, another lysosomal disease affecting the brain, in which disturbed cholesterol trafficking to lysosomes is associated with accumulation of glycosphingolipids and possibly sphingosine in neurons; intracellular calcium pools appear to be disturbed. Although at the time of writing, the FDA has not yet approved the agent, it remains a welcome treatment for patients with Niemann–Pick C disease who would otherwise have no options.

Pharmacological chaperone therapy (also see Chapter 22)

Mode of action

Molecular chaperones are designed to enhance the activity of unstable mutant forms of lysosomal enzymes by binding to the newly formed enzyme molecule and promoting its intracellular delivery to the site of action in the lysosome – thus preventing premature destruction. The chaperone molecules preferably have greater affinity at neutral pH; they bind to the active site and are usually inhibitors that dissociate from the enzyme under the acid conditions of the lysosome. Retention of a functional active site in the given mutant enzyme target is necessary for it to be a candidate for chaperone treatment.

General considerations

Clearly this therapeutic principle requires high penetration of the chaperone molecule within the target cells and tissues principally affected by the disease. Only selected disease-associated mutant proteins will respond – a requirement that may necessitate mutation-specific testing *in vitro* to confirm the chaperone effect. If they can prevent misfolding and mistrafficking of the protein, and improve lysosomal targeting, diffusible molecules that bind as specific inhibitors of the target mutant protein may be useful for treatment as pharmacological chaperones. Once in the low pH environment of the lysosome, the enzyme-inhibitor complex is predicted to be destabilized and thus free to bind more favourably to the natural substrate within the organelle. The pharmacological chaperone molecule needs to bind, temporarily stabilize – and then dissociate from its molecular target. Thus, ensuring the appropriate means of administration ("on" and "off" times) – allowing for binding and dissociation according to the pharmacokinetics of the given chaperone agent and biosynthetic rate of the mutant protein target – is of critical importance. Although the chaperone molecule will be designed to interact with a specific enzyme, each mutant enzyme–chaperone combination will be unique to patients with the same mutation, in whom the abundance, stability and intralysosomal activity of the enzyme are to be enhanced.

Application to specific diseases

Amicus Therapeutics is developing orally available small molecules as pharmacological chaperones for treating diseases including lysosomal disorders and related conditions. The company has conducted preclinical studies evaluating the combination of pharmacological chaperones and enzyme therapy for Fabry disease and Pompe disease as well as preclinical studies examining the use of pharmacological chaperones for the treatment of Parkinson disease. Here the object is to increase the activity of β-glucocerebrosidase and so accumulation of alpha-synuclein in the brain of patients with Parkinson disease, linked to mutant forms of β-glucocerebrosidase, as first recognized in Gaucher disease.

Fabry disease

The lead investigational drug developed by Amicus, Amigal™ (the iminosugar, 1-deoxygalactonojirimycin – "migalastat HCl2") is under investigation in Phase 3 as a pharmacological chaperone with a potential therapeutic action on mutant α-galactosidases A in Fabry disease. A trial to compare ERT and chaperone therapy for Fabry disease is under way.

Gaucher disease

Amicus started clinical testing in a Phase 1 study of the AT2101 Plicera™ (isofagomine – "afegostat tartrate") in 2006. All patients showed an increase in white-cell glucocerebrosidase activity but only 1 of the 18 patients who completed the study had improved disease parameters. Afegostat tartrate was generally well tolerated and no serious adverse events occurred. However, at the time of writing the trial has been discontinued for lack of general efficacy.

Pompe disease

After completing Phase 1 studies of AT2220 (1-deoxynojirimycin HCl) in healthy volunteers in 2008, Amicus initiated a Phase 2 clinical trial in patients with adult Pompe disease. This trial involved initial treatment with a high dose of AT2220: two patients experienced muscle weakness and withdrew. The events were categorized as serious and probably related to the agent and in 2009 Amicus suspended trial enrolment and received a clinical trial hold from the FDA (US Food and Drug Administration).

Preliminary results of preclinical research in Pompe mice showed that 1-deoxynojirimycin HCl consistently decreased the content of glycogen in several tissues, including heart, diaphragm and skeletal muscles. Apparently encouraged by these preclinical results, the company aims to evaluate the use of the iminosugar AT2220 in combination with enzyme therapy. Amicus plans to report additional data from these studies, but at the time of writing no further information is forthcoming about the further clinical development of 1-deoxynojirimycin HCl as a pharmacological chaperone in human Pompe disease.

β-Galactosidase deficiency (Morquio type B; GM1 gangliosidosis)

Morquio B disease is caused by heterogeneous mutations in the gene encoding lysosomal acid β-galactosidase. N-octyl-4-epi-β-valienamine has pharmacological chaperone activity on nascent mutant β-galactosidase proteins and it appears that > 20% disease-related mutant proteins are likely to respond to this iminosugar-related agent. The outcomes of clinical trials planned to investigate this promising question in GM1 gangliosidosis are thus awaited with interest. N-octyl-4-epi-β-valienamine is a potentially informative chaperone molecule for investigation in β-galactosidase deficiency and possibly also for some mutant forms of acid β-glucocerebrosidase in patients with Gaucher disease.

Substrate removal

Mode of action

Another stratagem is to dissolve the accumulated toxin within the lysosome. The use of cysteamine, to disperse cystine deposits in cystinosis by forming soluble mixed-thiols, is an example of this approach to substrate removal. Cysteamine also disrupts thioester linkages, which are not broken down in CLN1 due to a deficiency of palmitoyl-protein thioesterase (PPT1), providing a rationale for the use of cysteamine in CLN1. Also in this category are cyclodextrins, which are being explored in patients with Niemann–Pick disease type C. Cyclodextrins can chelate cholesterol and have been shown to decrease the pathological intralysosomal accumulation of cholesterol in cells. Cyclodextrins also chelate other molecules, including steroid hormones and cations; they thus have several potential modes of action in Niemann–Pick disease type C and other lysosomal disorders.

Cystinosis (see Chapter 17)

Cystinosis, a life-threatening condition, affects about 1 in 100,000 persons and is caused by genetic defects in a lysosomal protein, cystinosin, a membrane transporter of cystine. Excess free cystine causes intracellular crystal formation in most tissues, with early effects on the kidney tubule and cornea. Infants affected by nephropathic cystinosis have growth retardation and renal tubular disease causing a Fanconi syndrome and later kidney failure. The kidney disorder causes critical loss of phosphate and other minerals leading to dehydration, acidosis and hypophosphatemic rickets. Corneal crystal deposits are usually apparent by the age of one year; they cause photophobia and impaired vision. Systemic cystinosis causes end-stage renal failure in childhood: long-term complications include thyroid failure, male hypogonadism, cerebellar and pyramidal signs with impaired cognition and pseudo-bulbar palsy, encephalopathy and stroke-like episodes with radiological changes in the brain. Benign intracranial hypertension has also been reported. Myocardial and pulmonary disease occurs in older survivors.

Management of cystinosis

Hitherto, treatment of cystinosis was limited to treating metabolic acidosis due to the Fanconi syndrome and replenishing electrolytes and key nutrients lost in the urine; early-onset chronic renal failure was inevitable. The availability of phosphocysteamine and preparations of topical and systemic (oral) cysteamine, together with advances in contemporary renal transplantation, have greatly improved the outlook and quality of life in patients with this otherwise disabling and fatal lysosomal disease.

Without treatment, painful erosions of the cornea and neovascularization in the periphery of the iris occur.

Dehydration and salt depletion should be avoided, especially during febrile illnesses accompanied by vomiting or diarrhoea. Urinary potassium and bicarbonate losses should be restored with regular oral supplements; active vitamin D analogues with additional phosphate and appropriate monitoring will prevent osteodystrophy. Thyroid function should be monitored and thyroid failure should be treated. Long-term studies suggest that judicious use of angiotensin converting-enzyme inhibitors correlates with better outcomes in nephropathic cystinosis.

Indomethacin appears to mitigate dehydration in patients with nephropathic cystinosis and functioning kidneys, in which it decreases glomerular filtration rate and improves tubular sensitivity to endogenous antidiuretic hormone. Rigorous follow-up is required for its use because, as a non-steroidal anti-inflammatory agent, indomethacin causes glomerular injury and in the long term frequently causes peptic ulceration. (The latter may be ameliorated by eradication of Helicobacter pylori infection and co-prescription of a proton-pump inhibitor.) If indomethacin is to be used, renal glomerular function should be monitored carefully and any symptoms indicating peptic ulcer disease must be explored. Without proven clinical efficacy, carnitine – the plasma and tissue content of which is decreased by excess urinary loss – may be given with the intention of improving oxidative metabolism and muscle function.

Since stunted growth is the rule, recombinant human growth hormone should be considered to improve growth velocity in affected children with nephropathic cystinosis. Use of this agent before renal failure ensues is effective and safe and does not accelerate the decline in renal function; however, the hormone has limited benefit in young patients treated by renal dialysis.

Kidney transplantation greatly prolongs survival and improves life-quality in patients with cystinosis: donor kidney tissue is not subject to recurrent injury due to intracellular cystine crystal deposition. However, the procedure has no effect on the systemic manifestations of cystinosis in other organs; thus after transplantation, specific therapy with cysteamine or phosphocysteamine (see below) must be continued.

Specific therapies

Cysteamine, and the pro-drug phosphocysteamine, are aminothiols which enter lysosomes and in a thiol–disulphide interchange reaction convert cystine into the soluble cysteine monomer; the diffusible mixed cysteine–cysteamine adduct is formed. In patients with cystinosis, cysteamine reduces cystine accumulation in some cells (e.g. leukocytes, muscle and liver cells) and its early introduction delays the onset of renal failure.

Cysteamine is available as the hydrochloride, bitartrate – and as a sodium salt of phosphocysteamine. Some investigators and patients have suggested that cysteamine bitartrate and phosphocysteamine are better tolerated with superior bioavailability over cysteamine hydrochloride; neither benefit has been clearly shown – at least in healthy subjects.

Topical therapy

Cysteamine (mercaptamine 0.11–0.5% w/v) eye drops are available as a non-proprietary topical treatment for preventing and treating the ocular symptoms due to crystalline deposits in the cornea (cystine keratopathy); in the UK this is available as a manufactured special. The agent may be prepared extraneously, according to good manufacturing practice, elsewhere.

Systemic therapy

Cysteamine (as mercaptamine bitartrate, Cystagon™, Orphan Europe SARL) has been authorized since 1997. Starting doses should be one-quarter to one-sixth of the expected maintenance dose and increased gradually over 4–6 weeks to avoid intolerance. Phosphocysteamine is a pro-drug which provides phosphate and one third of the molar equivalent by weight of cysteamine; in the UK this is available as a manufactured special, it may be prepared extraneously, according to good manufacturing practice, elsewhere. Cysteamine bitartrate (in the delayed release preparation, Cystagon™) is supplied by Raptor Pharmaceuticals.

Monitoring

Cysteamine therapy should be initiated promptly once nephropathic cystinosis has been diagnosed by clinical signs *and* biochemical studies (leucocyte cystine assay above 2 nmol hemicystine/mg protein). The goal of therapy is to keep leucocyte cystine concentrations < 1 nmol hemicystine/mg protein and monitoring is used to adjust the dose with determinations 5 to 6 hours after dosing; monthly measurements are recommended at the start of treatment and every 3–4 months when the dose has been established. The dose should be raised if the drug is tolerated and the leucocyte cystine concentration remains above 1 nmol hemicystine/mg protein.

Cysteamine and phosphocysteamine are malodorous sulfhydryl compounds: they cause gastrointestinal disturbances and an unpleasant odour in the patient. Compliance is a major issue in the management of cystinosis.

Given the striking prolongation of life and improved life-quality now achievable for patients with cystinosis, it is important to add that cysteamine and its congeners are teratogens and should not be administered to pregnant women or nursing mothers.

Therapeutic outcomes

The outcome of cysteamine treatment in 246 children with cystinosis in three principal clinical trials is available. Cysteamine maintains growth, which is stunted in untreated patients but growth velocity may not allow a catch up for age. Renal tubular function was unaffected by treatment. The severity of dysphagia has been correlated with the severity of muscular disease attributable to cystinosis and has been reported to decrease with the duration of specific therapy with cysteamine. Long-term follow-up studies from a single centre over more than 20 years confirm the benefit of promptly initiating cysteamine therapy as well as the clear survival advantage of early diagnosis to mitigate the effects of the condition on the kidney and other organs.

Neuronal Ceroid Lipofuscinosis , infantile variant – CLN1 disease (see Chapter 18)

Cysteamine is undergoing trials in another lysosomal disease, acute infantile neuronal ceroid lipofuscinosis (CLN1 disease), which is due to a deficiency of lysosomal palmitoyl–protein thioesterase (PPT1). The deficiency of PPT1 impairs the cleavage of thioester linkages in palmitoylated proteins, preventing their hydrolysis by lysosomal proteinases. The accumulation of lipid-modified proteins (constituents of ceroid) in lysosomes is associated with neurodegeneration. The agent phosphocysteamine, which is lysosomotrophic, mediates the depletion of intralysosomal ceroid deposits in lymphoblasts derived from CLN1 patients, and may reduce apoptotic cell death. The possibility that related drugs, such as phosphocysteamine, may have a therapeutic action role in CLN1 merits further exploration but to date no convincing evidence of clinical benefit is available.

Cyclodextrin and Niemann–Pick C

Cyclodextrins, which have long been employed as carriers of drugs and as cyclic oligosaccharides with amphipathic properties, have steroid-binding properties that can be used to manipulate the cellular cholesterol content. Their potential application to Niemann–Pick disease type C has emerged from a chance observation that cyclodextrin alone prolonged the life of Niemann–Pick C mice. It is rapidly advancing from the level of preclinical trials in experimental animal models of the disease to clinical trials in patients with the current sanction of the US Food and Drug Administration (FDA). In 2009, the FDA approved intravenous infusions of hydroxy-propyl-β-cyclodextrin as an investigational new drug for 6-year-old identical twins. Subsequently orphan drug status was granted for a branded preparation of cyclodextrin, hydroxy-propyl-β-cyclodextrin, which was designated a treatment for Niemann–Pick type C disease. Further approval has been given for intrathecal administration, and direct injection into the brain will be considered in an attempt to arrest the neurodegeneration characteristic of this disease. The results of these ongoing trials in the twins and other patients are eagerly awaited.

Conclusions

Discoveries made in the late 1960s through to 1980s provided the basis for development of what is now known as targeted enzyme-replacement therapy for lysosomal diseases. From a practical viewpoint, it was the astonishing therapeutic success of macrophage-targeted β-glucocerebrosidase manufactured by the Genzyme corporation for Gaucher disease that stimulated revolutionary in-house investment in treatments for other lysosomal diseases and committed commercial competition from other biopharmaceutical companies. However, despite their promise, and much welcome investment in accompanying clinical research and services, licensed enzyme therapies have in the main been less radically life-changing for patients with diseases where the therapeutic targeting involves receptor-mediated systems not predicated on the avid mannose lectin system. There is nonetheless little doubt that the initiatives have radically altered the commercial perspective of orphan drug development and provide a step-up in revenue and activity for the whole field.

For the future there is no place for despondency: the example of three competing enzyme therapies for Gaucher disease, two for Fabry disease and several enzyme therapies in late-stage development for ultra-rare diseases such as Niemann–Pick type B, Morquio disease and α-mannosidosis, is inspiring. Moreover, other agents with distinct modes of action are either approved (miglustat for Niemann–Pick type C and Gaucher disease in addition to cysteamine preparations for cystinosis) or licensed and in advanced development (eliglustat for Gaucher disease and congeners with therapeutic potential for several glycosphingolipidoses, including those that affect the brain). Moreover, the success of any emerging therapy can only enhance confidence and the commitment to credible investment into the drugs of the future: selective substrate inhibitors and pharmacological chaperones, as well as other striking innovations – including the clinical development of gene therapy.

References

1 Hoogerbrugge P, Brouwer O, Bordigoni P, *et al*. Allogeneic bone marrow transplantation for lysosomal storage diseases. The European Group for Bone Marrow Transplantation. *Lancet* 1995; **345**: 1398–1403.

2 Staba S, Escolar M, Poe M, *et al*. Cord-blood transplants from unrelated donors in patients with Hurler's syndrome. *N Engl J Med* 2004; **350**: 1960–1969.

3 Giugliani R, Federhen A, Rojas MV, *et al*. Mucopolysaccharidosis I, II, and VI: Brief review and guidelines for treatment. *Genet Mol Biol* 2010; **33**: 589–604.

4 Wraith JE. Limitations of enzyme replacement therapy: current and future. *J Inherit Metab Dis* 2006; **29**: 442–447.

5 Herskhovitz E, Young E, Rainer J, *et al*. Bone marrow transplantation for Maroteaux-Lamy syndrome (MPS VI): long-term follow-up. *J Inherit Metab Dis* 1999; **22**: 50–62.

6 Giugliani R, Harmatz P, Wraith JE. Management guidelines for mucopolysaccharidosis VI. *Pediatrics* 2007; **120**: 405–418.

7 Krivit W, Peters C, Shapiro EG. Bone marrow transplantation as effective treatment of central nervous system disease in globoid cell leukodystrophy, metachromatic leukodystrophy, adrenoleukodystrophy, mannosidosis, fucosidosis, aspartylglucosaminuria, Hurler, Maroteaux-Lamy, and Sly syndromes, and Gaucher disease type III. *Curr Opin Neurol* 1999; **12**: 167–176.

8 Broomfield AA, Chakrapani A, Wraith JE . The effects of early and late bone marrow transplantation in siblings with alpha-mannosidosis. Is early haematopoietic cell transplantation the preferred treatment option? *J Inherit Metab Dis* 2010 Feb 18. (E-pub in advance)

9 Escolar ML, Poe MD, Provenzale JM, *et al*. Transplantation of umbilical-cord blood in babies with infantile Krabbe's disease. *N Engl J Med* 2005; **352**: 2069–2081.

10 Van Patten SM, Hughes H, Huff MR, *et al*. Effect of mannose chain length on targeting of glucocerebrosidase for enzyme replacement therapy of Gaucher disease. *Glycobiology* 2007; **17**: 467–478.

11 Mistry PK, Wraight EP, Cox TM. Delivery of proteins to macrophages: implications for treatment of Gaucher's disease. *Lancet* 1996; **348**: 1555–1559.

12 Rohrbach M, Klein A, Köhli-Wiesner A, *et al*. CRIM-negative infantile Pompe disease: 42-month treatment outcome. *J Inherit Metab Dis* 2010; **33**: 751–757.

13 van der Ploeg AT, Clemens PR, Corzo D, *et al*. A randomized study of alglucosidase alfa in late-onset Pompe's disease. *N Engl J Med* 2010; **362**: 1396–1406.

Further reading

14 Brady RO. Enzyme replacement for lysosomal diseases. *Annu Rev Med* 2006; **57**: 283–296.

15 Desnick RJ, Brady R, Barranger J, *et al*. Fabry disease, an under-recognized multisystemic disorder: expert recommendations for diagnosis, management, and enzyme replacement therapy. *Ann Intern Med* 2003; **138**: 338–346.

16 Desnick RJ, Schuchman EH. Enzyme replacement and enhancement therapies: lessons from lysosomal disorders. *Nat Rev Genet* 2002; **3**: 954–966.

17 Grewal S, Wynn R, Abdenur JE, *et al*. Safety and efficacy of enzyme replacement therapy in combination with hematopoietic stem cell transplantation in Hurler syndrome. *Genet Med* 2005; **7**: 143–146.

18 Güngör D, de Vries JM, Hop WC, *et al*. Survival and associated factors in 268 adults with Pompe disease prior to treatment with enzyme replacement therapy. *Orphanet J Rare Dis* 2011; **6**: 34.

19 Harmatz P, Giugliani R, Schwartz I, *et al*. Enzyme replacement therapy for mucopolysaccharidosis VI: a phase 3, randomized, double-blind, placebo-controlled, multinational

study of recombinant human N-acetylgalactosamine 4-sulfatase (recombinant human arylsulfatase B or rhASB) and follow-on, open-label extension study. *J Pediatr* 2006; **148**: 533–539.

20 Kishnani PS, Corzo D, Nicolino M, *et al*. Recombinant human acid [alpha]-glucosidase: major clinical benefits in infantile-onset Pompe disease. *Neurology* 2007; **68**: 99–109.

21 Madra M, Sturley SL. Niemann-Pick type C pathogenesis and treatment: from statins to sugars. *Clin Lipidol* 2010; **5**: 387–395.

22 Meikle PJ, Hopwood JJ, Clague AE, Carey WF. Prevalence of lysosomal storage disorders. *JAMA* 1999; **281**: 249–254.

23 Nesterova G, Gahl WA. Cystinosis. In: Pagon RA, *et al*. (eds.), *GeneReviews* [Internet]. Seattle (WA): University of Washington, Seattle; 1993–2001 Mar 22 [updated 2011 Aug 11].

24 Neufeld EF. From serendipity to therapy. *Annu Rev Biochem* 2011; **80**: 1–15.

25 Saftig, P. *Lysosomes*. Springer-Verlag, New York Inc., 2005; 195 pp.

26 Schiffmann R, Ries M, Askari H, *et al*. Pathological findings in a patient with Fabry disease who died after 2.5 years of enzyme replacement. *Virchows Arch* 2006; **448**: 337–343.

27 Sly WS. Enzyme replacement therapy for lysosomal storage disorders: successful transition from concept to clinical practice. *Mol Med* 2004; **101**: 100–104.

28 von Figura K, Hasilik A. Lysosomal enzymes and their receptors. *Annu Rev Biochem* 1986; **55**: 167–193.

29 Wraith JE, Clarke LA, Beck M, *et al*. Enzyme replacement therapy for Mucopolysaccharidosis I: a randomized, double-blinded, placebo-controlled, multinational study of recombinant human alpha-L-iduronidase (laronidase). *J Pediatr* 2004; **144**: 581–588.

CHAPTER 21

Central Nervous System Aspects, Neurodegeneration and the Blood–Brain Barrier

David J. Begley[1] and Maurizio Scarpa[2]

[1] Institute of Pharmaceutical Science, Kings College London, London, UK
[2] Department of Paediatrics, University of Padova, Padova, Italy

Introduction

Of the 50 or more described lysosomal storage diseases (LSDs) the majority are neuronopathic and associated with profound neurodegeneration. The blood–brain barrier (BBB) is created by the vascular bed of the central nervous system (CNS) and very closely regulates the composition of the brain extracellular fluid. The blood–brain barrier is a vital issue in neuronopathic LSDs as substrate reduction, chaperone and enzyme replacement therapies must obtain access to the CNS in order to treat the neurological aspects of the disease. It has been shown that the BBB is compromised in a number of the neuronopathic LSDs, especially those with an early onset. Dysfunction of the BBB and a compromise of its regulatory role in CNS homeostasis may contribute to the CNS pathology and neurodegeneration.

The LSDs are a unique model in which to study neurodegeneration. In fact, although the accumulation of intermediate degradation products is due to a single gene defect, this affects the whole cellular metabolic system causing neuronal death apoptosis or necrosis at advanced stages of the disease. CNS pathology causes mental retardation and progressive neurodegeneration that ultimately ends in an early death. Many of these features are also found in adult neurodegenerative disorders, such as Alzheimer, Parkinson or Huntington diseases. A lysoso-mal involvement in the pathogenesis of these disorders has been described. Improved knowledge of secondary events will have an impact on diagnosis, staging and the follow-up of affected children. Importantly, new insights may provide indications about possible advances in treatment and disease reversal.

CNS storage and neuropathology

A common characteristic of many LSDs is the onset and relentless progression of neurodegenerative signs and symptoms. This neurodegeneration may start early in life or not manifest until later, depending on the LSD and the nature of the enzyme deficit. The cascade of events that leads to neurodegeneration and the neuropathology is not simple and is certainly not related solely to the primary storage product. Many secondary storage products, such as gangliosides, accumulate and may be a principal cause of CNS damage. Abnormal inflammatory responses are also present in the brains of LSD patients and the microglia are "activated" and show abnormal activity and secretion of cytokines.

Many of the LSDs exhibit, as part of their CNS manifestation, increases in oxidative stress, alterations in calcium homeostasis, autophagy and altered lipid trafficking in addition to neuronal, glial and other CNS

Lysosomal Storage Disorders: A Practical Guide, First Edition. Edited by Atul Mehta and Bryan Winchester.

© 2012 John Wiley & Sons, Ltd. Published 2012 by John Wiley & Sons, Ltd.

cell accumulation of the primary storage product. Primary and secondary events have a profound impact on the morphology and function of neural cells, producing alteration in dendritic processes with the generation of meganeurites and axonal spheroids together with somatic swelling. Meganeurites are huge axon hillock enlargements containing typical storage bodies, which often exceed the volume of adjacent perikarya. Meganeurites are probably associated with an increased expression of GM2-ganglioside, which probably acts as a neurite growth promoting factor or as an acceptor molecule for growth factors which influence the cells. Axonal spheroids are enlargements distal to the axon initial segment region. While meganeurites contain storage material consistent with the specific defective lysosomal hydrolase, and their morphology is therefore considered disease-specific, axonal spheroids contain a distinctly different array of materials with ultrastructural features (tubulovesicular profiles, mitochondria and dense and multivesicular-type bodies) that are the same across many types of storage disorders. While there is quite a clear understanding of possible mechanisms underlying the genesis of ectopic dendrites on cortical pyramidal neurons in LSDs, little is known regarding the functional consequences of this event. Asymmetrical synapses are known to occur on these dendrites and this input is likely to injure the neuron function. Evidence suggests that lysosomal storage impairs autophagy, and relies on the hypothesis that storage may interfere with lysosomal contribution to the autophagic process resulting in accumulation of polyubiquitinated proteins and dysfunctional mitochondria ultimately leading to apoptosis.

This becomes relevant since it has been hypothesized that treatment might be achieved by controlling autophagy. The lysosome is not an isolated "waste disposal" organelle within the cell, but is in communication with all the major cell domains. Mitochondrial abnormalities have been shown in many LSDs suggesting a common cause. As mitochondria are essential in the production of energy via ATP and lipid biosynthesis, alteration in their function causes activation of an ER stress response, mitochondrial apoptotic signalling, or both triggering cell death under physiologic or pathologic conditions. Depletion of ER calcium-stores or elevation of cytosolic calcium levels, can activate different biochemical pathways such as the cytoplasmic apoptotic pathway mediated by ER-localized caspase activity that in turn induces a form of ER stress, known as the "unfolded protein response" (UPR). The UPR system is aimed at minimizing protein production in the ER and increasing production of the chaperone proteins that can facilitate correct folding of the unfolded or misfolded proteins. It has been suggested that UPR may represent a common mediator of apoptosis in both neurodegenerative and non-neurodegenerative LSDs.

Calcium is a fundamental component of eukaryotic cells and plays a major role in cell homeostasis as an intracellular mediator. Excitable cells respond by alterations in cell signaling pathways, through calcium modulation. A high calcium concentration is toxic to neurons so at rest the cytosolic calcium concentration is maintained at low levels by the concerted action of specialized channels, a calcium pump, calcium-dependent enzymes, and calcium-binding proteins. These mechanisms are localized in the cytosol, ER and mitochondria, the three compartments that control the traffic of calcium across the plasma membrane or into intracellular stores. In neurons, calcium is stored mainly in the ER where it is pumped from the cytosol by the sarco/endoplasmic reticulum calcium ATPase (SERCA) and from which it is released back into the cytosol through two types of channel, one of which is a ryanodine receptor. Altered calcium homeostasis is one of the most common pathological features of lysosomal storage in LSDs. It has been described in several LSDs, including Gaucher disease.

Like calcium homeostasis, iron homeostasis is also essential in the CNS and furthermore it appears to play a role in the pathogenesis of neurodegenerative disease including Parkinson and Alzheimer diseases if altered. The exact mechanism by which iron causes this pathogenic consequence is still not clear. A recent study on murine models of GM1- and GM2-gangliosidoses, both of which are characterized by progressive depletion of iron in brain tissue, showed alterations in iron homeostasis. Progress in the understanding of such complex processes will open, together with a better comprehension of the development of the LSD phenotype, the application of new potential synergistic therapies to be coupled to the actual gold standard treatment, such as enzyme replacement therapy (ERT).

Normal function of the blood–brain barrier

The BBB enables the creation of an unique fluid environment for the brain which is extremely stable and much more tightly controlled than the extracellular

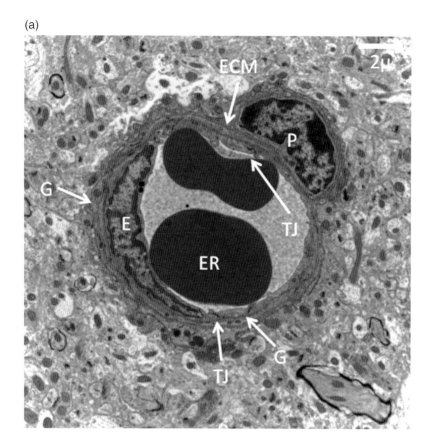

(a)

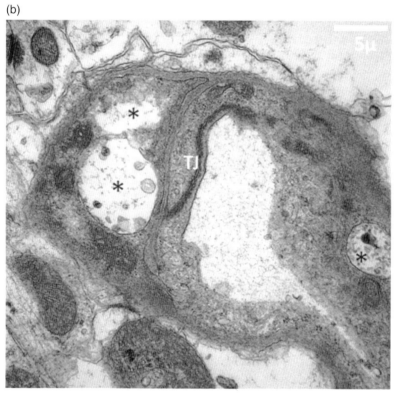

(b)

fluid (ECF) of the soma. Regulation of the ionic composition of the brain ECF and cerebrospinal fluid (CSF) needs to be precisely controlled in order to allow the maintenance of stable resting potentials and the generation of reliable action potentials. The background concentrations of the multiple CNS neurotransmitters is also tightly regulated to reduce background noise at synapses in order to maintain the complex neural integrative processes that the CNS must perform. Also the total protein content of CSF is very low and is only 0.5% of that of plasma. The protein content of the CSF in foetal life is much higher and this promotes neurogenesis, gliogenesis and vasculogenesis. Some of these foetal proteins are transported into the brain and others are synthesized within the cerebral compartment. Once the brain is fully developed CSF proteins levels fall in early life in order to promote brain cellular structural stability, which is vital for correct and predictable CNS function.

A major role of the BBB is neuroprotection, as it protects the brain from blood-borne neurotoxins, which may be endogenous metabolites or acquired from the environment (Figure 21.1). The BBB is essentially formed by the endothelial cells of the cerebral capillaries which are the major exchange surface area (up to 20 m² in the human) between the blood and the brain. The endothelial cells also form tight junctions between the individual cells of the capillary wall which are robust enough to prevent even the diffusion of small ions through the paracellular pathway and can create an electrical resistance *in vivo* of at least 2,000 $\Omega.cm^2$ across the endothelium. The fact that simple aqueous paracellular diffusion of solutes is prevented by the tight junctions means that all solutes entering or leaving the brain must cross the cerebral endothelium by a transcellular route.

Thus physicochemical interactions with the plasma membrane and glycocalyx of the endothelial cells and the presence of transport systems embedded in the membranes of endothelial cells facing the blood and brain will determine the permeability properties of the BBB. The blood–brain barrier possesses a spectrum of solute carriers (SLCs) which transport essential small molecular weight nutrients into the brain and several members of the ATP binding cassette (ABC) transporters, principally P-glycoprotein (PgP/MDR), breast cancer-related protein (BCRP) and a number of the multidrug resistance proteins (MRPs). These ABC transporters are energy-dependent and can transport solutes out of the brain against a concentration gradient.

Therapeutic delivery across the blood–brain barrier

The presence of tight junctions in the BBB between the endothelial cells will prevent the paracellular diffusion, via an aqueous pathway, of virtually any hydrophilic solute irrespective of molecular size. Table 21.1 summarizes the mechanisms by which therapeutics may cross the blood–brain barrier.

Small molecular weight entities, groups A to D, may show a variety of interactions with the BBB. Molecules that have a significant polar surface area and are not lipophilic (Group A) are generally excluded from the brain as, there is no paracellular pathway. Further, they are unable to dissolve in the lipid of the cell membrane from the water phase because of the Gibbs free energy required and consequently cannot cross the BBB by simple diffusion. These exclusion rules also apply to many polar metabolites that the brain requires and thus the substrate-specific solute carriers (SLCs) are embed-

Figure 21.1 Blood–brain barrier in mouse.

(a) Cerebral capillary, site of the blood–brain barrier, in a normal adult C57B6 mouse containing two erythrocytes (ER). E, endothelial cell, with nucleus clearly visible; TJ, tight junctional complexes; P, pericyte; ECM, extracellular matrix surrounding the capillary which has a different composition from that of the parenchymal matrix. The pericytes are responsible for secreting and re-modelling this perivascular extracellar matrix of which heparan sulfate and dermatan sulfate are major components; G, glial end feet. (Courtesy of Dr Anja Zensi.)

(b) Cerebral capillary from a symptomatic 8- to 10-month-old MPS IIIA mutant mouse showing significant pathology. *Large inclusion bodies in endothelial cell and the pericyte are probably late endosomes/lysosomes, loaded with the major storage product, heparan sulphate. The profile of the capillary is partially collapsed and the lumen is constricted. The borders of the extracellular matrix appear corrugated compared to the wild-type mouse. The cytoplasm of the endothelial cell is thickened and will present a greater diffusional barrier than in the normal mouse. The tight junctional complex appears normal and can be shown experimentally to effectively close the paracellular pathway to sucrose (MW 342.3), even at this late stage of the disease. (Courtesy of Dr Larisa Mihoreanu.)

Table 21.1 Solute transport at the blood–brain barrier.

Group	Penetration	Physico-chemical characteristics	Examples	Comments
A	Poor	Low MW Ionised at physiological pH Low lipid solubility (logD7.4 <1.0) Polar (Polar surface area >80 Å^2)	Atenolol Sumatriptan Amantidine	Many drugs used to treat peripheral conditions with little CNS penetration or action
B	Good	Low MW Ionised at physiological pH Low lipid solubility (logD7.4 <1.0) Polar (Polar surface area >80 Å^2) Subject to transport/facilitation	L-dopa Gabapentin Baclofen Simvastin metabolites	Drugs which have useful central actions, often discovered serendipitously
C	Good	Low MW Lipid soluble (logD7.4 <1.0) Polar (Polar surface area < 80 Å^2)	Diazepam Pergolide Sertraline	Drugs commonly used to treat central nervous diseases with good penetration not subject to significant ABC efflux
D	Poor	Low–medium MW Lipid soluble(logD7.4 >1.0) Subject to ABC efflux (N + O > 8, acid pKa > 4, MW > 400, high aromatic density, branching molecules with rotatable bonds, high hydrogen bonding capacity	Cyclosporin Loperamide Ivermectin Vincristine	A large number of centrally active drugs may be placed in this category, their CNS penetration can be greatly reduced by ABC efflux activity but if sufficiently potent can still have significant CNS activity. Others may become frankly neurotoxic if ABC activity is reduced/inhibited (eg ivermectin/vincristine)
E	Poor to moderate	High MW Proteins Trojan Horses Gene vectors	Monoclonal antibodies Growth factors Enzyme replacement therapy	Require receptor-mediated transcytotic mechanism with the addition of appropriate binding domains can be used to deliver large drug vectors such as liposomes and nanoparticles.

ded in the cell membranes of the endothelial cells that will transport essential metabolites across the barrier. These SLC transporters may simply facilitate diffusion or may be exchangers or be secondarily active in that they are powered by an ion-gradient. Importantly the expression of the carrier proteins can be different in the blood-facing and brain-facing membranes of the endothelial cells so that transport for specific substrates has a polarity either into or out of the brain. Furthermore, some small molecular weight therapeutics are sufficiently similar to an endogenous metabolite as to be recognized by these transporters and are carried into the brain (Group B). Generally this transport of drugs has been serendipitously discovered, for example with L-dopa, and only occasionally has been deliberately designed into the molecule as is the case with gabapentin. Molecules which are more lipid-soluble at physiological pH (Group C) can intercalate with the cell membrane and passively cross the BBB by simple diffusion. For these passively diffusing molecules, greater lipid solubility tends to enhance the rate of their brain penetration. However, a number of the more lipid soluble molecules are substrates for the ABC transporters and are actively ejected from the cerebral endothelium with little consequent brain penetration (Group D). Lipid-soluble molecules, which have a larger molecular weight (more than 8 nitrogen or oxygen atoms in their structure), tend to be acidic, have a more complex planar or branched structure, are likely to be substrates for the P-glycoprotein and breast cancer-related protein which are probably the major ABC effluxers in all mammals. The Multidrug Resistance Proteins (MRPs) are a futher group of ABC transporters. The substrates of ABC transporters may actually be removed from the cell membrane before they fully enter the endothelial cell. The degree to which molecules disturb the structure of the cell membrane, and the time they spend in the cell membrane (dwell-time), may relate to their likelihood of being a substrate for an ABC transporter and their chance of being recognized by the transporters. The MRPs tend to prefer substrates that have already undergone Phase 1 metabolism and are conjugated, for example sulfated or glucuronidated. This renders them less membrane-permeant and they are simply pumped out of the endothelial cells by the MRPs. The currently used substrate reduction therapeutics (SRTs) and chaperones all tend to be low molecular weight substances and their brain penetrance will be subject to the above considerations.

Large molecular weight substances cannot cross the cell membrane directly in addition to being excluded at the BBB by tight junctions from the paracellular pathway. They are dependent on internalization into the cell by an endocytic mechanism (Group E). If a large molecule is to enter brain tissue it must undergo a process of transcytosis, where it is trafficked across the endothelial cell, to be released on the brain side by an exocytic event. The mechanism of transcytosis across tight cell layers is still poorly understood but the best described is that of receptor-mediated transcytosis (RMT) where a protein or macromolecule binds to a cell surface receptor on the blood-side of the endothelium and this initiates a vesicular internalization of the ligand, endocytosis. To access the brain this vesicle must be directed away from the lysosomal pathway within the endothelial cell and the vesicle must fuse with the contraluminal cell membrane and release its contents on the brain side. Electron microscopical studies indicate that many of these receptor-mediated endocytic vesicles are of the clathrin-coated variety and it is possible that this coating is responsible for trafficking them across the cell, thus avoiding the lysosomal compartment. Most endothelial cells show a high level of endocytic activity and a large variety of macromolecules will initiate these receptor-mediated events. A crucial difference in the cerebral endothelium compared to peripheral endothelium is that the number of observable endocytic events is much fewer and a smaller variety of receptors capable of initiating transcytosis are expressed on the luminal BBB surface (blood-facing) and hence fewer macromolecules are capable of being endocytosed and subsequently transcystosed. For example, albondin (p60), which will bind and internalize albumin, is expressed on peripheral endothelial cells but not on the BBB. A cardinal feature of intrauterine BBB formation seems to be the down-regulation of many of the receptors that will initiate RMT at the BBB, either before birth or perinatally. Thus the cerebral endothelium will only endocytose and transcytose the macromolecules that the brain really requires from the periphery for its normal function. Examples of where RMT remains at the BBB are mechanisms for transferrin, lipoprotein (Apo/LRP1-2), insulin and advanced glycosylation end products (RAGE). However, it remains controversial in a number of cases as to whether the whole receptor–ligand complex is transcytosed or just the important payload (e.g. iron in the case of transferrin) and released at the brain side. Very significantly, the mannose-6-phosphate (M6P) and mannose receptors appear to be absent in the BBB after the neonatal period and thus enzyme replacement therapies (ERTs) are excluded from the brain even when administered at high dose. Strategies for getting enzyme across the barrier (Figure 21.2) will need to rely on molecular constructs that retain enzyme activity but also contain a binding domain, which will allow RMT at the BBB (see Chapter 22). Fortunately neurones and glial cells appear to retain a M6P-dependent uptake mechanism for lysosomal enzymes.

Development of the blood–brain barrier

Contrary to popular belief the blood–brain barrier is well developed at birth especially with respect to proteins and macromolecules. In the mouse the BBB begins to establish between E11 and E17 during vasculogenesis and identifiable tight junctional structures and proteins are present at E10 in the mouse and E11 in the rat, thereby providing a barrier to polar and large molecules. Thus, tight junction formation is a primary event in vasculogenesis in the brain. These tight junctions are effective by E21 in the rat and they exhibit the high electrical resistance characteristic of the BBB. In mammals that are born in a relatively immature state, such as the rat and mouse, some maturation of the BBB may of course still occur post-natally. However, the vascular space marker, mannitol, has a brain volume of distribution that is identical in both the one week-old and the adult rat.

An RT-PCR signal for the ABC transporter mdr2 is present in the mouse brain and mdr1a, mdr1b and mdr2 all exhibit strong signals by E18. Mdr1a (Pgp) is present in the BBB of the rat and can be detected with

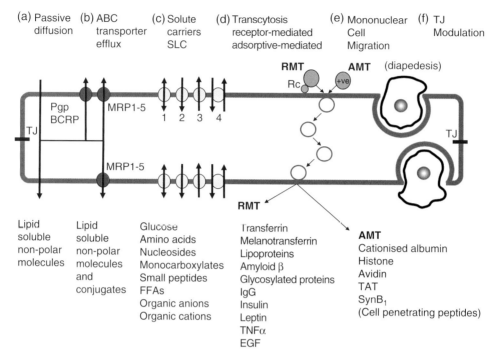

Figure 21.2 Routes of transport across the BBB.

(a) Passive diffusion of solutes through the cell membrane and across the endothelium.

(b) Active efflux carriers (ABC cassette transporters) intercept some of passively penetrating solutes and pump them out of the endothelial cell either as they diffuse through the cell membrane itself or from the cytoplasm. Pgp and BCRP are strategically placed in the luminal membrane of the BBB endothelium whereas MRPs 1–5 are inserted into both the luminal and abluminal membranes.

(c) Carrier-mediated influx via solute carriers (SLCs) may be passive or secondarily active and can transport many essential polar molecules such as glucose, amino acids and nucleosides into the CNS. The solute carriers may: (1) be bi-directional with the direction of transport being dictated by the substrate concentration gradient; (2/3) be unidirectional either into or out of the cell; (4) involve an exchange of one substrate for another or be driven by an ion gradient. The direction of transport is also reversible depending on concentration gradients.

(d) Receptor-mediated transcytosis (RMT) requires receptor activation and can transport a variety of macromolecules, such as peptides and proteins, across the cerebral endothelium. Adsorptive-mediated transcytosis (AMT) is induced in a non-specific manner by negatively charged macromolecules and can also transport across the endothelium. Both RMT and AMT appear to be vesicular-based systems that carry their macromolecular content across the endothelial cells.

(e) Transport of leukocytes across the BBB by a process of diapedesis through the endothelial cells close to the tight junctional regions. The junction-associated molecules (JAM) and the cell surface protein CD99 interact with the leukocytes to initiate diapedesis.

(f) Tight junction modulation can also occur either endogenously within the cell association or be induced pharmacologically, in which molecular re-arrangement of the proteins of the tight junctions is induced, resulting in a whole or partial opening of the paracellular aqueous diffusional pathway.

(Reproduced from Begley DJ. Structure and function of the blood–brain barrier. In: Toutitou E, Barry BW (eds.), *Enhancement in Drug Delivery*. Boca Raton: CRC Press, 2007: p. 585, with permission from Taylor & Francis.)

immunoblotting at P7 and gives a maximal signal at P28. The human BBB is probably just as, if not more, effective at birth and the tight junction proteins occludin and claudin-5 are present from 14 weeks gestation. Studies in human stillbirths and perinatal deaths have demonstrated a tight BBB to the dye, trypan blue, which, if perfused intravascularly, from the start of the second trimester, encounters a barrier comparable to that of the adult. Thus, the suggestion that the effectiveness of ERT, if given intravenously from birth, is due to a leaky and immature BBB is patently false. It is most likely to be the result of a residual mannose-6-phosphate dependent transcytotic system still present in the neo-natal barrier which is subsequently down-regulated. This is certainly the case in the rodent, in which these studies have been performed.

Damage to the blood–brain barrier in lysosomal storage diseases

In some of the LSDs the blood–brain barrier is clearly compromised and extravasation of plasma proteins and large molecular weight tracers can be demonstrated. In mouse models of Sandhoff disease, GM1-gangliosidosis and juvenile Batten disease, leakage of large molecular weight tracers at the BBB can be shown, whereas in mouse models of late-onset Tay–Sachs and mucopolysac-charidosis IIIA the barrier appears to remain intact to both large and small molecular weight tracers even at late stages of the disease. As the BBB has such a major role in brain homeostasis and neuroprotection, it may be resistant to opening in many LSDs. Thus frank leakage is only apparent in the diseases with an early onset of neuropathology, and the LSDs with a more attenuated course show less or no BBB leakage. Clearly, if the function of the BBB is seriously compromised, this can in itself cause CNS damage and pathology and add to the burden of neurodegeneration via mechanisms such as neuroexcitatory apoptosis and gliosis. Certainly there is some evidence that the transport properties of the BBB and transporter expression may be altered in some LSDs although the tight junction may remain intact.

Bibliography

Abbott NJ, Patabendige AA, Dolman DE, *et al.* Structure and function of the blood–brain barrier. *Neurobiol Dis* 2010; **37**: 13–25.

Begley DJ, Pontikis CC, Scarpa M. Lysosomal storage diseases and the blood brain barrier. *Curr Pharm Des* 2008; **14**: 1566–1580.

Begley DJ. ABC transporters and the blood–brain barrier. *Curr Pharm Design* 2004; **10**: 1295–1312.

Begley DJ. Delivery of therapeutic agents to the central nervous system: the problems and the possibilities. *Pharmacol Therapeut* 2004; **104**: 29–45.

Begley DJ. Stucture and function of the blood–brain barrier. In: Toutitou E, Barry BW (eds.), *Enhancement in Drug Delivery*. Boca Raton: CRC Press, 2007: pp. 575–559.

Bellettato CM, Scarpa M. Pathophysiology of neuropathic lysosomal storage disorders. *J Inherit Met Dis* 2010; **33**: 347–362.

Cox TM, Cachon-Gonzalez MB. The cellular pathology of lyso-somal diseases. *J Pathol* 2012; **226**: 241–256.

d'Azzo A, Tessitore A, Sano R. Gangliosides as apoptotic signals in ER stress cell response. *Cell Death Diff* 2006; **13**: 404–414.

Engelhardt B. Ontogeny of the blood–brain barrier. In: Dermietzel R, *et al.* (eds), *Blood–Brain Barriers*, Vol. 1. Weinheim: Wiley-VCH, 2006: pp. 11–39.

Farfel-Becker T, Vitner EB, Pressey SN, *et al.* Spatial and tempo-ral correlation between neuron loss and neuroinflammation in a mouse model of neuronopathic Gaucher disease. *Hum Mol Genet* 2011; **20**: 1375–1386.

Harris H, Rubinsztein DC. Control of autophagy as a therapy for neurodegenerative disease. *Nat Rev Neurol* 2011; **8**(2): 108–17.

Killedar S, Dirosario J, Divers E, *et al.* Mucopolysaccharidosis IIIB, a lysosomal storage disease, triggers a pathogenic CNS autoimmune response. *J Neuroinflam* 2010; 7: 39–47.

Kiselyov K, Muallem S, Mitochondrial Ca2+ homeostasis in lys-osomal storage diseases. *Cell Calcium* 2008; **44**: 103–111.

Moos T, Morgan EH. The metabolism of neuronal iron and its pathogenic role in neurological disease: Review. *Ann NY Acad Sci* 2004; **1012**: 14–26.

Platt FM, Walkley SU (eds.). *Lysosomal Disorders of the Brain*. Oxford University Press, 2004.

Schultz ML, Tecedor L, Chang M, Davidson BL. Clarifying lyso-somal storage diseases. *Trends Neurosci* 2011; **34**: 401–410.

Settembre C, Fraldi A, Jahreiss L, *et al.* A block of autophagy in lysosomal storage disorders. *Hum Mol Genet* 2008; **17**: 119–129.

Urayama A, Grubb JH, Sly WS, Banks WA. Mannose 6-phosphate receptor-mediated transport of sulphatase across the blood–brain barrier in the neonatal mouse. *Molec Ther* 2008; **16**: 1261–1266.

Vitner EB, Platt FM, Futerman AH. Common and uncommon pathogenic cascades in lysosomal storage diseases. *J Biol Chem* 2010; **20**: 20423–20427.

Walkley SU. Cellular pathology of lysosomal storage disorders. *Brain Pathol* 1998; **8**: 175–193.

Walkley SU. Pathogenic cascades and brain dysfunction. In: Platt FM, Walkley SU (eds.), *Lysosomal Disorders of the Brain*. Oxford University Press, 2004: pp. 32–49.

Wei H, Kim SJ, Zhang Z, *et al.* ER and oxidative stresses are com-mon mediators of apoptosis in both neurodegenerative and non-neurodegenerative lysosomal storage disorders and are alleviated by chemical chaperones. *Hum Mol Genet* 2008; **17**: 469–77.

Xilouri M, Stefanis L. Autophagic pathways in Parkinson disease and related disorders. *Expert Rev Mol Med* 2011; **13**: e8 doi:10.1017/S1462399411001803

CHAPTER 22

Emerging Treatments and Future Outcomes

T. Andrew Burrow and Gregory A. Grabowski

The Division of Human Genetics, University of Cincinnati, Department of Pediatrics and Cincinnati Children's Hospital Medical Center, Cincinnati, OH, USA

Introduction

Over the past two decades, treatments for the lysosomal storage diseases (LSDs) have advanced rapidly and now provide several safe and effective specific therapies (see Chapter 20). These advances have been based on two fundamental concepts: (i) re-establishment of substrate metabolism to a level that is consistent with lack of progression and/or a return to health; and (ii) early intervention to prevent development of tissue damage, i.e. avoidance of irreversible and/or self-propagating disease manifestations.

The knowledge of the pathophysiology of LSDs has evolved with our appreciation of the integration of the lysosomal apparatus into the entire cellular function. This evolution has been from the simplistic notion of "constipated" dysfunctional storage cells to a complex disruption of the lysosomal system including cascades of abnormal calcium homeostasis, oxidative stress, inflammation, autophagy, endoplasmic reticulum stress, and autoimmune responses [1]. These conditions are more appropriately considered as lysosomal system disorders (Figure 22.1).

The need for early intervention derives from the progressive nature of the tissue/cellular involvement in LSDs. Initially, tissues in LSD patients are minimally involved but progress through several stages: (i) disruption of substrate flux with pathogenic alterations of the lysosomal system before microscopic pathology; (ii) gross progressive accumulation of primary substrates, cellular dysfunction and secondary substrates (e.g. GM_2 ganglioside in MPS I), and initiation of inflammatory processes; (iii) progressive tissue damage and disease-independent propagation of aberrant inflammatory/anti-inflammatory processes (fibrosis, inflammation, and/or cellular death) even after lysosomal enzyme reconstitution.

These stages can be grossly divided into two major end-stage effects:

1 Space occupying lesions impacting cell/tissue structures by localized destruction and systemic release of effectors (e.g. cytokines and chemokines) or cell death. The prototype is accumulation of Gaucher cells in tissues.

2 Malformational or disruptive events molecularly mediated by storage materials that radically alter cellular function and/or organ development, e.g. dysplastic skeletal development in the MPS diseases.

For emerging LSD therapies to be successful, the stages of pathological involvement require elucidation. Essential to stage-specific therapies is the improvement of substrate metabolism in target cells by providing recombinant enzymes, pharmacologic enhancers or "molecular chaperones", and substrate synthesis inhibition. Each could slow the rate of disease progression. In the pre-pathologic stage, adjunctive therapies likely would be unnecessary in the presence of sufficient metabolic reconstitution; MPS and glycosphingolipid storage diseases in the CNS have minimal early inflammatory responses. Therapeutic targeting of several brain cell types could prevent the excess accumulation of toxic

Lysosomal Storage Disorders: A Practical Guide, First Edition. Edited by Atul Mehta and Bryan Winchester.
© 2012 John Wiley & Sons, Ltd. Published 2012 by John Wiley & Sons, Ltd.

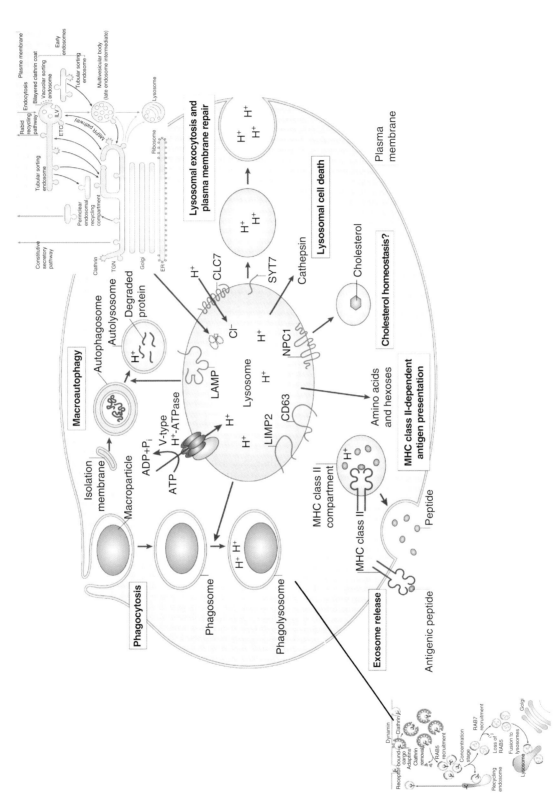

Figure 22.1 Figure of cell demonstrating the complex pathophysiological mechanisms involved in the lysosomal system disorders. (Adapted from Saftig P and Klumperman J. Nat Rev Mol Cell Biol 2009; 10: 623–635, with permission from the Nature Publishing Group.)

substrates and blunt or obviate microglial-assisted inflammatory responses. Lysosomal membrane instability [2], induced by excess toxic substrates, likely initiates inflammation. During the mid-stages, adjunctive anti-inflammatory agents and accumulated substrate reduction may be essential for halting disease progression and facilitating reversal. Disease reversibility in different organs and tissues will be dependent on the cell renewal potential (liver, bone marrow) or its absence (neurons or podocytes). In the MPS diseases, neurons can die, but the major pathology appears to be reversible substrate accumulation. In neuronopathic Gaucher disease, Krabbe disease, and the ceroidlipofuscinoses, neuronal death is primary and likely irreversible.

Late stage approaches will be directed toward controlling self-propagating events resulting from tissue damage; these continue despite alleviation of the primary metabolic abnormality. Anti-inflammatory, anti-autophagocytic, or lysosomal membrane stabilization could be considered. Multiple therapies should be considered at most disease stages as tissue damage will likely have already occurred at the time of diagnosis.

The CNS and skeletal system will be the focus since they represent major unmet medical needs with current inadequate treatment. About two-thirds of the LSDs have primary CNS involvement. The selectively impermeable blood brain barrier is a major hurdle, but understanding the unique initial neuropathophysiologies is critical to future success. The emphasis for CNS LSDs should focus on pre-pathologic initial (enzyme deficiency correction) and propagating mechanism, i.e. prevention. Early intervention is based on accurate prognostic prediction and validated biomarkers; these will not be addressed.

Current approaches to the treatment of LSD skeletal disease (e.g. Gaucher disease, MPS types I, II, and VI) are inadequate. Little attention has been focused on the direct and indirect pathophysiological consequences of specific cell types in which storage materials preferentially accumulate (i.e. macrophages in Gaucher disease; chondrocytes in mucopolysaccharidosis type 1) and the particular microenvironments in which these cells are localized.

Approaches to CNS Enzyme Delivery

The blood–brain barrier (BBB) is impermeable to large proteins, and direct intrathecal (IT) or intraventricular routes for enzyme delivery are being evaluated in animal models, e.g. MPS I (dog), MPS IIIA (mouse), and Krabbe disease (mouse). Results show gradients of non-uniform enzyme distribution across the CNS, and clearance of the

lysosomal storage material within glial and neuronal cells; improved survival and function resulted [3–5]. Intrathecal human trials are underway for MPS I, MPS II, and MPS IIIA. Reformulation of the IT therapeutic was essential for some. Indwelling devices for IT administration and direct infusions into cerebrospinal fluid present obvious risks to patients, including infection, and risks related to surgical procedures.

The differences in CSF circulation between humans and animals have not been fully delineated, nor have the potential effects of the disease itself and distribution of the IT enzyme. In human trials, knowledge of the disease stage at the start of treatment is essential because irreversible damage will limit potential efficacy. Currently available approaches for assessing the CNS are inadequate. For example, LSD neurological manifestations, (i.e. subtle MRI white matter aberrations) can be presymptomatic. Thus, a critical threshold may be exceeded before diagnosis/treatment.

Similarly in bone, threshold levels of disease may be exceeded and full recovery may not be possible. In Gaucher disease, osteonecrosis or lytic lesions have not been convincingly reversed. For both the CNS and bone involvement, early preventive therapy is an emerging field.

Alternative Enzyme Variants for CNS Targeting

Molecular Trojan horses, endogenous peptides or monoclonal antibodies attached to enzymes, or genes, can ferry the therapeutic across biological barriers, e.g. the BBB, via receptor-mediated transport [6]. Several receptor-mediated transcytotic mechanisms for BBB transport have been targeted, e.g. those for insulin, tumour necrosis factor α, and apolipoprotein E [7].

Chinese hamster ovary (CHO) cells [8] were engineered to produce a fusion protein of a genetically engineered monoclonal antibody (MAb) against the human insulin receptor (HIR) and iduronate-2-sulfatase (IDS), (MAbHIR)-IDS, which could be delivered to lysosomes of MPS II fibroblasts via the insulin receptor. In adult rhesus MPS II monkeys, (MAbHIR)-IDS showed a >20-fold greater uptake than IDS alone indicating the potential for CNS delivery of an intravenous injected macromolecule.

The intravenous or ventrical injection of viruses expressing fusion proteins of the HIV Tat protein transduction domain linked to β-glucuronidase into MPS VII mice improved the distribution of β-glucuronidase compared with viruses expressing non-Tat containing enzyme [9]. The Tat-fusion β-glucuronidase also showed greater tissue delivery and reduction in storage material than the unmodified enzyme [9]. The CNS distributions of these and other fusion proteins need detailed characterization to ensure that sufficient active enzyme reconstitution occurs globally rather than regionally. Other targeting peptides may be found, but the fusion proteins must retain activity and not have increased immunogenicity.

Nanotechnology refers to use of materials or devices that interact with biological systems at a molecular level [10] to enhance delivery to, or uptake by target cells, and/ or reduce toxicity of the free drug to non-target organs [11]. Enzymes, drugs (e.g. substrate reduction therapeutics), and genes can be encapsulated into nanoparticles of various compositions [11]. Such flexibility can facilitate more selective delivery to many tissues or to sequestered tissues, i.e. bone and CNS, as well as a protection of the biopharmaceutical from denaturation. For example, calcium alginate microspheres encapsulating glucocerebrosidase (the enzyme deficient in Gaucher disease) showed improved delivery to bone [12]. The enzyme retained full activity and had sustained release. Clinical efficacy remains to be demonstrated. Inflammatory and toxic effects of nanotherapy do occur and will require more complete study [11].

Gene/Cell Based Interventions

Gene-based therapies provide potential for a stable, long-term CNS and non-CNS LSD treatment. The goal of gene-based approaches is cell-specific reconstitution of enzyme/proteins using gene-corrected cell replacement or by metabolic cross-correction due to enzyme secretion and uptake into non-gene-corrected cells. Importantly, thresholds for correction must be exceeded. Ideally, the gene-corrected cells would be recipient derived, genetically altered, and returned to the same individual to avoid immunologic rejection.

Gene addition, gene correction/alteration, and gene knock-ins, viral and liposomal vectors, and *in vivo* or *ex vivo* techniques are being investigated. The DNA may be integrated into the host's DNA, or can function episomally outside of the genome [13]. Based on viral tropism, vectors can be directed to specific organ (i.e. liver, brain), specific cell types (i.e. hematopoietic cells), or multiple organs. A variety of recombinant non-pathogenic retroviruses (RNA viruses) or adenoviruses (DNA viruses) have been used as delivery vectors: the former randomly integrate into the genome of dividing cells, whereas the latter are episomal (non-integrating). Current vectors, including lenti- and adeno-associated (AAV) viruses, genomi-

cally integrate into non-dividing cells. Specific serotypes of AAV have differential tropism, whereas lentiviruses have less specificity. Direct intravenous, intraventricular, or intracerebral injections of vectors and/or their gene-altered stem cells have been explored for treatment of CNS disease. In neonatal mice, intravenous therapy has been successful based on the permeability of the BBB early in life. For visceral organs, hematopoietic stem cells containing the added integrated genes have been vehicles to produce the "internal factories" for metabolic cross correction in various organs. Similarly, neuronal stem cells containing such genes show promise when directly administered to the CNS. For example, gene therapy of the MPS IIIB mouse model evaluated the effects of intracranial injection of viral–vector-mediated gene delivery on the neuropathology of the disease [14, 15]. The studies in a larger animal model, feline α-mannosidosis, provide impressive evidence that early CNS treatment using AAV can be therapeutic [16]. The larger primate brains make it unlikely that focal vector injections will result in adequate amounts of secreted enzyme reaching CNS areas distant from the injection site. Transduction of the vascular endothelium (with secretion of the enzyme product basolaterally) was proposed as an approach to providing widespread enzyme distribution [17]. A modified human adenovirus vector, targeting the human transferrin receptor was used to successfully enter brain vascular endothelial cell cultures. Such techniques may allow for more widespread distribution of enzyme and, potentially, greater efficacy of the therapy. The composition of the vectors, the promoters used, optimization of expression, and the need for *in vivo* selection of corrected cells have been extensively reviewed and are beyond the scope of this review. However, these are important factors that allow for better specificity in the treatment of the LSDs.

A phase I clinical trial investigating intracranial injections of AAV type 2-mediated gene transfer of CLN2 cDNA was performed in 10 children with late infantile neuronal ceroidlipofuscinosis [18], a uniformly fatal, neuronal loss disease. In participants with significantly advanced disease, significant slowing of neurologic decline was suggested. The potential for greater therapeutic effects will need to be evaluated in individuals much earlier in the course of their disease.

Development of vectors with specific tropism and expression of the corrective enzyme/protein at therapeutic levels in specific cell types remains a challenge. Vectors with generalized distribution are in development; specific vectors may require disease- and/ or cell-specific tailoring. Persistent gene expression for a lifetime is needed for therapeutic benefit. Viewed from the perspective of drug development, gene therapeutics require evaluations of their pharmacokinetic/dynamic and specific exposure properties. Also, typical adverse events and hypersensitivity reactions to the vector or produced enzyme/protein must be investigated as highly immunogenic proteins are a risk for patients who express little if any protein. Finally, insertion of the vectors for stable integration can lead to endogenous activation of oncogenes insertional mutagenesis. These risks must be weighed against the nature of the diseases being treated.

Induced pluripotent stem cells (iPSCs) provide a potential way to avoid immunological and insertional mutagenesis issues with viral vectors. Induced pluripotent stem cells are recipient-derived genetically altered or transformed stem cells. This approach should avoid Graft vs Host or HVG reactions. Additional data are needed, however, since iPSCs transferred into genetically matched mice have shown immune rejection whereas embryonic stem cells did not [19]. This is quite controversial and further research and validation are essential. iPSCs approaches include (i) *ex vivo* transduction with vectors that produce the needed product; and more intriguingly, (ii) the site-directed correction of a specific locus in iPSC prior to transplantation. For example, iPSCs from skin fibroblasts of mice with sickle cell anemia underwent *ex vivo* homologous recombination to repair the genetic defect [18]. The corrected hematopoietic stem cells were transplanted into the affected, sickle donor mice with improvement of red blood cells and body weight, breathing, and renal medullary blood flow. This is proof-of-concept of iPSC-derived stem cells for the treatment of genetic conditions. This is a rapidly evolving field that holds the promise of specific cell therapies via individualized approaches.

Insertion of specific genes into iPSCs provides potential sources for endogenous enzyme/protein production for individual patients. This approach would facilitate metabolic cross correction *in vivo*, e.g. hematopoietic or neuronal stem cells, following transplantation of "corrected cells". All the considerations of ET for adverse events apply to this approach, except that the corrected cells continuously produce a potentially immunogenic therapeutic. Volitionally-controlled expression systems will be needed to address this potential issue. The genes inserted into the "corrected cells" would contain elements that respond to small molecules that would permit the turning of expression on or off by administering those non-toxic small molecules/drugs, e.g. tetracycline derivatives. Depending on the nature (on or off switch) of the inserted control elements, the corrective gene's expres-

sion would either be facilitated or inhibited, resulting in the desired change in enzyme/protein production.

Augmentation of mRNA Translation/ Natural Enzyme Function

An emerging class of agents includes drugs that alter the endogenous enzyme activity(s), e.g. antisense oligonucleotides, RNA interference (RNAi), and chaperones [enzyme enhancement therapy (EET)].

Antisense oligonucleotide treatment for conditions with splice-site mutations (and others) are conceptually based on the binding to and blocking of mutationally-created aberrant splice sites, thereby facilitating restoration of normal splicing and generation of a wild-type protein [20]. The cryptic splice site in Niemann–Pick disease type C fibroblasts was targeted with resultant restoration of normal splicing [20]. This approach also has the potential for excluding one or more exons to restore an open reading frame caused by a frame shift, or forcing use of alternative splice sites [21]. A minority of disease-causing mutations are splice junction defects and in these rare diseases therapeutics would be mutation-specific in rare diseases. This represents an important potential therapy for patients with LSDs.

Premature stop codon mutations may account for 18-25% of the mutant alleles in MPS I and neuronal ceroid lipofuscionosis [22]. In selected ethnic/demographic groups, such mutations are commonly identified e.g. the Q70X and W402X mutations occur in approximately 35 and 37% of MPS I patients of European descent, respectively [23]. Read-through of stop codons could alleviate the nonsense-mediated RNA decay and residual enzyme could be made. The three stop codons used in humans (UAA, UAG, and UGA) demonstrate differential degrees of natural read-through potential that can be differentially targeted. When fibroblasts from a MPS I patient, who was a compound heterozygote for Q70X and W402X, were treated with gentamycin, α-L-iduronidase enzyme activity was increased and reductions in glycosaminoglycan accumulation were observed [24].

This approach may result in small increases in enzyme activity but that may be sufficient to attenuate the phenotypic features of selected diseases. Also, these drugs are small and may have a greater distribution space than the ERT proteins [22]. Efficacy may be limited to patients with premature stop codons, and the scope of toxic side effects requires investigation.

RNA interference can suppress the functions of a specific genes [25]. Similar to "substrate reduction therapy" with miglustat or eliglustat (Chapter 20), miRNA specific for glucosylceramide synthase, the enzyme that synthesizes glucosylceramide, could diminish its production. RNA interference has the potential for greater specificity with fewer off-target effects.

Enzyme enhancement therapy seeks to augment the residual mutant enzyme by improving its stabilization, compartmentalization, and/or catalytic capacity. The major approaches have used potent inhibitors of specific lysosomal enzymes [26] as pharmacological chaperones, since such agents have significant corrective effects in cultured cells. However, clinical trials in Gaucher and Fabry diseases have not shown significant therapeutic effects (see Chapter 20). The potentially drug-related (deoxynojirmycin) exacerbation of late-onset Pompe disease through inhibition of lysosomal α-glucosidase needs to be considered. Of additional fundamental concern is the potential mutational dependency of effect, as is evident from *ex vivo* studies showing only some mutant enzymes with large responses [27]. Finally, the imino sugars can have off target effects [28].

Indirect therapies

Inflammatory processes occur in most LSDs and contribute to their pathophysiology. Consequently, anti-inflammatory drugs have been proposed as a potential treatment modality for LSD. Numerous studies evaluating anti-inflammatory therapy, particularly in animal LSD models, have shown potential benefit [29, 30]. When used alone, anti-inflammatory therapies will be an ineffective treatment approach for LSDs, but they may be useful adjuncts in their management. Additional studies in humans are needed.

Intriguingly, heat shock protein 70 (HSP70) was shown to stabilize lysosomal membranes by binding to an endolysosomal anionic phospholipid bis(monoacylglycero) phosphate (BMP), an essential co-factor for lysosomal sphingomyelin metabolism. Acid sphingomyelinase-deficient fibroblasts exposed to recombinant Hsp70 showed improved enzyme activity and stabilization of the lysosomes [2]. This study suggests a new class of agents for LSD treatment, lysosomal membrane stabilizers.

Combination therapies

The complex pathophysiology of LSDs and phenotypic variability challenge the potential for single agents to effectively treat all components of LSD. Combination therapies allow for a more personalized care program for patients. An exploratory study in Gaucher disease type 1

showed visceral improvement with combined ERT and miglustat treatment, but not in hemoglobin or platelet levels [31]. Gaucher mouse models suggest a synergistic effect of ERT and eliglustat [32]. Other combinations and/or transitions between various therapies when rigorously evaluated may show significant enhancements of stage-specific safety or efficacy. This may be particularly true for CNS and skeletal disease.

Conclusions

More thorough understanding of the pathophysiology of individual LSDs, particularly their tissue/organ differences, should reveal additional direct or adjunctive therapeutic targets. However, access to current and future therapies is hindered by cost and geography. These major challenges remain and should be the focus of future research. The rarity of each LSD will continue to challenge the potential for less costly agents. The development of small molecular substrate synthesis inhibitors or EETs may address the geographic boundaries.

References

1 Vitner EB, Platt FM, Futerman AH. Common and uncommon pathogenic cascades in lysosomal storage diseases. *J Biol Chem* 2010; **285**: 20423–7.

2 Kirkegaard T, Roth AG, Petersen NH, Mahalka AK, Olsen OD, Moilanen I, et al. Hsp70 stabilizes lysosomes and reverts Niemann–Pick disease-associated lysosomal pathology. *Nature* 2010; **463**: 549–53.

3 Kakkis E, McEntee M, Vogler C, Le S, Levy B, Belichenko P, et al. Intrathecal enzyme replacement therapy reduces lysosomal storage in the brain and meninges of the canine model of MPS I. *Mol Genet Metab* 2004;**83**:163–74.

4 Lee WC, Tsoi YK, Troendle FJ, DeLucia MW, Ahmed Z, Dicky CA, et al. Single-dose intracerebroventricular administration of galactocerebrosidase improves survival in a mouse model of globoid cell leukodystrophy. *FASEB J* 2007;**21**:2520–7.

5 Savas PS, Hemsley KM, Hopwood JJ. Intracerebral injection of sulfamidase delays neuropathology in murine MPS-IIIA. *Mol Genet Metab* 2004;**82**:273–85.

6 Boado RJ, Zhang Y, Xia CF, Wang Y, Pardridge WM. Genetic engineering of a lysosomal enzyme fusion protein for targeted delivery across the human blood–brain barrier. *Biotechnol Bioeng* 2008;**99**:475–84.

7 Begley DJ, Pontikis CC, Scarpa M. Lysosomal storage diseases and the blood–brain barrier. *Curr Pharm Des* 2008;**14**:1566–80.

8 Lu JZ, Boado RJ, Hui EK, Zhou QH, Pardridge WM. Expression in CHO cells and pharmacokinetics and brain uptake in the Rhesus monkey of an IgG-iduronate-2-sulfatase fusion protein. *Biotechnol Bioeng* 2011;**108**:1954–64.

9 Xia H, Mao Q, Davidson BL. The HIV Tat protein transduction domain improves the biodistribution of beta-glucuronidase expressed from recombinant viral vectors. *Nat Biotechnol* 2001;**19**:640–4.

10 Modi G, Pillay V, Choonara YE, Ndesendo VM, du Toit LC, Naidoo D. Nanotechnological applications for the treatment of neurodegenerative disorders. *Prog Neurobiol* 2009;**88**:272–85.

11 De Jong WH, Borm PJ. Drug delivery and nanoparticles: applications and hazards. *Int J Nanomedicine* 2008;**3**:133–49.

12 Barrias CC, Lamghari M, Granja PL, Sa Miranda MC, Barbosa MA. Biological evaluation of calcium alginate microspheres as a vehicle for the localized delivery of a therapeutic enzyme. *J Biomed Mater Res A* 2005;**74**:545–52.

13 Kay MA. State-of-the-art gene-based therapies: the road ahead. *Nat Rev Genet* 2011;**12**:316–28.

14 Cressant A, Desmaris N, Verot L, Brejot T, Froissart R, Vanier MT, *et al.* Improved behavior and neuropathology in the mouse model of Sanfilippo type IIIB disease after adeno-associated virus-mediated gene transfer in the striatum. *J Neurosci* 2004;**24**:10229–39.

15 Fu H, Samulski RJ, McCown TJ, Picornell YJ, Fletcher D, Muenzer J. Neurological correction of lysosomal storage in a mucopolysaccharidosis IIIB mouse model by adeno-associated virus-mediated gene delivery. *Mol Ther* 2002;**5**:42–9.

16 Vite CH, McGowan JC, Niogi SN, Passini MA, Drobatz KJ, Haskins ME, *et al.* Effective gene therapy for an inherited CNS disease in a large animal model. *Ann Neurol* 2005;**57**(3):355–64.

17 Xia H, Anderson B, Mao Q, Davidson BL. Recombinant human adenovirus: targeting to the human transferrin receptor improves gene transfer to brain microcapillary endothelium. *J Virol* 2000;**74**:11359–66.

18 Worgall S, Sondhi D, Hackett NR, Kosofsky B, Kekatpure MV, Neyzi N, *et al.* Treatment of late infantile neuronal ceroid lipofuscinosis by CNS administration of a serotype 2 adeno-associated virus expressing CLN2 cDNA. *Hum Gene Ther* 2008;**19**:463–74.

19 Zhao T, Zhang ZN, Rong Z, Xu Y. Immunogenicity of induced pluripotent stem cells. *Nature* 2011;**474**:212–5.

20 Rodriguez-Pascau L, Coll MJ, Vilageliu L, Grinberg D. Antisense oligonucleotide treatment for a pseudoexon-generating mutation in the NPC1 gene causing Niemann–Pick type C disease. *Hum Mutat* 2009;**30**:E993-E1001.

21 Perez B, Rodriguez-Pascau L, Vilageliu L, Grinberg D, Ugarte M, Desviat LR. Present and future of antisense therapy for splicing modulation in inherited metabolic disease. *J Inherit Metab Dis* 2010;**33**:397–403.

22 Brooks DA, Muller VJ, Hopwood JJ. Stop-codon read-through for patients affected by a lysosomal storage disorder. *Trends Mol Med* 2006;**12**:367–73.

23 Bunge S, Kleijer WJ, Steglich C, Beck M, Zuther C, Morris CP, *et al.* Mucopolysaccharidosis type I: identification of 8 novel mutations and determination of the frequency of the two common alpha-L-iduronidase mutations (W402X and Q70X) among European patients. *Hum Mol Genet* 1994;**3**:861–6.

24 Keeling KM, Brooks DA, Hopwood JJ, Li P, Thompson JN, Bedwell DM. Gentamicin-mediated suppression of Hurler syndrome stop mutations restores a low level of alpha-L-iduronidase activity and reduces lysosomal glycosaminoglycan accumulation. *Hum Mol Genet* 2001;**10**:291–9.

25 Angaji SA, Hedayati SS, Poor RH, Madani S, Poor SS, Panahi S. Application of RNA interference in treating human diseases. *J Genet* 2010;**89**:527–37.

26 Asano N, Ishii S, Kizu H, Ikeda K, Yasuda K, Kato A, *et al.* In vitro inhibition and intracellular enhancement of lysosomal alpha-galactosidase A activity in Fabry lymphoblasts by 1-deoxygalactonojirimycin and its derivatives. *Eur J Biochem* 2000;**267**:4179–86.

27 Steet RA, Chung S, Wustman B, Powe A, Do H, Kornfeld SA. The iminosugar isofagomine increases the activity of N370S mutant acid beta-glucosidase in Gaucher fibroblasts by several mechanisms. *Proc Natl Acad Sci USA* 2006;**103**:13813–8.

28 Sun Y, Ran H, Liou B, Quinn B, Zamzow M, Zhang W, *et al.* Isofagomine in vivo effects in a neuronopathic Gaucher disease mouse. *PLoS One.* 2011;**6**:e19037.

29 Arfi A, Richard M, Gandolphe C, Bonnefont-Rousselot D, Therond P, Scherman D. Neuroinflammatory and oxidative stress phenomena in MPS IIIA mouse model: the positive effect of long-term aspirin treatment. *Mol Genet Metab* 2011;**103**:18–25.

30 Smith D, Wallom KL, Williams IM, Jeyakumar M, Platt FM. Beneficial effects of anti-inflammatory therapy in a mouse model of Niemann–Pick disease type C1. *Neurobiol Dis* 2009;**36**:242–51.

31 Elstein D, Dweck A, Attias D, Hadas-Halpern I, Zevin S, Altarescu G, *et al.* Oral maintenance clinical trial with miglustat for type I Gaucher disease: switch from or combination with intravenous enzyme replacement. *Blood* 2007;**110**:2296–301.

32 Marshall J, McEachern KA, Chuang WL, Hutto E, Siegel CS, Shayman JA, *et al.* Improved management of lysosomal glucosylceramide levels in a mouse model of type 1 Gaucher disease using enzyme and substrate reduction therapy. *J Inherit Metab Dis* 2010;**33**:281–9.

CHAPTER 23

Newborn, High Risk and Carrier Screening for Lysosomal Storage Disorders

Gabor E. Linthorst and Carla E.M. Hollak

Department of Internal Medicine, Endocrinology and Metabolism, Academic Medical Center, Amsterdam, The Netherlands

Cases study A

A 4 year-old male child was diagnosed with Mucopolysaccharidosis I, Hurler type (MPS-1 H). At the time of diagnosis psychomotor retardation was already present, which deteriorated while being treated with enzyme replacement therapy (ERT). Family screening revealed that a 6 month old female sibling had also been diagnosed with MPS-IH. Before the onset of symptoms she was treated with ERT and scheduled to undergo hematopoietic stem cell transplantation (HSCT). After HSCT, her psychomotor skills were normal, but she developed a kyphosis at the age of 7 years.

Cases study B

A 54 year-old female was found to have severe left ventricular hypertrophy. Following a cardiac MRI, Fabry disease was suggested by the radiologist. A mutation (A143T) in the alfagalactosidaseA (aGal A) gene was detected and family screening revealed that her three sons (all in their mid twenties) also have this mutation. Two of the young males have substantial left ventricular hypertrophy but no other symptoms of Fabry disease. Subsequently, a diagnosis of atypical (or late onset) Fabry disease was made in all four subjects. Biochemical analysis in the three males revealed significant residual aGalA activity (up to 40% of normal) and absence of elevated globotriaosylceramide (Gb3) in plasma and urine and normal plasma lysoGb3, casting doubt on the diagnosis of Fabry disease. Additional genetic analysis demonstrated that the index case and the two sons with LVH had a mutation in the cardiac myosin binding protein C gene, the gene most frequently involved in left ventricular hypertrophy.

Introduction

The lysosomal storage disorders (LSDs) comprise a very heterogeneous group of diseases with regard to onset and diversity of symptoms. The heterogeneity and the low prevalence of individual LSDs can hamper early recognition and diagnosis. It is not uncommon that more than a decade passes before a proper diagnosis is finally made [1]. LSDs are generally progressive disorders and early diagnosis may be important for treatment decisions and genetic counselling. Therefore, screening in high-risk populations and carrier screening have been employed and newborn screening is the subject of intense debate. On the other hand newborn screening is already available in some countries. The most well known and earliest example of successful screening for LSDs comes from carrier screening for Tay–Sachs disease. In the early 1970s identification of carriers became feasible using enzymatic assays, later followed by mutation analysis. A joint program resulted in

Lysosomal Storage Disorders: A Practical Guide, First Edition. Edited by Atul Mehta and Bryan Winchester.
© 2012 John Wiley & Sons, Ltd. Published 2012 by John Wiley & Sons, Ltd.

Table 23.1 Outcome of screening studies for Fabry disease in different cohorts.

Cohort	No. of studies	Prevalence	
		Males	Females
Renal dialysis	12 M/6 F	0.33% (CI 0.20–0.47)	0.10%(CI 0.0–0.19)
Left ventricular hypertrophy	4	0.9–5.3%	1.11–13%
Young stroke	2	0–4.2%	0–2.1%

Data summarized from Linthorst *et al.* [6].

a dramatic decrease in the incidence of Tay–Sachs disease in the Ashkenazi Jewish population [2]. More recently, with the development of enzyme replacement therapy (ERT) and hematopoietic stem cell transplantation (HSCT), screening has focused on early identification of individuals who may benefit from timely intervention, i.e. before irreversible damage has occurred. For example, there is broad consensus that MPSIH (Hurler disease) patients should receive HSCT before the age of 2.5 years [3].

However, for most LSDs the limited data on the natural course, especially of the attenuated forms, as well as the paucity of long-term follow-up data on the effectiveness of different treatments, hamper wide implementation of screening. Nevertheless, the developments and the technical advances in biochemical and genetic testing have resulted in several efforts towards expanded carrier, high risk and newborn screening.

Carrier screening

The purpose of carrier screening is to advise couples about the risk for recessive diseases in their offspring. In the Ashkenazi Jewish population, this has become an accepted way of preventing severe genetic diseases. Following this success, the approach has been expanded to other ethnic groups. Increasing knowledge on diversity in clinical expression may cause some concerns. For example, the Tay–Sachs heterozygote detection program at New York University Medical Center, New York, was expanded in January 1994 to include carrier testing for Gaucher disease. Since the most common form of Gaucher disease may exhibit very mild symptoms, carrier testing for this disorder does not necessarily prevent severe disease. Despite these concerns, the American College of Medical Genetics (ACMG) recently recommended carrier screening not only for Tay–Sachs and Gaucher disease

but also for mucolipidosis type IV and Niemann–Pick disease type A in high risk groups [4]. While the lack of unequivocal genotype–phenotype relationships may hamper adequate predictions and counselling, the ethical discussion has fallen behind the advancement in genome sequencing programs and availability of commercial kits to screen young couples for many inherited disorders, including several LSDs.

High risk population screening

High-risk population screening involves the screening of patients with specific symptoms that could be caused by a LSD but where a LSD had not been considered. This has occurred particularly for Fabry disease after the introduction of ERT. Nakao *et al.* were the first to demonstrate an increased prevalence of Fabry disease (7/230, 3%) in males with left ventricular hypertrophy (LVH) [5]. This observation has led to additional screening studies in patients with unexplained LVH, but also in patients with end stage renal disease, young stroke and other symptomatic cohorts (summarized in Table 23.1, adapted from [6]). To our knowledge there are currently no systematic high-risk screening studies published for other lysosomal storage disorders.

Newborn screening

Early diagnosis of LSDs can avoid diagnostic odysseys and may result in timely initiation of treatment, which can be of great importance to patients and their families. For some disorders, early recognition of the disease and appropriate therapy can result in more favourable outcomes. This is particularly true for HSCT in some neurological LSDs such as Krabbe disease and MPS-1 H, although late complications can occur (see also case A). In infantile Pompe disease, early initiation of ERT is lifesaving, while irreversible skeletal complications may be prevented by early initiation of ERT in Gaucher disease. In Fabry disease, end organ damage is generally irreversible. These considerations form the rationale for the implementation of newborn screening programs. However, the long-term outcomes of HSCT and the effectiveness of pre-symptomatic initiation of ERT have not been fully elucidated. It is conceivable that therapeutic failure is perhaps too quickly ascribed to delayed intervention. Currently pilot programs for Fabry and Pompe disease are being employed in Taiwan and the state of Washington, USA. In some other US States Fabry, Pompe, Krabbe, Niemann–Pick A and Gaucher disease have been added to the newborn screening programs. Recently, the AMCG Working Group on diagnostic confirmation of LSDs has published an excellent educational guideline for the diagnostic approach and management of these LSDs [7].

Methodological issues of screening

A wide range of laboratory tests have been used to detect the presence of an LSD in a given population (be it newborn or a symptomatic cohort). Chamoles *et al.* [8] were the first to demonstrate that blood spots can be used to measure a variety of different lysosomal enzymes with artificial substrates. Other methods, which are still experimental, include multiplexing techniques to measure several lysosomal enzymes at once and the detection of accumulated substrate in blood or urine samples. Despite the tremendous technical progress, many challenges remain. For example, enzymatic analysis may fail to detect some individuals (e.g. females with Fabry disease) or may detect patients with a pseudodeficiency, who will never develop disease (e.g. arylsulfatase A deficiency without pathologic evidence of storage) [7]. Confirmation and interpretation by skilled biochemical laboratories is needed to avoid misdiagnosis. Undoubtedly, the most promising technique that will have a profound impact on screening is whole genome or next generation sequencing. While this technique is currently predominantly used to identify the genetic cause of well-defined phenotypes, the rapidly declining costs of whole genome sequencing may ultimately result in its use as a screening tool. While this technique may circumvent the aforementioned issues with false-negative or false-positive results regarding enzyme activity analysis, it may create uncertainty when (new) mutations with unknown clinical significance are identified (see case B).

Considerations of screening

In order for a disease to be included in a neonatal screening program, several criteria need to be met. While Wilson and Jungner's criteria in 1968 (listed in Box 23.1) still form the basis of the decision to include diseases in a newborn screening program, these have been subject to intense debate. In 2006, the AMCG issued a report that newborn screening could be justified for family and societal benefits, even if there is no direct benefit for the screened infant. In countries outside the US, some disorders are included when adequate supportive care has been shown to have a profound effect on life expectancy and quality of life (e.g. cystic fibrosis). The same debate is ongoing for LSDs and will require input from patient groups and various specialties, including ethicists, biochemists and medical specialists.

One of the major concerns is the detection of late-onset variants or genetic variants of unknown clinical significance. As stated previously, the phenotypic spectrum of LSDs is broad and ranges from severe disease with early childhood mortality to late-onset disease with limited morbidity. Neonatal screening will identify patients from this entire spectrum. In order to distinguish those patients with LSDs who benefit from early treatment, a reliable prediction of the phenotype is mandatory. Genotyping can be helpful in some cases but in general genotype/phenotype correlation is poor in most LSDs [7]. Variants with uncertain clinical phenotypes will be identified and

---

Box 23.1 **Criteria for successful newborn screening set out by Wilson and Jungner in 1968**

1 The condition should be an important health problem.
2 There should be a treatment for the condition.
3 Facilities for diagnosis and treatment should be available.
4 There should be a latent stage of the disease.
5 There should be a test or examination for the condition.
6 The test should be acceptable to the population.
7 The natural history of the disease should be adequately understood.
8 There should be an agreed policy on whom to treat.
9 The total cost of finding a case should be economically balanced in relation to medical expenditure as a whole.
10 Case-finding should be a continuous process, not just a "once and for all" project.

Table 23.2 Outcome of newborn screening studies.

Disease	Study	Country/ no. screened	Prevalence (overall, classical, late-onset)	Comment
Fabry disease[a]	Spada et al. [11]	Italy 37.104	1:3.092 1:3.373 1:37.104	First ever LSD screening study in newborns
	Hwu et al. [12]	Taiwan 90,288	1:1236 1:22750 1:1390	High incidence of specific Chinese late onset mutation
	Lin et al. [13]	Taiwan 57,451	1:1368 1:57,451 1:1.401	Only one third of affected grandfathers with Chinese late-onset mutation had signs of LVH
Pompe disease	Chien et al. [14]	Taiwan 132,538	1.33.134	Complicated by high incidence of pseudodeficiency
Krabbe's disease	Caggana et al. [15]	USA 260,000	1:65,000	Two subjects were transplanted in the newborn period

[a]Results for Fabry disease only shown for males.

it is likely that the number of these uncertain or late-onset variants identified through screening will become the majority of the diagnosed subjects (as is clear from Table 23.2). An early diagnosis in a patient with unclear or late onset disease may cause anxiety, lead to societal problems such as higher premiums for health insurance and create loss of an unconcerned carefree life. Societal support for early detection of adult onset diseases is mixed [9] and has not been investigated for detection of abnormalities of uncertain significance. In addition to these concerns, much has to be learned about the long-term effectiveness of treatments, both for the classical as well as late-onset variants. Gradually, it has become clear that many LSDs are not cured by the currently available strategies. For example, pre-symptomatic bone marrow transplantation in Krabbe disease may not prevent motor disability, speech difficulties and growth failure [10]. Larger, collaborative studies are needed to explore these outcomes, and these need to be incorporated in the ethical discussions.

Conclusions

There is an increased interest in screening high-risk cohorts or newborns for LSDs. Screening for LSDs may indeed shorten the prolonged period of time before a diagnosis is made on clinical grounds. The progressive nature of these disorders results in precious time being lost as irreversible symptoms may develop. Yet to make sure that these positive results will not be nullified by the

detection of many more individuals with uncertain risk for disease, further studies on the natural course of most LSDs are needed. This could include a well understood genotype/phenotype correlation or the availability of predictive biomarkers. In addition, better and long-term outcome data of treatments are a prerequisite.

References

1 Mehta A, Ricci R, Widmer U, Dehout F, Garcia de Lorenzo A, Kampmann C, et al. Fabry disease defined: baseline clinical manifestations of 366 patients in the Fabry Outcome Survey. *Eur J Clin Invest* 2004;**34**:236–242.

2 Scott SA, Edelmann L, Liu L, Luo M, Desnick RJ, Kornreich R. Experience with carrier screening and prenatal diagnosis for 16 Ashkenazi Jewish genetic diseases. *Hum Mutat* 2010;**31**:1240–1250.

3 de Ru MH, Boelens JJ, Das AM, Jones SA, van der Lee JH, Mahlaoui N, et al. Enzyme replacement therapy and/or hematopoietic stem cell transplantation at diagnosis in patients with mucopolysaccharidosis type I: results of a European consensus procedure. *Orphanet J Rare Dis* 2011;**6**:55.

4 Gross SJ, Pletcher BA, Monaghan KG, Professional Practice and Guidelines Committee. Carrier screening in individuals of Ashkenazi Jewish descent. *Genet Med* 2008;**10**:54–56.

5 Nakao S, Takenaka T, Maeda M, Kodama C, Tanaka A, Tahara M, et al. 080395 An Atypical Variant of Fabry's Disease in Men. *New Engl J Med* 2000;**21**:1–6.

6 Linthorst GE, Bouwman MG, Wijburg FA, Aerts JMFG, Poorthuis BJHM, Hollak CEM. Screening for Fabry disease in

high-risk populations: a systematic review. *J Med Genet* 2010;**47**:217–222.

7 Wang RY, Bodamer OA, Watson MS, Wilcox WR, ACMG Work Group on Diagnostic Confirmation of Lysosomal Storage Diseases. Lysosomal storage diseases: diagnostic confirmation and management of presymptomatic individuals. *Genet Med* 2011;**13**:457–484.

8 Chamoles NA, Blanco M, Gaggioli D. Fabry disease: enzymatic diagnosis in dried blood spots on filter paper. *Clin Chim Acta* 2001;**308**:195–196.

9 Hasegawa LE, Fergus KA, Ojeda N, Au SM. Parental Attitudes toward Ethical and Social Issues Surrounding the Expansion of Newborn Screening Using New Technologies. *Public Health Genomics* 2011;**14**:298–306.

10 Escolar ML, Poe MD, Yelin K, Kurtzberg J. Long-term developmental follow-up of babies treated for infantile Krabbe disease with unrelated cord blood transplantation. *Mol Genet Metab* 2008;**93**:21.

11 Spada M, Pagliardini S, Yasuda M, Tukel T, Thiagarajan G, Sakuraba H, *et al.* High incidence of later-onset fabry disease revealed by newborn screening. *Am J Hum Genet* 2006;**79**:31–40.

12 Hwu W, Chien Y, Lee N, Chiang S, Dobrovolny R, Huang A, *et al.* Newborn screening for Fabry disease in Taiwan reveals a high incidence of the later-onset GLA mutation c.936 + 919 G > A (IVS4 + 919 G > A). *Human Mutat* **30**:1397–405.

13 Lin H-Y, Chong K-W, Hsu J-H, Yu H-C, Shih C-C, Huang C-H, *et al.* High incidence of the cardiac variant of Fabry disease revealed by newborn screening in the Taiwan Chinese population. *Circulation Cardiovasc Genetics* 2009;**2**:450–456.

14 Chien YH, Chiang SC, Zhang XK, Keutzer J, Lee NC, Huang AC, *et al.* Early Detection of Pompe Disease by Newborn Screening is Feasible: Results From the Taiwan Screening Program. *Pediatrics* 2008;**122**:e39–e45.

15 Caggana M, Saavedra C, Wenger D, Helton L, Orsini J. Newborn screening for Krabbe disease in New York state: Experience from the first year. *Mol Genet Metab* 2008; **93**:17.

CHAPTER 24

The Patient Perspective on Rare Diseases

Alastair Kent[1], Christine Lavery[2], and Jeremy Manuel[3]

[1] Genetic Alliance UK, London, UK
[2] Society for Mucopolysaccharide Diseases, Amersham, UK
[3] European Gaucher Alliance, Dursley, UK

Introduction

The arrival of a newborn baby is a time of excitement and change. The first question asked by the new parents is "Is my baby alright?" Fortunately, for the great majority the answer is "Yes". Sadly, in a small number of cases the answer is "No", often precipitating a medical emergency during which the needs of the parents may be pushed aside in the rush to intervene; parents are often left feeling marginalised and at a loss.

Advances in screening technologies and improvements in antenatal care mean that, for a growing number of diseases and disorders, a diagnosis can be made during pregnancy. This gives expectant parents the opportunity to find out about the condition detected and make more informed choices among the options available to them. However, despite rapid advances in research, and greatly increased understanding of the care and support women and their (potential) children need to maximise their chances of having a healthy baby, it remains the case that many babies with serious life-limiting conditions remain undetected for considerable periods of time, leaving parents struggling to understand what has happened and how to cope with the consequences. This is particularly the case if the disease in question is rare. In these circumstances, obtaining a timely and accurate diagnosis, accessing appropriate services and receiving adequate support can be a time-consuming and uncertain process.

The scale of the problem

This is not a trivial issue. Families affected by rare diseases can sometimes feel marginalised, almost as if "rare" equates with "unimportant" in terms of the priorities of the health care system. And while it may indeed be the case that, on its own, any one rare disease may only affect a handful of families in the UK, the fact that there are so many different rare diseases [over 6000 identified (and rising) as new diagnostic tools are developed] means that, paradoxically, rare diseases are not actually uncommon.

It has been estimated that rare diseases, as defined throughout the European Union as those with a prevalence of 5 in 10000 or fewer [1], affect up to 1 in 17 of the population. This means that in the UK there are around 3.5 million people who live with the daily consequences that arise from serious, lifelong, often degenerative and sometimes lethal rare conditions. Quite apart from the personal and family impact for those directly affected, this represents a serious public health issue and a significant challenge to health care systems across the globe in terms of resource allocation. However, because those affected by rare diseases are seen in terms of their individual tragedy rather than as a collective need, their impact on the system is rarely appreciated by planners and service providers.

Addressing an issue of this magnitude might reasonably be expected to be seen as a priority by commissioners and those responsible for strategic decisions in health

Lysosomal Storage Disorders: A Practical Guide, First Edition. Edited by Atul Mehta and Bryan Winchester.
© 2012 John Wiley & Sons, Ltd. Published 2012 by John Wiley & Sons, Ltd.

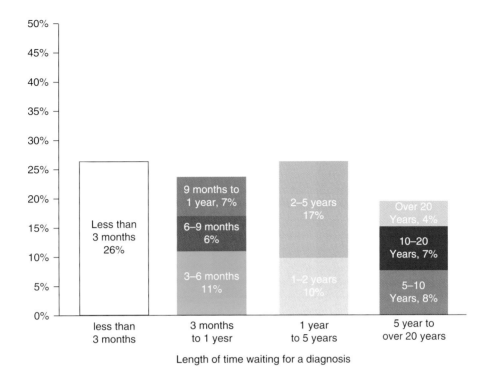

Figure 24.1 Chart: "How long did you/your family member have to wait for a final diagnosis following the onset of disease symptoms?" *Source*: Rare Disease UK survey on patients and family experiences of rare diseases. (http://www.raredisease.org.uk/documents/RDUK-Family-Report.pdf). Reproduced with permission from Genetic Alliance UK.

care. A recent survey by Rare Diseases UK of almost 600 families affected by over 100 different rare diseases [2] indicated that this does not seem to be the case. Families reported long delays before establishment of a diagnosis, with a significant minority waiting more than 5 years, and some never receiving a diagnosis at all. Equally disturbing is the fact that many patients receive a wrong diagnosis, sometimes more than once.

Given that 80% or more of rare diseases are genetic, arising from changes in a specific gene, this is an issue affecting whole families and across generations. Misdiagnosis means that potentially treatable conditions remain untreated, while others may be treated for conditions they do not have. This is unlikely to help alleviate symptoms; it wastes resources and allows potentially avoidable harm to continue.

Even when a correct diagnosis is made, the situation is not straightforward. Families with rare diseases often report significant difficulties in getting access to information about their condition that they can understand, and act upon in ways that will allow them to gain and retain a degree of control over their lives to the extent that they

wish and that is possible given the realities of their condition and the wider context in which they live their lives.

Facing the challenges

Most rare diseases are complex. They affect different body systems and often have psychological as well as physical consequences. A small but growing number of rare diseases can be treated. For example, enzyme replacement therapy (ERT) has been developed for a few inborn errors of metabolism, but despite these examples of progress, it remains the case that the vast majority remain untreatable. In such cases, practical help with the day to day management of the different issues that arise can be invaluable in helping families to cope.

Peer to peer support, and the collected experience of what works (and what may not) is usually and effectively channelled through patient support organisations. Many of these have developed from the initial experiences of patients and affected families, and have evolved into highly effective providers of information, advice and support. One area where patient organisations have

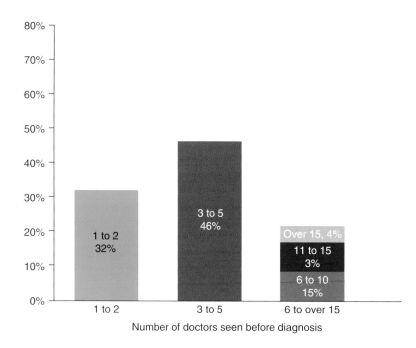

Figure 24.2 Chart: "How many doctors did you/your family member see before the final diagnosis was made?" *Source*: Rare Disease UK survey on patients and family experiences of rare diseases. (http://www.raredisease.org.uk/documents/RDUK-Family-Report.pdf). Reproduced with permission from Genetic Alliance UK.

been particularly effective and influential is the inborn errors of metabolism, including the Lysosomal Storage Disorders (LSDs).

The LSD Patient Organisation Collaborative was set up in the UK in 2008 by six founding members, each a pre-existing patient body representing patients with an LSD [Association for Glycogen Storage Disease; Batten Disease Family Association; Gauchers Association; MPS Society; Niemann–Pick Disease Group (UK); Representing Krabbe Leukodystrophy: Save Babies through Screening Foundation (UK)] to undertake joint promotion and a shared understanding of LSDs, to advance standards of care for LSD patients and to enhance the well-being of those affected. Their focus is to stimulate interest and work in partnership where groups can discuss matters of common interest, and establish criteria for the development and dissemination of good practice in looking after patients.

This collaborative effort has built upon the significant experience of individual organisations that have for many years provided specific disease information resources, family conferences, regional conferences, disease-specific expert meetings, focus groups and workshops. Some of the Associations, for example the MPS Society and the Niemann–Pick Disease Group UK, provide an individual advocacy service, which focuses on all aspects of social care and daily living, as well as palliative needs and pre- and post-bereavement.

Access to treatment

Even when a therapy that will improve the quality of life and the life expectancy of a patient exists (and in so doing provides additional valuable benefits for relatives, carers and the wider community), it is by no means certain that those who need it will be able to receive it. Novel therapies are often developed after extensive research and a long process of clinical development. A particular consideration in the case of rare diseases is that the number of affected patients is small, and the natural history of the disease is frequently poorly characterised. The effectiveness of therapy may appear uncertain to those charged with the responsibility of maximising health gain, particularly as the cost per patient is often high. Consequently health authorities and funding agencies may be reluctant to authorise prescription and payment for novel therapies for rare diseases. In addition, doctors may lack awareness of the disease entities, and even if they succeed in establishing a diagnosis, they may be unaware of new possibilities for intervention. Patient organisations have been proactive in helping to secure the development of and access to new treatments for their member families and to all those affected and in need.

Novel therapies are the result of detailed and extensive work by key stakeholders operating across professional, clinical, academic and commercial barriers. Patient organisations have worked for many years to fill in the gaps in the understanding of the conditions that affect their members. They have raised money to fund research, worked closely with interested academics and clinicians to plan and develop basic research strategies and secure the patient and family involvement to enable this to succeed. When the time was right they have collaborated with industry and the statutory regulators to progress the clinical development, production and licensing of new therapies, and then they have had to use their powers of persuasion and representational skills to sometimes cajole often reluctant health authorities to pay for these new treatments.

A United Kingdom perspective

The first enzyme therapy to become available was Ceredase, a purified form of natural β-glucocerebrosidase, which was approved by the FDA in the United States in 1991 for Gaucher disease. The enzyme was extracted and purified from human placentas and offered the first specific treatment for an LSD. A recombinant form of the enzyme, Cerezyme, was approved in 1994.

Patients and their doctors wanted access to this treatment but lack of approval outside the United States, as well as its very high cost, made access a real challenge. In the UK, the newly formed (1991) Gauchers Association developed a strategy with patients and their families, whereby their doctors who wanted to prescribe the treatment and were willing to take responsibility for the unlicensed products, did so on a "Named Patient Basis". As each local health authority needed to approve and pay for the treatment, there was considerable resistance, often citing the excuse that the drug was "experimental" as it was not licensed at that point in the UK. Patients and their families worked together and involved the support of their elected parliamentary representatives (Members of Parliament). Patient groups provided data and other evidence to medical officers of health authorities to challenge their negative attitude toward these treatments, and in some cases, media exposure was used to exert further pressure.

In 1996, an application by physicians to the Department of Health resulted in designated funding being allocated for initially three (in 1997), and the following year for a fourth, national specialist centre to carry out the assessment and management of patients with Gaucher disease. By May 2000, 171 Gaucher patients were attending these four national centres. However, the cost of the enzyme therapy remained under the control of Local Health Authorities (by then termed Primary Care Trusts), which

meant that equity of provision throughout the UK was not achieved. The term 'post code prescribing' has been used to describe this unsatisfactory state of affairs.

A further challenge faced Gaucher patients in 2001 when the Department of Health wanted to "de-designate" the four Gaucher centres. Patients were aware of the impact of special designation, and fearing such a return would result in a deterioration of access to treatment, the Gauchers Association teamed up with doctors at the National Centres and strongly argued that those few patients with a rare condition required a centralised specialist service where they could be seen by experts, as had been the case under the terms of the original designation. Patients described their experiences of designated specialist centres as the "NHS at its very best" – misdiagnosis, doctors who knew nothing about their condition, or inappropriate treatment, previously common experiences for so many, were now things of the past.

The Gauchers Association was able to partner with physicians and successfully lobby the Government that, not only should the specialised service for Gaucher patients be retained, but also that it would be beneficial to extend this to cover to the cost of treatment of other rare lysosomal conditions. These meetings coincided with the efforts of other groups representing patients with LSDs, who were similarly campaigning vigorously to receive specialist designation.

To address the funding pressure on individual local health bodies, 'risk sharing' consortia grew up, whereby a number of neighbouring Primary Care Trusts came together to share the considerable cost burden of newly diagnosed patients. Whilst this was beneficial to those in control of local budgets, it did involve a considerable amount of time and input both from the doctors and their teams, as well as patient advocates: decision making could be slow and was not always positive for many LSD patients.

In August 2001, ERT for Fabry disease was licensed in Europe. This was followed by ERT for MPS I in June 2003, MPS VI in January 2006 and MPS II in March 2007.

However, in 2003, across Europe, hope became despair for many patients as funding was refused for many of these new life-saving treatments. In the UK, individual Primary Care Trusts were unprepared for the battle ahead, and all too frequently, patient organisations were told by their members, "I have an ultra orphan disease, I meet the clinical criteria for enzyme replacement therapy but no one will fund my ERT" or "My local health funder cannot make a decision to fund ERT as there is no national policy".

New therapies had already been developed and licensed for use. Patients and their families understood that it could take years to develop a new therapy, but not, once a treatment option was developed, why access was blocked. In December 2003, when doctors from the expert centres for LSDs, together with patient representatives, met with Members of Parliament, it was agreed that a meeting with the Minister of Health was needed.

In addition, in January 2004, the MPS society started investigating the legal options for members who were being refused ERT. A legal firm specialising in discrimination and human rights agreed to take up individual cases of children who met the clinical criteria for treatment and who were eligible for public funding. In March 2004, the MPS society and two medical experts met with the Minister of Health, who agreed to look at the issues raised. The message to the Minister was clear, "Time is neither a healer nor on the patient's side; they just get worse and worse".

Whilst maintaining political awareness, the MPS Advocacy Team in 2004 supported 15 Fabry and MPS I patients in their challenges to health authorities by demanding judicial review of the failure of due process. This action was financially costly with respect to the public purse, but was nothing in comparison to the cost suffered by affected children, young adults and their parents, who found themselves living this nightmare. One never imagines a situation where parents literally have to beg for their child's treatment.

In July 2004, the Department of Health announced specialist commissioning for all LSDs. However, as with the original Gaucher service, this specialist commissioning did not include the cost of ERT. The breakthrough came in October 2004 when the Department of Health reaffirmed specialist commissioning for LSDs, and that from April 2005, it would include the cost of ERT in England, but not in other parts of the UK, who make their own independent decisions about such funding.

The current situation in the UK, 2012

In the UK, each patient organisation works closely with the eight nationally designated LSD specialist centres. These centres are designated and financially supported by central government. They are staffed by specialist physicians and scientists, who work alongside nurses, genetic counsellors and other health care professionals, to provide state of the art multidisciplinary care for patients and families affected by LSDs. The centres have a key role in the diagnosis of LSDs, co-ordination and provision of specific and sup-

portive therapy, and research into the pathophysiology of the diseases and the development of improved treatments. Patient organisations support outreach clinics throughout the UK where members of the patient organisation will often be present to offer additional support. These clinics provide an excellent opportunity to explore advocacy needs and provide a 'listening ear', particularly to newly diagnosed families. Most patients receive treatment in their own homes, administered either by themselves, family members, or by qualified staff providing domiciliary support. The clinics are also a conduit for bringing families together and for sharing experiences. The economic outlook in 2012 is grim, both in the UK and elsewhere in the world, and this situation is constantly under threat of 'rationalisation', 'analysis of cost-effectiveness' and other initiatives aimed at reducing the cost of care incurred by the state. Of course, patients with rare diseases, and the organisations representing them, must be prepared to play their part towards improving the cost-effectiveness of their treatment during these stringent times. However, a centralised system, such as that operating in the UK, has the potential to negotiate very good terms from the pharmaceutical industry and from the providers of home care.

Since June 2009, there has been a worldwide shortage of some enzyme formulations as a direct result of production difficulties encountered by Genzyme Corporation. The UK is well placed to meet this challenge as there is an infrastructure in place which allows patients to have a voice. The physicians, funding agencies and industry representatives agreed to reduce deliveries of enzyme therapies, prioritise patients according to need, and introduce new treatments which were often (initially at least) unlicensed. These challenges are currently still being embraced. This experience has evidenced the absolute necessity that patient organisations must partner with physicians, carers and all others who hold patients' interests at heart, to ensure that the patient's perspective is powerfully vocalised at all times and in all arena.

A European perspective

Other European government responses have been wide-ranging, and to some degree surprising, with Norway and Sweden very slow to recognise the need to fund ERT. In Poland, a country with one of the lowest expenditures per capita on health in the EU, the Polish MPS Society used extraordinary patient power to successfully persuade their government that, apart from death, there is no alternative to supporting access to ERT for their members. They were successful. Even today for those who live in Scotland or Wales (parts of the UK which have devolved responsibility for health services) and are diagnosed with a LSD, achieving funded ERT is a challenge. In addition, there is evidence that in some European countries the health authorities will fund treatment for children, but once the patient reaches the age of 18, funding is no longer available.

The Gaucher patient community in Europe came together to form the European Gaucher Alliance (EGA) to help and support all patient groups in their efforts to access treatment in their respective countries either by providing information, help with lobbying central government or local authorities, or by seeking humanitarian aid where treatment was otherwise inaccessible. The EGA has grown to include 31 countries in 2012 and has worked with others to secure humanitarian support through Genzyme's (the manufacturer of Cerezyme) charitable activity for over 100 Gaucher patients.

In parallel with these activities, patient organisations have also provided training and professional development opportunities for interested doctors, nurses and other medical professionals, and worked in partnership with medical and scientific leaders to develop centres of expertise that have the critical mass to secure ongoing improvements in the understanding of their disease and improvements in the lives of those affected.

It is certainly true that the decision by the Department of Health to commission the clinical management and treatment of LSDs on a nationwide basis in England has transformed accessibility to ERT and brought about regional equity. Clinical specialists and representatives of the patient organisations have been involved in drawing up and agreeing the clinical and treatment guidelines for Gaucher, Fabry, MPS I, MPS II and MPS VI. These guidelines play an important role in ensuring transparent and fair decision-making in deciding on treatment options.

The founding principle of the National Health Service in the UK was that access to treatment should be based on need, not on the ability to pay, accident of geography or some other non-clinical factor. Nowhere does it say that patients with rare diseases should have lesser expectations from their health systems than those with more common conditions. Health authorities need to generate and implement a systematic strategy to ensure that patients with rare diseases and their families receive the services and support they need in a timely, appropriate and user friendly way.

The elements of such a strategy have recently been articulated in a Communication from the European Commission [1] and a Recommendation from the Council of Health Ministers [3]. These two documents call upon Member States to articulate plans or strategies by 2013 to improve services and support and improve access to health care for patient and families with rare diseases. The elements of such a plan or strategy would be:-

• Prompt access to accurate diagnosis and the development of screening programmes to secure universal early detection for rare conditions.

• Accurate, comprehensive and comprehensible information, advice and counselling for patients and families with rare diseases.

• Integrated service provision between disciplines and across institutional boundaries, including support for the development of centres of expertise.

• Creation of a research infrastructure that facilitates the investigation of currently poorly understood conditions and the development of responses to the needs thus identified.

• Structural arrangements for the planning and commissioning of services that are sustainable, equitable and which cut across budgetary silo boundaries, where expenditure in one area secures benefits in another, but institutional barriers prevent a holistic overview from being considered, in order to secure high quality, cost and clinically effective care.

Conclusion

The journey for a patient with a rare disease and their family often starts with bewilderment, fear, and the hope that, whatever the precipitating signs and symptoms are, there will be a simple explanation that will reveal that the fear is unfounded and the problem will go away. If this is not possible, then the hope is for a cure or for effective prevention. Too often this is either currently unachievable or the options (such as antenatal testing and the offer of termination of pregnancy) are unacceptable. The need then is for information, care, support and effective relief of symptoms, linked to the hope that comes from knowing that research is being undertaken and that things may change for the better for future generations, even if improvements come too late for those currently affected.

Patients, patient support groups, doctors, scientists, industry, planners, policy makers, regulators and politicians all have a role to play in making this happen.

Through partnership, mutual recognition and respect, the effective provision of integrated high quality care and support that reflects both clinical possibility and current scientific understanding will become increasingly the norm. However, this will not happen if we all sit on our hands and wait for someone else to do something. As our experience has shown, the challenge for all of us is to work together towards the achievement of this shared goal, and bring it into being sooner rather than later.

References

1 http://eur-lex.europa.eu/LexUriServ/LexUriServ.do?uri= COM:2008:0679:FIN:EN:

2 http://www.raredisease.org.uk/documents/RDUK-Family-Report.pdf

3 http://eur-lex.europa.eu/LexUriServ/LexUriServ.do?uri=OJ: C:2009:151:0007:0010:EN:PDF

4 Mehta A, Lewis S, Laverey C. Treatment of lysosomal storage disorders (Editorial). BMJ 2003; **327**: 462–463.

Index

Note: Page numbers in italics refer to Figures; those in bold to Tables

Lysosomal Storage Disorders: A Practical Guide, First Edition. Edited by Atul Mehta and Bryan Winchester.
© 2012 John Wiley & Sons, Ltd. Published 2012 by John Wiley & Sons, Ltd.